Recurrent Implantation Failure

Jason M. Franasiak • Richard T. Scott Jr.
Editors

Recurrent Implantation Failure

Etiologies and Clinical Management

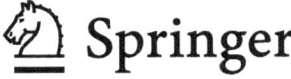 Springer

Editors
Jason M. Franasiak
Reproductive Medicine Associates of NJ
Thomas Jefferson University
Basking Ridge, NJ
USA

Richard T. Scott Jr.
Reproductive Medicine Associates of NJ
Thomas Jefferson University
Basking Ridge, NJ
USA

ISBN 978-3-030-10137-4   ISBN 978-3-319-71967-2   (eBook)
https://doi.org/10.1007/978-3-319-71967-2

Printed on acid-free paper

This Springer imprint is published by the registered company Springer International Publishing AG part of Springer Nature
The registered company address is: Gewerbestrasse 11, 6330 Cham, Switzerland

To my wife, Kaitlin, who is my constant. Without your love and support, this book would not have been possible.

Jason M. Franasiak

Preface

We are fortunate to practice reproductive medicine during a time of unprecedented success when it comes to assisted reproductive technology. With the advent of comprehensive chromosomal screening, the contribution of aneuploidy to implantation failure has been all but eliminated. Still, though, euploid embryos fail to implant. Why is that? The dwindling rate of implantation failure makes the remaining cases a particular challenge for both practitioners and their patients. The very workup for recurrent implantation failure, let alone available treatment options, often remains elusive.

This text is unique in its multifaceted approach to thinking about these challenging cases. It starts with a foundational look at the signaling between the embryo and endometrium, which leads to the management of embryo and endometrial synchrony. The pathologic nature of implantation failure is then explored with an eye toward the gamete and embryo to the maternal anatomy, immune, and hematologic system. The neuroendocrine system is considered as well as the psychological impact recurrent implantation failure has on patients. Novel theories such as the female reproductive tract microbiome are also discussed. The text is designed for clinicians and researchers in the field of reproductive endocrinology and infertility patients as a guide not only for clinical care but also for encouraging much needed research in the area.

We live in an exciting time in reproductive medicine. With ever improving technology that is becoming both widely available and cost-effective, there are more tools than ever at our fingertips to address the most challenging problems that confront our patients. It is incumbent upon practitioners and researchers alike to understand the capabilities and impact of various treatments, both proven and experimental, for implantation failure. We hope this book offers some answers as well as raises unaddressed questions as we strive to better our patient care.

Basking Ridge, NJ, USA   Jason M. Franasiak, MD, HCLD

Basking Ridge, NJ, USA   Richard T. Scott Jr., MD, HCLD

Contents

Contributors

Diana Alecsandru, MD, PhD Rey Juan Carlos University, IVI RMA-Madrid, Madrid, Spain

Baris Ata, MD Department of Obstetrics and Gynecology, Koc University School of Medicine, Istanbul, Turkey

Sarah L. Berga, MD Department of Obstetrics and Gynecology, Wake Forest School of Medicine, Winston-Salem, NC, USA

Andrea Mechanick Braverman, PhD Sidney Kimmel Medical College of Thomas Jefferson University, Philadelphia, PA, USA

J. David Wininger, PhD Department of Obstetrics and Gynecology, Wake Forest School of Medicine, Winston-Salem, NC, USA

Jeffrey L. Deaton, MD Department of Obstetrics and Gynecology, Wake Forest School of Medicine, Winston-Salem, NC, USA

Eric J. Forman, MD, HCLD Reproductive Endocrinology and Infertility, Columbia University, New York, NY, USA

Chelsea Fox, MD Department of Obstetrics and Gynecology, Greenville Health System, Greenville, SC, USA

Jason M. Franasiak, MD, HCLD Sidney Kimmel Medical College, Thomas Jefferson University Philadelphia, PA, USA

IVI-RMA of New Jersey, Basking Ridge, NJ, USA

Juan A. Garcia-Velasco, MD, PhD Rey Juan Carlos University, IVI RMA-Madrid, Madrid, Spain

Julian Gingold, MD Department of Gynecology and Obstetrics, Cleveland Clinic, Cleveland, OH, USA

Jeffrey M. Goldberg, MD Department of Gynecology and Obstetrics, Cleveland Clinic, Cleveland, OH, USA

James M. Hotaling, MD, MS, FECSM Center for Reconstructive Urology and Men's Health, Division of Urology, University of Utah, Salt Lake City, UT, USA

Erika Johnston-MacAnanny, MD Department of Obstetrics and Gynecology, Wake Forest School of Medicine, Winston-Salem, NC, USA

Daniel J. Kaser, MD Sidney Kimmel Medical College, Thomas Jefferson University Philadelphia, PA, USA

IVI-RMA of New Jersey, Basking Ridge, NJ, USA

Sorena Keihani, MD Center for Reconstructive Urology and Men's Health, Division of Urology, University of Utah, Salt Lake City, UT, USA

Bruce A. Lessey, MD, PhD Department of Obstetrics and Gynecology, Greenville Health System, Greenville, SC, USA

Natalia Llarena, MD Department of Gynecology and Obstetrics, Cleveland Clinic, Cleveland, OH, USA

Inmaculada Moreno, PhD Research Department, Igenomix, Valencia, Spain

Department of Obstetrics and Gynecology, School of Medicine, Stanford University, Stanford, CA, USA

Scott Morin, MD Sidney Kimmel Medical College, Thomas Jefferson University Philadelphia, Philadelphia, PA, USA

IVI-RMA of New Jersey, Basking Ridge, NJ, USA

Jeremy B. Myers, MD, FACS Center for Reconstructive Urology and Men's Health, Division of Urology, University of Utah, Salt Lake City, UT, USA

Shelby A. Neal, MD Sidney Kimmel Medical College, Thomas Jefferson University Philadelphia, PA, USA

IVI-RMA of New Jersey, Basking Ridge, NJ, USA

Bonnie Patel, MD Department of Obstetrics and Gynecology, Wake Forest School of Medicine, Winston-Salem, NC, USA

Catherine Racowsky, PhD, HCLD Department of Obstetrics and Gynecology, Brigham and Women's Hospital, Harvard Medical School, Boston, MA, USA

Richard T. Scott, MD, HCLD Sidney Kimmel Medical College, Thomas Jefferson University Philadelphia, PA, USA

IVI-RMA of New Jersey, Basking Ridge, NJ, USA

Emre Seli, MD Department of Obstetrics Gynecology and Reproductive Sciences, Yale School of Medicine, New Haven, CT, USA

Yimin Shu, MD Department of Obstetrics and Gynecology, Wake Forest School of Medicine, Winston-Salem, NC, USA

Carlos Simon, MD, PhD Department of Pediatrics, Obstetrics and Gynecology, University of Valencia/INCLIVA, Spain, Igenomix, Valencia, Spain

Department of Obstetrics and Gynecology, Stanford University, Stanford, CA, USA

Department of Obstetrics and Gynecology, Baylor College of Medicine, Houston, TX, USA

Keren Sofer, PsyD Independent Practice, Philadelphia, PA, USA

Robert N. Taylor, MD, PhD Department of Obstetrics and Gynecology, Wake Forest School of Medicine, Winston-Salem, NC, USA

Nathan Treff, PhD Rutgers University School of Medicine, Newark, NJ, USA

Genomic Prediction, Newark, NJ, USA

Shannon D. Whirledge, PhD Department of Obstetrics, Gynecology and Reproductive Sciences, Yale University School of Medicine, New Haven, CT, USA

Alexandra Wilson, MD Department of Obstetrics and Gynecology, Wake Forest School of Medicine, Winston-Salem, NC, USA

Jie Yu, MD Department of Obstetrics and Gynecology, Wake Forest School of Medicine, Winston-Salem, NC, USA

Rebekah S. Zimmerman, PhD, FACMG Icahn School of Medicine at Mount Sinai, New york, NJ, USA

Chapter 1
Signaling Between Embryo and Endometrium: Normal Implantation

Chelsea Fox and Bruce A. Lessey

Pregnancy has been one of life's great mysteries and captivated both the scientific and artistic realms (Fig. 1.1). The endometrium is where life begins, and a receptive endometrium lies at the crossroads of menstruation and pregnancy. In a perfect world, the peak of receptivity of the endometrial lining is achieved synchronously with the arrival into the uterine cavity of a healthy blastocyst that can then adhere, attach and invade, and grow protected until parturition. However, for human reproduction in particular, it is not always a perfect world; for every successful pregnancy, there are many fertilized eggs that either implant and fail as clinical or subclinical pregnancies or never are able to interact with the endometrium, resulting in infertility. Issues involving embryo quality and chromosome number and diseases that can impair normal endometrial receptivity have the potential to alter the outcome of pregnancy in devastating ways. The endometrium is a specialized, almost immortal, tissue that regenerates again and again with the sole purpose of continuing the survival of our species. In this chapter, we will review a global overview of normal implantation and what is known about the signaling components of embryo and endometrial interactions. Our current understanding of implantation also provides a better appreciation for why pregnancies fail.

Timing of Implantation

Normal implantation occurs in the mid-secretory phase of the menstrual cycle and requires synchronous development of the endometrium, oocyte, and subsequent embryo. Events leading to a successful pregnancy begin several months ahead of time with recruitment of the cohort of oocytes that will mature and ovulate some

C. Fox, MD • B.A. Lessey, MD, PhD (✉)
Department of Obstetrics and Gynecology, Greenville Health System, Greenville, SC, USA
e-mail: cfox@ghs.org; blessey@ghs.org

© Springer International Publishing AG 2018
J.M. Franasiak, R.T. Scott Jr. (eds.), *Recurrent Implantation Failure*,
https://doi.org/10.1007/978-3-319-71967-2_1

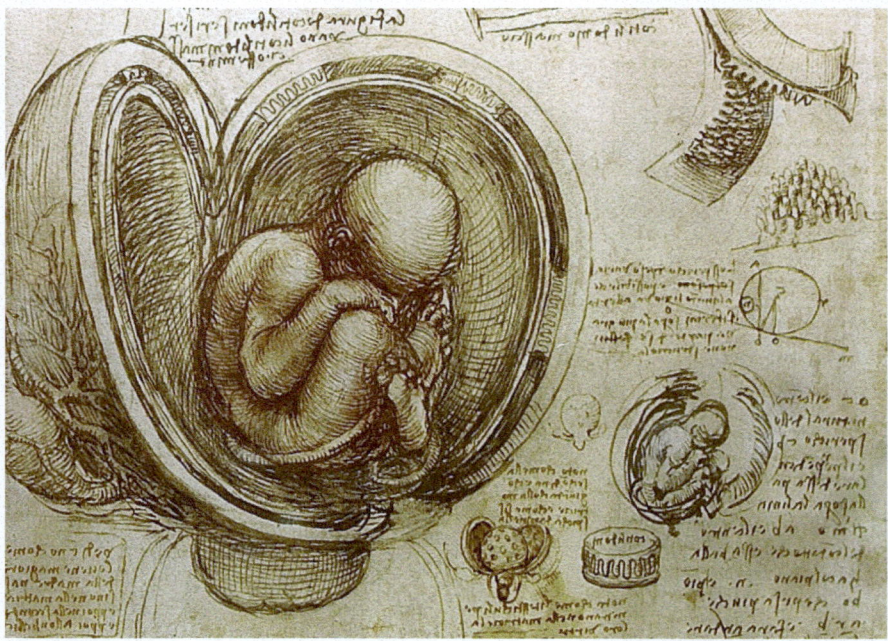

Fig. 1.1 Anatomical depiction of a human pregnancy by Leonardo da Vinci, circa 1510

months hence. In the month of implantation, at the time of menstruation, progesterone levels fall with the demise of the corpus luteum. It has been suggested that menstruation is more than simply a decline in ovarian steroids [1]; there is evidence that menstruation is an active and complex process with purposeful blockade of progesterone action through induction of inflammatory mediators leading to progesterone resistance [2]. With an abrupt and active loss of progesterone support coupled with the concomitant rise in ovarian estrogen, the upper layers of the endometrial (the functionalis layer) are sloughed but rapidly repaired and reconstituted without scarring, from underlying stroma and epithelial fragments [3]. This remarkable process of renewal can occur up to 400 times in a woman's lifetime.

The cessation of bleeding and repair of the endometrial lining is an estrogen-dependent process and occurs as the negative hypothalamic and pituitary feedback is released after the fall in progesterone. In response to rising follicle-stimulating hormone (FSH), a cohort of ovarian follicles begins to develop, releasing increasing amounts of estradiol into the circulation. In response to rising estrogen concentrations, the endometrium produces more estrogen receptors (ER), allowing proliferation and thickening, ultimately achieving a trilaminar appearing layer by ultrasound by the time ovulation occurs. In natural cycles, the dominant follicle is selected as that follicle has adequate FSH receptors to grow despite falling gonadotropin levels in the mid-proliferative phase of the menstrual cycle.

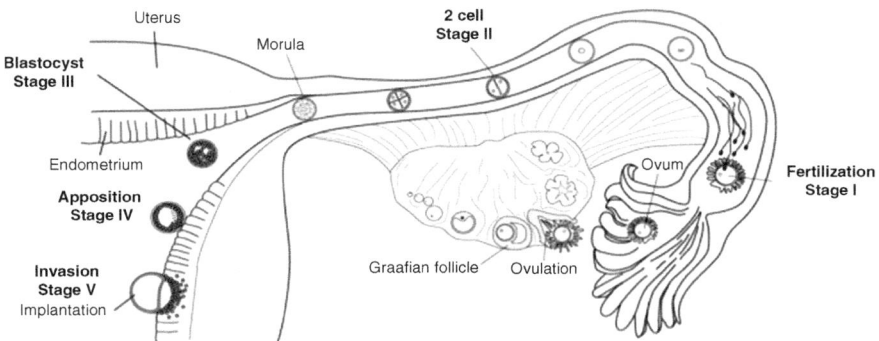

Fig. 1.2 Stages of implantation correspond to and are largely driven by ovarian steroids from the developing follicle and subsequent corpus luteum that forms. Development and progression of the embryo is synchronously timed to endometrial development, such that both embryo and endometrium become receptive toward each other at the proper time

In response to positive feedback to rising estrogen, an ovulatory LH peak from the pituitary triggers release of the mature oocyte(s). As shown in Fig. 1.2, the release of the egg results in collapse and consolidation of the vacated follicular cyst, with subsequent development of the corpus luteum and a rise in serum progesterone. Progesterone is essential for the success of a pregnancy. Unlike estrogen that stimulates endometrial cell proliferation, progesterone transforms the thickened endometrium into a secretory structure and induces a host of factors essential for embryonic survival, attachment, and invasion. Meanwhile, the released oocyte is picked up by the fimbria and transported along the fallopian tube where it is fertilized by waiting sperm. The newly formed embryo undergoes progressive development from zygote to 8-cell embryo to blastocyst during its transit down the fallopian tube culminating in its discharge into the uterine cavity. By the time it arrives, under optimal conditions, the endometrium has developed into a receptive surface with the appropriate glandular secretions, adhesion moieties, and vascular changes required to support a pregnancy.

Implantation is a complex network of events happening synchronously in the embryo and endometrium that culminates with the envelopment of the blastocyst within a *decidualized* endometrial stroma. The stages of early implantation have been divided into three phases: apposition, attachment, and invasion. When implantation occurs, this process is rapid, with apposition, attachment, and invasion happening within hours rather than days.

In one of the early morphologic studies on the timing of implantation, hysterectomy specimens were obtained from volunteers who agreed to try and become pregnant prior to surgery to remove the uterus. In this remarkable and usual study, 34 embryos were found within luteal phase hysterectomy specimens. Based on the time of hysterectomy relative to the last menstrual period, 8 embryos were found free-floating within the uterine cavity, while the remaining 26 embryos were in various stages of implantation and had begun to complete the invasion process [4, 5]. Based on these findings, the timing of implantation appeared to occur around cycle day 19 to 20 of an idealized menstrual cycle. The timing of implantation based on assisted reproductive technology cycles has tended to agree with these results [6–8]. In vitro studies have tried to record these events as well, with mixed success [9, 10].

Implantation begins with the hatching of the embryos out of its zona pellucida about 1–3 days after the morula enters the uterine cavity (Fig. 1.2). Apposition of the hatched blastocyst to the uterine epithelium usually occurs 2–4 days after the morula has entered the cavity. By this point, the blastocyst, as it is now called, has differentiated into an inner cell mass (ICM) that subsequently forms the embryo and the trophectoderm which will give rise to the placenta. Importantly, hatching from its protective shell exposes a variety of adhesive molecules expressed on the outer surface of the embryo, complementing those on the endometrial epithelium and later the decidualized stroma. Penetration of the embryo through the uterine epithelium and basal lamina occurs quickly, allowing in the invasion of cytotrophoblast inside the uterine vasculature [11]. This clogging of the arterioles of the maternal endometrium reduces hemostatic pressure on the implanting blastocyst but also means that blood supply to the embryo is limited until the end of the first trimester [12].

The Endometrium

The endometrium is composed of a mucosal layer within the myometrial layers of the uterus. The female reproductive tract is derived from the urogenital ridge, which arises from paired mesodermal (paramesonephric) tubes that form from the longitudinal invaginations of the coelomic epithelium [13]. The early uterus is lined by a simple cuboidal epithelium that subsequently becomes columnar and pseudostratified. Beneath this epithelial layer is a dense mesenchymal layer that becomes the endometrial stroma as well as the surrounding myometrium. What later will become the glandular epithelium invaginates from buds arising in the luminal epithelium, growing into the underlying stroma.

By mid-gestation, the uterus has the appearance of the adult organ. After delivery, with the fall in maternal steroids, the endometrium may have an initial menstruation event, but then regresses to an inactive state, where it will remain until puberty and the rise in ovarian steroid secretions. With the initiation of cyclic menstrual cycles, the endometrium will undergo repetitive stages of development in response to follicular estrogen followed by ovulatory progesterone. These changes are predicated on the timely induction of cognate steroid receptors for both estrogen and progesterone, which orchestrate the genomic activation of thousands of endometrial genes. In the event that pregnancy does not occur, the endometrium breaks down and then is rapidly rebuilt until pregnancy is established. This process of menstruation, proliferation, and regeneration occurs without scarring and speaks to the seeming immortality of the endometrium, a structure that continues to proliferate throughout the woman's life without deterioration.

Endometrial Receptivity

Anyone who studies the endometrial cycles and implantation, in particular, recognizes that the endometrium is non-receptive through much most of its cyclic changes. Our understanding of endometrial function comes largely from early animal studies on implantation [14–17]. Over 65 years ago, Noyes and colleagues described the histological changes that the endometrium undergoes during its cyclic development from menses to menses [18]. Within this 28-day menstrual cycle, receptivity toward the embryo only occurs for 3–5 days. The endometrium is unique as one of the few tissues into which an embryo will not attach and grow, except for a narrow period of uterine receptivity [19, 20]. This putative "window" of implantation, as first suggested by Finn [16], has been demonstrated in both animal models [17, 21] and in humans [6, 7].

As interest in the role of the endometrium in blastocyst attachment and invasion has increased, a great deal of research has been done to identify biomarkers of a receptive endometrium. Significant progress has been made in this field although the majority of potential biomarkers require further randomized studies in order to test their validity and clinical usefulness. The ideal biomarker is accurate, reproducible, and sensitive but should be able to be obtained by noninvasive means [22]. Potential sources of noninvasive biomarkers may include urine, saliva, vaginal fluid, cervical mucus, vaginal epithelial smears, blood, ultrasound, and basal body temperature measurement [23, 24].

Histologic Dating

The traditional "gold standard" for comparison of methods assessing the quality of luteal function remains histologic dating described by Noyes et al. in 1950 [18]. Use of this method leads to the description of the luteal phase defect (LPD) in which infertility and early pregnancy loss were thought to occur as a consequence of delayed endometrial maturation secondary to inadequate corpus luteum progesterone (P) production [25]. Since the 1950s, the clinical usefulness of histologic dating has been challenged off and on, due to methodological flaws noted in the original study as well as high inter-and intra-observer variation of histologic interpretation [26, 27]. The major flaw identified in the Noyes study is all of the endometrial samples were obtained from women with infertility, not from normally cycling parous controls. A subsequent prospective, randomized observational study reexamined histologic dating criteria in 130 regularly cycling, fertile women [26]. This landmark study concluded that endometrial dating does not have the accuracy or precision necessary to diagnose a luteal phase defect or guide clinical management of infertility. Furthermore, a prospective study of 847 subjects compared the endometrial biopsies of fertile and infertile patients. The pathologists, blinded to fertility status and menstrual day of biopsy, were not able to reliably discriminate between the two patient populations, and the authors recommended against the use of histo-logic dating in the routine evaluation of infertility [28].

Adhesion Molecules

At implantation, the trophectoderm of the embryo and the endometrial luminal epi-thelium acquire mutual adhesiveness [29]. Changes in cellular motility occur in response to adhesion and intracellular signaling. Embryos begin to exhibit a high rate of protrusion formation [30]. Sutherland captured the intrusive behavior of mouse embryos, with trophoblast cells probing out until finding a cleavage plane to intrude into the uterine wall [31]. The basis for this adhesion and signaling is complex and has been reviewed elsewhere [32–34] but represents an unsettled area of research as to the primary or most important adhesion molecule for embryo implantation.

Structural changes have also been found to occur on the luminal epithelium throughout implantation and thought to play a pivotal role in attachment. Pinopodes are cell membrane prominences on the apical cell membrane of the endometrial luminal epithelium. First identified in 1958 [35], they have since been investigated as potential biomarkers for endometrial receptivity. While their timing of expression appears to coincide with the window of implantation (WOI) [36, 37], not all studies agree. Pinopodes have been studied extensively by electron microscopy [37–39], and their appearance appears to be cycle dependent and under the control of proges-terone [40]. They are visible by light microscopy as well [41] and are decorated with both endometrial integrins as well as osteopontin (OPN), two candidate biomarkers of embryo/endometrial attachment (Fig. 1.3a) [42]. Bentin-Ley has cap-tured human embryos attaching to cultured endometrium, in vitro, seeming to show a preference for areas containing pinopode structures (Fig. 1.3b; [43]). Aplin has

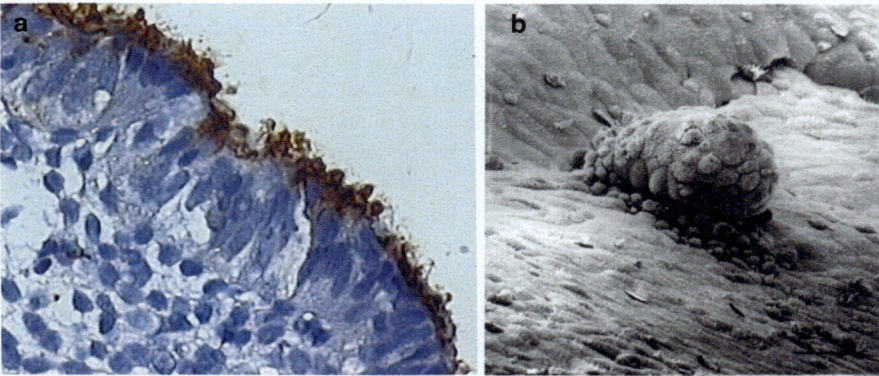

Fig. 1.3 Pinopodes or endometrial uterodomes are present at the time of implantation and sites of integrin and OPN expression (**a**). Human embryos can be seen attaching to these structures using in vitro culture and electron microscopy (**b**) (used with permission by Human Reproduction)

used similar techniques with mouse and human embryos and demonstrated the increased expression of OPN and integrin $\alpha\upsilon\beta3$ at the site of attachment [44]. They also showed that decreased attachment occurred if either OPN or the integrin was artificially downregulated. Despite the association between pinopode expression and the WOI, the clinical usefulness of their expression has been criticized. Arguments against the use of pinopodes as a biomarker of endometrial receptivity include their brief time of expression, the subjective nature of scoring them, and subsequent studies which have failed to show their temporal expression within the WOI [45–47].

Integrins are transmembrane glycoproteins which function as cell adhesion molecules (CAMs). They are formed from alpha and beta subunits which function as cell surface ligands between the embryo and the endometrium. Several integrins have been found to be only expressed during the WOI suggesting a role a possible biomarker for endometrial receptivity [48–50]. In humans, low expression of certain integrins has been linked to infertility [51, 52]. Furthermore, multiple studies have described abnormally low or absent levels of integrins, particularly the $\alpha\upsilon\beta3$ integrin, in inflammatory disease states associated with implantation failure such as endometriosis, polycystic ovarian syndrome, and hydrosalpinges [52–55].

Extracellular matrix proteins such as fibronectin and laminin are secreted by the endometrium under progesterone control [56]. These proteins have been found to interact with integrins and likely play a role in limiting trophoblastic invasiveness [57–59]. Damsky et al. [58, 60] have shown cells at the maternal-fetal interface switch their integrin phenotype expression at least twice during trophoblastic invasion. Fisher went on to show the importance of the $\alpha\upsilon\beta3$ integrin, a fibronectin receptor, as part of the mimicry cytotrophoblast uses to masquerade as endothelial cells and invade maternal vascular during early implantation [61]. High maternal levels of fibronectin have been associated with fetal growth restriction, hypertensive disorders, and abnormal umbilical artery Doppler in the third trimester of pregnancy [59]. These findings not only shed light on the well-orchestrated events that must occur in normal implantation, but they also provide a foundation to study disease processes where trophoblastic invasion is either insufficient or excessive (i.e., placenta accreta, preeclampsia, choriocarcinoma).

Selectins are carbohydrate-binding proteins known to mediate interactions between leukocytes and endothelium in the vasculature [62]. These proteins help facilitate leukocyte capture by L-selectin expression on the endothelial surface allowing "rolling adhesion" to slow the leukocyte to an eventual stop at the appropriate location. Genbacev et al. found selectin expression was also present at the maternal-fetal interface increases during the window of receptivity where it may play a similar role [63]. Studies suggest that L-selectin expression was increased in both the uterine epithelial cells and on the trophoblast cells suggesting these adhesion interactions may help slow the embryo down as it approaches the site of implantation [64]. The loss of L-selectin has been shown to occur in women with infertility [65, 66] suggesting that this class of molecules remains a promising area of interest.

Mucin 1 (MUC-1), a glycoprotein, is found at many secretory epithelial sites throughout the body where it forms a mucin coating. In the endometrium, its expression is increased during the luteal phase and WOI where it is produced and secreted by the luminal epithelium [67]. MUC-1 has displayed both adhesive and anti-adhesive properties in various studies [32, 68, 69] suggesting a complex balance in its role in implantation. In humans, MUC-1 was found at the implantation site, but not at the surface of pinopodes possibly to allow the blastocyst to preferentially bind to these specialized structures [70].

Growth Factors and Cytokines

Several growth factors including insulin-like growth factor (IGF), heparin-binding epidermal growth factor (HB-EGF), and vascular endothelial growth factor (VEGF) have been identified whose expression in the endometrium coincides with the window of implantation [51, 72–75].

The two subtypes of insulin-like growth factors, IGF-I and IGF-II, appear to both play a role in implantation and placentation. IGF expression appears to correlate with estrogen concentration with IGF-I expressed primarily during the proliferative phase and IGF-II expression seen in the secretory endometrium [51]. IGF-I has been implicated in a variety of functions including endometrial proliferation [51, 71], placental function [72], and enhancement of embryo development and quality [73, 74]. IGF-II expression is seen at both the maternal-fetal interface in early human pregnancy and by the trophoblastic cells in early intrauterine pregnancies. The spatial expression of IGF at the decidual-trophoblastic interface suggests these peptides may function as mediators of trophoblastic invasion; however, the mechanism of this action remains unknown [75].

Heparin-binding epidermal growth factor (HB-EGF) expression within the uterus has been shown in both human and mouse models to occur in a cycle-dependent manner with its maximal expression occurring at the window of implantation [76]. Furthermore, immunohistochemistry staining for HB-EGF on endometrial biopsies have shown the coexistence of pinopodes with HB-EGF expression [77, 78]. HB-EGF is also expressed in early pregnancy on both the villous and extravillous trophoblastic tissue suggesting a role implantation and trophoblastic invasion [79]. Studies have shown its expression is associated with increased rates of embryo hatching and development and can also promote trophoblastic growth in vitro [80, 81]. Thus, HB-EGF appears to function in communication between the early embryo and endometrium although further studies are needed to clarify its exact role in implantation.

Vascular endothelial growth factor (VEGF) is a key regulator of angiogenesis throughout the body. VEGF is produced by both the embryo and endometrium during implantation highlighting its potential role in angiogenesis and vasodilation at the implantation site [78]. Interestingly, VEGF expression is increased in pre-eclampsia [82]. It is hypothesized that this increase occurs as a result of inadequate angiogenesis at the placentation site wherein VEGF is upregulated in a compensatory fashion. VEGF has also been studied in assisted reproduction. Elevated levels of VEGF appear to be markers of follicular hypoxia and suboptimal embryo development [83]. Dorn et al. found that higher serum concentrations of VEGF on the day of oocyte retrieval were correlated with IVF outcome; however, the mechanism behind these findings has not yet been elucidated [84].

Matrix Metalloproteinases

Matrix metalloproteinases (MMPs) comprise a family of zinc-dependent extracellular matrix (ECM)-degrading endopeptidases. MMPs, secreted by the cytotrophoblast, appear to play a key role in matrix degradation during trophoblastic invasion [85]. They can be classified into four subfamilies based on their substrate specificity and structure: gelatinases, collagenases, stromelysins, and a subfamily containing MMP-14, MMP-15, MMP-16, and MMP-17 [85]. Animal models suggest MMP-2 and MMP-9 (members of the gelatinase subfamily) have the most important role in ECM degradation and trophoblastic invasion [86–91]. Similar to MMPs, ADAMTS (a disintegrin and metalloproteinase with thrombospondin motifs) are also proteolytic enzymes that likely contribute to the invasive properties of the blastocyst [92]. In particular, ADAM-TS5 is highly expressed by day 7 embryos with decreased expression thereafter suggesting this enzyme may play a role in proteolytic processing during the peri-implantation phase [85, 92]. MMP and ADAM are modulated locally by tissue inhibitors of metalloproteinases (TIMP). TIMP binds to and inhibits the active forms of MMP and ADAM within the extracellular space [85]. It appears the co-localization of MMP, ADAM, and TIMP at the maternal-fetal interface promotes implantation while also regulating the limits of trophoblastic invasion.

HOX Genes

The homeobox (*Hox*) genes encode transcription factors which guide embryologic development but have also been shown to regulate gene expression within the endometrium during the menstrual cycle [93]. The DNA-binding domains of these transcription factors are highly conserved across divergent organisms suggesting communal ancestry and genetic importance [94]. There are 39 *HOX* genes arranged in four parallel clusters (termed A, B, C, and D) [95]. *HOXA10* and *HOXA11* are expressed by endometrial glands and stroma at varying levels throughout menstruation [96]. Both genes are upregulated by 17β-estradiol and progesterone which are maximally expressed during the mid-secretory phase at the time of implantation. The spatial and temporal expression of *HOXA10* and *HOXA11* within the endometrium suggests a role in endometrial development, implantation, and maintenance of pregnancy [97]. Hox genes are known to mediate the expression of endometrial receptivity markers such as LIF, pinopodes, and integrin $\alpha v \beta 3$. Furthermore, diseases associated with subfertility such as polycystic ovarian syndrome (PCOS), hydrosalpinges, and endometriosis have also been associated with defects of *HOX* gene expression [98–100]. Unfortunately, much of the available research regarding *HOX* genes and endometrial receptivity involves mouse models. The possible role of gene therapy involving manipulation of *HOX* expression to enhance implantation is promising although further research is necessary.

Prostaglandins

An increase in endometrial vascular permeability has been proposed as an essential requirement for trophoblastic implantation and decidualization [15, 101]. Prostaglandins (PGs) have been identified as important mediators of this localized vascular response in addition to playing a critical role in the decidualization reaction in animal models [102–108].

PGs are produced from arachidonic acid through the cyclooxygenase (COX) pathway. The rate-limiting step in this conversion pathway is the enzyme COX which exists in two isoforms, COX-1 and COX-2. $PG-H_2$ is the common precursor for all prostaglandins produced from this pathway [$PG-E_2$, $PG-F_2$, $PG-D_2$, thromboxane A_2 ($TX-A_2$), and prostacyclin ($PG-I_2$)]. Uncertainty exists regarding the exact site of PG production although it appears both the blastocyst and the endometrium are able to produce PGs. Endometrial prostaglandin production changes throughout the menstrual cycle with increased $PG-F_2$ and $PG-E_2$ concentrations seen during the mid-luteal phase during the WOI [109–114]. This cyclical rise in PG production suggests a possible role in implantation. Furthermore, multiple studies using animal models have shown administration of nonsteroidal anti-inflammatory agents, such as indomethacin, inhibits prostaglandin synthesis which leads to inhibition or delay of decidualization and implantation [105, 115–118]. Additional studies have shown administration of exogenous PGs can overcome the effects of indomethacin on implantation [119, 120]. Despite substantial evidence to support the role of PGs in implantation and decidualization, significant knowledge gaps exist regarding the specific types of PGs involved as well as their specific mode of action.

Cytokines

Cytokines are a group of proinflammatory signaling proteins that control the immune response. They have also been implicated in playing an important role in mammalian implantation [121–123] and have been characterized as biomarkers as a noninvasive test of endometrial receptivity [124]. Implantation is associated with elevated levels of proinflammatory markers including cytokines, prostaglandins, and leukocytes [125]. Clinical findings have shown improved implantation rates when the endometrium is mechanically disrupted prior to embryo transfer in patients with recurrent pregnancy loss further supporting the importance of a proinflammatory environment during embryo implantation [121]. Proinflammatory cytokines identified at the maternal-fetal interface in early pregnancy include interleukin-1 (IL-1), interleukin-6 (IL-6), leukemia inhibitory factor (LIF), and numerous others [126, 127]. IL-1 exists as two subtypes, IL-1-α and IL-1-β. Both forms of IL-1 are under progesterone control although the receptor antagonist is not [128]. Animal experiments have shown IL-1 knockout mice are able to implant successfully, whereas implantation is impaired when their receptor is blocked with IL-1 receptor antagonist (IL-1ra) [125]. It is hypothesized that administration of IL-1ra causes downregulation of endometrial integrins leading to implantation failure [125].

LIF, an IL-6-like cytokine, is expressed by the human endometrium in a cycle-dependent manner with highest expression seen during the window of implantation [129]. LIF was one of the first cytokines shown to be essential for implantation of embryos in mice [130, 131] and in humans [132]. LIF affects trophoblastic differentiation, shifting the embryo toward a more adhesive phenotype [129, 133]. Studies of uterine flushings and endometrial biopsies of women with unexplained infertility and recurrent pregnancy loss have shown decreased expression of LIF when compared to fertile controls suggesting its role in implantation and establishment of pregnancy [134, 135]. Unfortunately, a recent randomized controlled trial (n = 149) using recombinant human LIF in patients with recurrent implantation failure did not show an improvement in implantation or pregnancy rates when compared to the placebo group [136]. Thus, further research is needed to investigate the complex implantation process in order to develop possible treatments to improve reproductive outcomes.

Theories of Endometrial Receptivity Defects

There remains much to understand about normal endometrial receptivity. The complexity of the process of implantation makes it also prone to dysfunction. Indeed, for every successful pregnancy culminating in live birth, there are a vast number of miscarriages, subclinical losses, and failed implantation events that preclude establishment of pregnancy [137]. We recently published a paradigm of endometrial receptivity defects that is focused on inflammation as the central defect [138]. As shown in Fig. 1.4, the activation of STAT3 by inflammatory cytokines, as seen in endometriosis, has been reported to recruit and stabilize hypoxia-induced factor 1-alpha (HIF1α) [139]. STAT3 also stabilizes a gene suppressor, BCL6 which is overexpressed in women with hydrosalpinges or endometriosis [140]. BCL6 appears to be a prime candidate as a cause of progesterone resistance along with SIRT1, which together have been shown to inhibit GLI1, which is involved in the progesterone-driven Indian Hedgehog pathway [141, 142]. Without progesterone working properly, progesterone-induced STAT5 [143] is not there to inhibit STAT3 [144]. Further, protein inhibitor of STAT3 (PIAS3) is also downregulated in

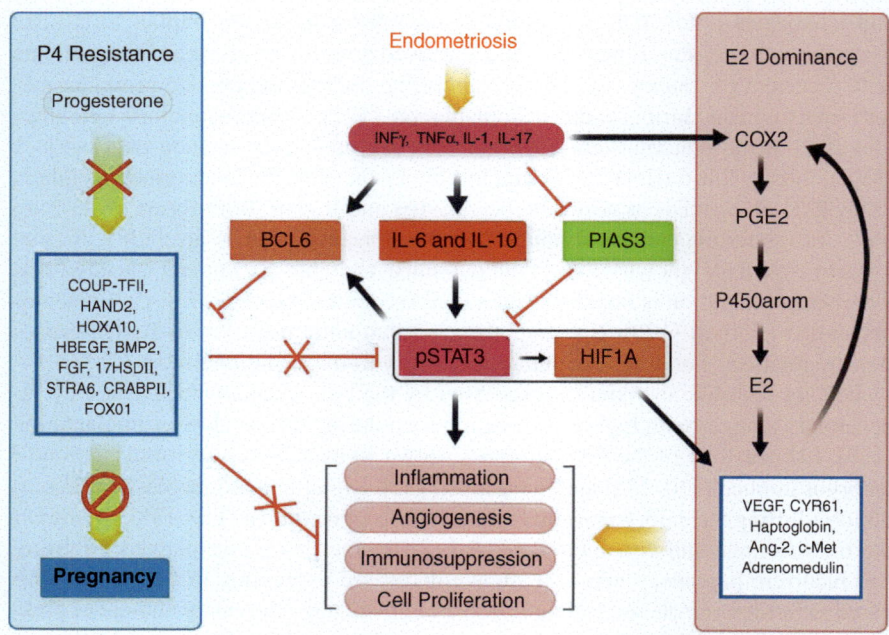

Fig. 1.4 Model of endometrial dysfunction in the setting of inflammatory conditions including endometriosis. Inflammatory cytokines such as interferon gamma (INFg), tumor necrosis factor alpha (TNFa), and interleukin-1 and interleukin-17 (IL-1 and IL-17) stimulate downstream events including interleukin-6 (IL-6) that activates STAT3 and HIF-1a. Mechanisms to destabilize STAT3 are inhibited through BCL6 and progesterone resistance and by overexpression of protein inhibitor of stat3 (PIAS3). Together the activation of STAT3 and HIF1a promotes inflammation, angiogenesis, and proliferation. Further, in the setting of progesterone resistance, pregnancy and normal implantation does not easily occur (Used with permission from Fertility and Sterility [138]) (Used with permission of Elsevier Inc.)

inflammatory conditions such as endometriosis [145], which results in further chronic activation of STAT3. This favors estrogen action and proliferation and contributes to cyclooxygenase 2 (COX2), prostaglandin production, aromatase expression, angiogenesis, and inflammation. We believe this model helps explain why pregnancy can be difficult in the setting of inflammation and conditions such as endometriosis. Finally, the oncogene KRAS is elevated in endometriosis and thought to drive this elevation in SIRT1, contributing to progesterone resistance [142].

Summary and Conclusions

An understanding of embryo implantation requires an extensive emersion into endocrinology, physiology, and cell biology. The concept of a window of implantation is a valid construct to frame the mechanisms of implantation and appreciate the temporal chain of events. Synchrony and cooperation between the embryo and endometrium appear critical to a successful pregnancy. Failure of implantation, while not covered by this introductory chapter, can be examined in the context of normal implantation and the molecular constraints required by synchrony and complex sequential events. There are multiple steps required for normal pregnancy to occur and conclude successfully. In the context of this book, many of those aspects will be discovered.

References

1. Evans J, Salamonsen LA. Inflammation, leukocytes and menstruation. Rev Endocr Metab Disord. 2012;13:277–88.
2. Lessey BA, Young SL. Homeostasis imbalance in the endometrium of women with implantation defects: the role of estrogen and progesterone. Semin Reprod Med. 2014;32:365–75.
3. Garry R, Hart R, Karthigasu KA, Burke C. A re-appraisal of the morphological changes within the endometrium during menstruation: a hysteroscopic, histological and scanning electron microscopic study. Hum Reprod. 2009;1:1–9.
4. Hertig AJ, Behrman SJ, Kistner RW. Implantation of the human ovum. In: Progress in infertility, vol. 1. Boston: Little, Brown, & Co.; 1975. p. 435.
5. Hertig AT, Rock J, Adams EC. A description of 34 human ova within the first 17 days of development. Am J Anat. 1956;98:435–93.
6. Navot D, Bergh P. Preparation of the human endometrium for implantation. Ann N Y Acad Sci. 1991;622:212–9.
7. Navot D, Bergh PA, Williams M, Garrisi GJ, Guzman I, Sandler B, Fox J, Schreiner-Engel P, Hofmann GE, Grunfeld L. An insight into early reproductive processes through the in vivo model of ovum donation. J Clin Endocrinol Metab. 1991;72:408–14.
8. Bergh PA, Navot D. The impact of embryonic development and endometrial maturity on the timing of implantation. Fertil Steril. 1992;58:537–42.
9. Bischof P, Aplin JD, Bentin-Ley U, Brannstrom M, Casslen B, Castrillo JL, Classen-Linke I, Critchley HO, Devoto L, D'Hooghe T, Horcajadas JA, Groothuis P, et al. Implantation of the human embryo: research lines and models. From the implantation research network 'fruitful'. Gynecol Obstet Investig. 2006;62:206–16.
10. Bentin-Ley U, Sjîgren A, Nilsson L, Hamberger L, Larsen JF, Horn T. Presence of uterine pinopodes at the embryo-endometrial interface during human implantation in vitro. Hum Reprod. 1999;14:515–20.
11. Norwitz ER, Schust DJ, Fisher SJ. Implantation and the survival of early pregnancy. N Engl J Med. 2001;345:1400–8.
12. Burton GJ, Jauniaux E, Charnock-Jones DS. Human early placental development: potential roles of the endometrial glands. Placenta. 2007;28(Suppl A):S64–9.
13. Lessey BA, Young SL. The structure, function and evaluation of the female reproductive tract. In: Strauss JFI, Barbieri RL, editors. Reproductive endocrinology: physiology, pathology and clinical management, vol. 7. Philadelphia: Saunders Elsevier; 2012. p. 192–235.
14. McLaren A, Michie D. Studies on the transfer of fertilized mouse eggs to uterine foster-mothers. J Exp Biol. 1954;33:394.
15. Psychoyos A. Hormonal control of ovoimplantation. Vitams Horm. 1973;31:201–56.
16. Finn CA, Martin L. The control of implantation. J Reprod Fertil. 1974;39:195–206.
17. Hodgen GD. Surrogate embryo transfer combined with estrogen-progesterone therapy in monkeys: implantation, gestation, and delivery without ovaries. JAMA. 1983;250:2167–71.
18. Noyes RW, Hertig AI, Rock J. Dating the endometrial biopsy. Fertil Steril. 1950;1:3–25.

19. Fawcett DW. The development of mouse ova under the capsule of the kidney. Anat Rec. 1950;108:71.
20. Kirby DR. The development of mouse blastocysts transplanted to the scrotal and cryptorchid testis. J Anat. 1963;97:119.
21. Beier HM. Oviducal and uterine fluids. J Reprod Fertil. 1974;37:221–37.
22. Campbell KL, Rockett JC. Biomarkers of ovulation, endometrial receptivity, fertilisation, implantation and early pregnancy progression. Paediatr Perinat Epidemiol. 2006;20(Suppl 1):13–25.
23. May KE, Villar J, Kirtley S, Kennedy SH, Becker CM. Endometrial alterations in endometriosis: a systematic review of putative biomarkers. Hum Reprod Update. 2011;17:637–53.
24. May KE, Conduit-Hulbert SA, Villar J, Kirtley S, Kennedy SH, Becker CM. Peripheral biomarkers of endometriosis: a systematic review. Hum Reprod Update. 2010;16:651–74.
25. Jones GS. Some newer aspects of management of infertility. JAMA. 1949;141:1123–9.
26. Murray MJ, Meyer WR, Zaino RJ, Lessey BA, Novotny DB, Ireland K, Zeng D, Fritz MA. A critical analysis of the accuracy, reproducibility, and clinical utility of histologic endometrial dating in fertile women. Fertil Steril. 2004;81:1333–43.
27. Practice Committee of the American Society for Reproductive M. Current clinical irrelevance of luteal phase deficiency: a committee opinion. Fertil Steril. 2015;103:e27–32.
28. Coutifaris C, Myers ER, Guzick DS, Diamond MP, Carson SA, Legro RS, McGovern PG, Schlaff WD, Carr BR, Steinkampf MP, Silva S, Vogel DL, et al. Histological dating of timed endometrial biopsy tissue is not related to fertility status. Fertil Steril. 2004;82:1264–72.
29. Schlafke S, Enders AC. Cellular basis of interaction between trophoblast and uterus at implantation. Biol Reprod. 1975;12:41.
30. Martin PM, Sutherland AE. Exogenous amino acids regulate trophectoderm differentiation in the mouse blastocyst through an mTOR-dependent pathway. Dev Biol. 2001;240:182–93.
31. Sutherland A. Mechanisms of implantation in the mouse: differentiation and functional importance of trophoblast giant cell behavior. Dev Biol. 2003;258:241–51.
32. Carson DD, Bagchi I, Dey SK, Enders AC, Fazleabas AT, Lessey BA, Yoshinaga K. Embryo implantation. Dev Biol. 2000;223:217–37.
33. Donaghay M, Lessey BA. Uterine receptivity: alterations associated with benign gynecological disease. Semin Reprod Med. 2007;25:461–75.
34. Cha J, Sun X, Dey SK. Mechanisms of implantation: strategies for successful pregnancy. Nat Med. 2012;18:1754–67.
35. Nilsson O. Ultrastructure of mouse uterine surface epithelium under different estrogenic influences. 5. Continuous administration of estrogen. J Ultrastruct Res. 1959;2:342–51.
36. Psychoyos A, Mandon P. Study of the surface of the uterine epithelium by scanning electron microscope. Observations in the rat at the 4th and 5th day of pregnancy. C R Acad Sci Hebd Seances Acad Sci D. 1971;272:2723–5.
37. Nikas G, Drakakis P, Loutradis D, Mara-Skoufari C, Koumantakis E, Michalas S, Psychoyos A. Uterine pinopodes as markers of the 'nidation window' in cycling women receiving exogenous oestradiol and progesterone. Hum Reprod. 1995;10:1208–13.
38. Psychoyos A, Nikas G. Uterine pinopodes as markers of uterine receptivity. Assist Reprod Rev. 1994;4:26–32.
39. Nikas G. Cell-surface morphological events relevant to human implantation. Hum Reprod. 1999;14(Suppl 2):37–44.
40. Martel D, Monier MN, Roche D, Psychoyos A. Hormonal dependence of pinopode formation at the uterine luminal surface. Hum Reprod. 1991;6:597.
41. Develioglu OH, Nikas G, Hsiu JG, Toner JP, Jones HW Jr. Detection of endometrial pinopodes by light microscopy. Fertil Steril. 2000;74:767–70.
42. Apparao KB, Murray MJ, Fritz MA, Meyer WR, Chambers AF, Truong PR, Lessey BA. Osteopontin and its receptor alphavbeta(3) integrin are coexpressed in the human endometrium during the menstrual cycle but regulated differentially. J Clin Endocrinol Metab. 2001;86:4991–5000.

43. Bentin-Ley U, Horn T, Sjîgren A, Sorensen S, Larsen JF, Hamberger L. Ultrastructure of human blastocyst-endometrial interactions in vitro. J Reprod Fertil. 2000;120:337–50.
44. Kang YJ, Forbes K, Carver J, Aplin JD. The role of the osteopontin-integrin alphavbeta3 interaction at implantation: functional analysis using three different in vitro models. Hum Reprod. 2014;29:739–49.
45. Acosta AA, Elberger L, Borghi M, Calamera JC, Chemes H, Doncel GF, Kliman H, Lema B, Lustig L, Papier S. Endometrial dating and determination of the window of implantation in healthy fertile women. Fertil Steril. 2000;73:788–98.
46. Quinn CE, Casper RF. Pinopodes: a questionable role in endometrial receptivity. Hum Reprod Update. 2009;15:229–36.
47. Usadi RS, Murray MJ, Bagnell RC, Fritz MA, Kowalik AI, Meyer WR, Lessey BA. Temporal and morphologic characteristics of pinopod expression across the secretory phase of the endometrial cycle in normally cycling women with proven fertility. Fertil Steril. 2003;79:970–4.
48. Lessey BA, Castelbaum AJ, Buck CA, Lei Y, Yowell CW, Sun J. Further characterization of endometrial integrins during the menstrual cycle and in pregnancy. Fertil Steril. 1994;62:497–506.
49. Reddy KV, Meherji PK. Integrin cell adhesion molecules in endometrium of fertile and infertile women throughout menstrual cycle. Indian J Exp Biol. 1999;37:323–31.
50. Achache H, Revel A. Endometrial receptivity markers, the journey to successful embryo implantation. Hum Reprod Update. 2006;12:731–46.
51. Hoozemans DA, Schats R, Lambalk CB, Homburg R, Hompes PG. Human embryo implantation: current knowledge and clinical implications in assisted reproductive technology. Reprod Biomed Online. 2004;9:692–715.
52. Lessey BA, Castelbaum AJ, Sawin SW, Sun J. Integrins as markers of uterine receptivity in women with primary unexplained infertility. Fertil Steril. 1995;63:535–42.
53. Lessey BA, Castelbaum AJ, Sawin SW, Buck CA, Schinnar R, Bilker W, Strom BL. Aberrant integrin expression in the endometrium of women with endometriosis. J Clin Endocrinol Metab. 1994;79:643–9.
54. Meyer WR, Castelbaum AJ, Somkuti S, Sagoskin AW, Doyle M, Harris JE, Lessey BA. Hydrosalpinges adversely affect markers of endometrial receptivity. Hum Reprod. 1997;12:1393–8.
55. Apparao KB, Lovely LP, Gui Y, Lininger RA, Lessey BA. Elevated endometrial androgen receptor expression in women with polycystic ovarian syndrome. Biol Reprod. 2002;66:297–304.
56. Zhu HH, Huang JR, Mazela J, Elias J, Tseng L. Progestin stimulates the biosynthesis of fibronectin and accumulation of fibronectin mRNA in human endometrial stromal cells. Hum Reprod. 1992;7:141–6.
57. Giudice LC. Potential biochemical markers of uterine receptivity. Hum Reprod. 1999;14(Suppl 2):3–16.
58. Damsky CH, Librach C, Lim KH, Fitzgerald ML, McMaster MT, Janatpour M, Zhou Y, Logan SK, Fisher SJ. Integrin switching regulates normal trophoblast invasion. Development. 1994;120:3657–66.
59. Karsdorp VH, Dekker GA, Bast A, van Kamp GJ, Bouman AA, van Vugt JM, van Geijn HP. Maternal and fetal plasma concentrations of endothelin, lipidhydroperoxides, glutathione peroxidase and fibronectin in relation to abnormal umbilical artery velocimetry. Eur J Obstet Gynecol Reprod Biol. 1998;80:39–44.
60. Damsky CH, Fitzgerald ML, Fisher SJ. Distribution patterns of extracellular matrix components and adhesion receptors are intricately modulated during first trimester cytotrophoblast differentiation along the invasive pathway, in vivo. J Clin Invest. 1992;89:210–22.
61. Zhou Y, Fisher SJ, Janatpour M, Genbacev O, Dejana E, Wheelock M, Damsky CH. Human cytotrophoblasts adopt a vascular phenotype as they differentiate - a strategy for successful endovascular invasion? J Clin Invest. 1997;99:2139–51.
62. Alon R, Feigelson S. From rolling to arrest on blood vessels: leukocyte tap dancing on endothelial integrin ligands and chemokines at sub-second contacts. Semin Immunol. 2002;14:93–104.

63. Genbacev OD, Prakobphol A, Foulk RA, Krtolica AR, Ilic D, Singer MS, Yan ZQ, Kiessling LL, Rosen SD, Fisher SJ. Trophoblast L-selectin-mediated adhesion at the maternal-fetal interface. Science. 2003;299:405–8.
64. Fazleabas AT, Kim JJ. Development. What makes an embryo stick? Science. 2003;299:355–6.
65. Foulk RA, Zdravkovic T, Genbacev O, Prakobphol A. Expression of L-selectin ligand MECA-79 as a predictive marker of human uterine receptivity. J Assist Reprod Genet. 2007;24:316–21.
66. Margarit L, Gonzalez D, Lewis PD, Hopkins L, Davies C, Conlan RS, Joels L, White JO. L-selectin ligands in human endometrium: comparison of fertile and infertile subjects. Hum Reprod. 2009;24:2767–77.
67. Hey NA, Graham RA, Seif MW, Aplin JD. The polymorphic epithelial mucin MUC1 in human endometrium is regulated with maximal expression in the implantation phase. J Clin Endocrinol Metab. 1994;78:337–42.
68. Hey NA, Aplin JD. Sialyl-Lewis x and Sialyl-Lewis a are associated with MUC1 in human endometrium. Glycoconj J. 1996;13:769–79.
69. Wesseling J, van der Valk SW, Hilkens J. A mechanism for inhibition of E-cadherin-mediated cell-cell adhesion by the membrane-associated mucin episialin/MUC1. Mol Biol Cell. 1996;7:565–77.
70. Lessey BA. Two pathways of progesterone action in the human endometrium: implications for implantation and contraception. Steroids. 2003;68:809–15.
71. Humbel RE. Insulin-like growth factors I and II. Eur J Biochem. 1990;190:445–62.
72. Murata K, Maruo T, Matsuo H, Mochizuki M. insulin-like growth factor-I (IGF-I) as a local regulator of proliferation and differentiation of villous trophoblasts in early pregnancy. Nihon Sanka Fujinka Gakkai Zasshi. 1994;46:87–94.
73. Oner J, Oner H. Immunolocalization of insulin-like growth factor I (IGF-I) during preimplantation in rat uterus. Growth Hormon IGF Res. 2007;17:271–8.
74. Rutanen EM. Insulin-like growth factors in endometrial function. Gynecol Endocrinol. 1998;12:399–406.
75. Van Sinderen M, Menkhorst E, Winship A, Cuman C, Dimitriadis E. Preimplantation human blastocyst-endometrial interactions: the role of inflammatory mediators. Am J Reprod Immunol. 2013;69:427–40.
76. Lessey BA, Gui Y, Apparao KB, Young SL, Mulholland J. Regulated expression of heparin-binding EGF-like growth factor (HB-EGF) in the human endometrium: a potential paracrine role during implantation. Mol Reprod Dev. 2002;62:446–55.
77. Stavreus-Evers A, Aghajanova L, Brismar H, Eriksson H, Landgren BM, Hovatta O. Co-existence of heparin-binding epidermal growth factor-like growth factor and pinopodes in human endometrium at the time of implantation. Mol Hum Reprod. 2002;8:765–9.
78. Smith SK. Angiogenesis and implantation. Hum Reprod. 2000;15(Suppl 6):59–66.
79. Leach RE, Khalifa R, Ramirez ND, Das SK, Wang J, Dey SK, Romero R, Armant DR. Multiple roles for heparin-binding epidermal growth factor-like growth factor are suggested by its cell-specific expression during the human endometrial cycle and early placentation. J Clin Endocrinol Metab. 1999;84:3355–63.
80. Das SK, Wang XN, Paria BC, Damm D, Abraham JA, Klagsbrun M, Andrews GK, Dey SK. Heparin-binding EGF-like growth factor gene is induced in the mouse uterus temporally by the blastocyst solely at the site of its apposition: a possible ligand for interaction with blastocyst EGF-receptor in implantation. Development. 1994;120:1071–83.
81. Martin KL, Barlow DH, Sargent IL. Heparin-binding epidermal growth factor significantly improves human blastocyst development and hatching in serum-free medium. Hum Reprod. 1998;13:1645–52.
82. Baker PN, Krasnow J, Roberts JM, Yeo KT. Elevated serum levels of vascular endothelial growth factor in patients with preeclampsia. Obstet Gynecol. 1995;86:815–21.
83. Barroso G, Barrionuevo M, Rao P, Graham L, Danforth D, Huey S, Abuhamad A, Oehninger S. Vascular endothelial growth factor, nitric oxide, and leptin follicular fluid levels correlate negatively with embryo quality in IVF patients. Fertil Steril. 1999;72:1024–6.

84. Dorn C, Reinsberg J, Kupka M, van der Ven H, Schild RL. Leptin, VEGF, IGF-1, and IGFBP-3 concentrations in serum and follicular fluid of women undergoing in vitro fertilization. Arch Gynecol Obstet. 2003;268:187–93.
85. Minas V, Loutradis D, Makrigiannakis A. Factors controlling blastocyst implantation. Reprod Biomed Online. 2005;10:205–16.
86. Alexander CM, Hansell EJ, Behrendtsen O, Flannery ML, Kishnani NS, Hawkes SP, Werb Z. Expression and function of matrix metalloproteinases and their inhibitors at the maternal-embryonic boundary during mouse embryo implantation. Development. 1996;122:1723–36.
87. Das SK, Yano S, Wang J, Edwards DR, Nagase H, Dey SK. Expression of matrix metalloproteinases and tissue inhibitors of metalloproteinases in the mouse uterus during the peri-implantation period. Dev Genet. 1997;21:44–54.
88. Maia-Filho VO, Rocha AM, Ferreira FP, Bonetti TC, Serafini P, Motta EL. Matrix metalloproteinases 2 and 9 and e-cadherin expression in the endometrium during the implantation window of infertile women before in vitro fertilization treatment. Reprod Sci. 2015;22:416–22.
89. Rechtman MP, Zhang J, Salamonsen LA. Effect of inhibition of matrix metalloproteinases on endometrial decidualization and implantation in mated rats. J Reprod Fertil. 1999;117:169–77.
90. Riley SC, Webb CJ, Leask R, McCaig FM, Howe DC. Involvement of matrix metalloproteinases 2 and 9, tissue inhibitor of metalloproteinases and apoptosis in tissue remodelling in the sheep placenta. J Reprod Fertil. 2000;118:19–27.
91. Salamonsen LA, Nagase H, Woolley DE. Matrix metalloproteinases and their tissue inhibitors at the ovine trophoblast-uterine interface. J Reprod Fertil Suppl. 1995;49:29–37.
92. Hurskainen TL, Hirohata S, Seldin MF, Apte SS. ADAM-TS5, ADAM-TS6, and ADAM-TS7, novel members of a new family of zinc metalloproteases. General features and genomic distribution of the ADAM-TS family. J Biol Chem. 1999;274:25555–63.
93. Taylor HS, Vanden Heuvel GB, Igarashi P. A conserved Hox axis in the mouse and human female reproductive system: late establishment and persistent adult expression of the Hoxa cluster genes. Biol Reprod. 1997;57:1338–45.
94. Kappen C, Schughart K, Ruddle FH. Early evolutionary origin of major homeodomain sequence classes. Genomics. 1993;18:54–70.
95. Schughart K, Kappen C, Ruddle FH. Mammalian homeobox-containing genes: genome organization, structure, expression and evolution. Br J Cancer Suppl. 1988;9:9–13.
96. Taylor HS, Arici A, Olive D, Igarashi P. HOXA10 is expressed in response to sex steroids at the time of implantation in the human endometrium. J Clin Invest. 1998;101:1379–84.
97. Taylor HS, Igarashi P, Olive DL, Arici A. Sex steroids mediate HOXA11 expression in the human peri-implantation endometrium. J Clin Endocrinol Metab. 1999;84:1129–35.
98. Cermik D, Selam B, Taylor HS. Regulation of HOXA-10 expression by testosterone in vitro and in the endometrium of patients with polycystic ovary syndrome. J Clin Endocrinol Metab. 2003;88:238–43.
99. Daftary GS, Taylor HS. Hydrosalpinx fluid diminishes endometrial cell HOXA10 expression. Fertil Steril. 2002;78:577–80.
100. Taylor HS, Bagot C, Kardana A, Olive D, Arici A. HOX gene expression is altered in the endometrium of women with endometriosis. Hum Reprod. 1999;14:1328–31.
101. Psychoyos A, Nikas G, Gravanis A. The role of prostaglandins in blastocyst implantation. Hum Reprod. 1995;10(Suppl 2):30–42.
102. Chakraborty I, Das SK, Wang J, Dey SK. Developmental expression of the cyclo-oxygenase-1 and cyclo-oxygenase-2 genes in the peri-implantation mouse uterus and their differential regulation by the blastocyst and ovarian steroids. J Mol Endocrinol. 1996;16:107–22.
103. Gupta A, Huet YM, Dey SK. Evidence for prostaglandins and leukotrienes as mediators of phase I of estrogen action in implantation in the mouse. Endocrinology. 1989;124:546–8.
104. Johnson DC, Dey SK. Role of histamine in implantation: dexamethasone inhibits estradiol-induced implantation in the rat. Biol Reprod. 1980;22:1136–41.
105. Kennedy TG. Evidence for a role for prostaglandins in the initiation of blastocyst implantation in the rat. Biol Reprod. 1977;16:286–91.

106. Lau IF, Saksena SK, Chang MC. Pregnancy blockade by indomethacin, an inhibitor of prostaglandin synthesis: its reversal by prostaglandins and progesterone in mice. Prostaglandins. 1973;4:795–803.
107. Malathy PV, Cheng HC, Dey SK. Production of leukotrienes and prostaglandins in the rat uterus during peri-implantation period. Prostaglandins. 1986;32:605–14.
108. Tawfik OW, Sagrillo C, Johnson DC, Dey SK. Decidualization in the rat: role of leukotrienes and prostaglandins. Prostaglandins Leukot Med. 1987;29:221–7.
109. Brumsted JR, Chapitis J, Deaton JL, Riddick DH, Gibson M. Prostaglandin F2 alpha synthesis and metabolism by luteal phase endometrium in vitro. Fertil Steril. 1989;52:769–73.
110. Ishihara O, Tsutsumi O, Mizuno M, Kinoshita K, Satoh K. Metabolism of arachidonic acid and synthesis of prostanoids in human endometrium and decidua. Prostaglandins Leukot Med. 1986;24:93–102.
111. Maathuis JB, Kelly RW. Concentrations of prostaglandins F2alpha and E2 in the endometrium throughout the human menstrual cycle, after the administration of clomiphene or an oestrogen-progestogen pill and in early pregnancy. J Endocrinol. 1978;77:361–71.
112. Salamonsen LA, Findlay JK. Regulation of endometrial prostaglandins during the menstrual cycle and in early pregnancy. Reprod Fertil Dev. 1990;2:443–57.
113. Singh EJ, Baccarini I, Zuspan FP. Levels of prostaglandins F-2alpha and E-2 in human endometrium during the menstrual cycle. Am J Obstet Gynecol. 1975;121:1003–6.
114. van der Weiden RM, Helmerhorst FM, Keirse MJ. Influence of prostaglandins and platelet activating factor on implantation. Hum Reprod. 1991;6:436–42.
115. Evans CA, Kennedy TG. The importance of prostaglandin synthesis for the initiation of blastocyst implantation in the hamster. J Reprod Fertil. 1978;54:255–61.
116. Hoos PC, Hoffman LH. Effect of histamine receptor antagonists and indomethacin on implantation in the rabbit. Biol Reprod. 1983;29:833–40.
117. Kennedy TG, Gillio-Meina C, Phang SH. Prostaglandins and the initiation of blastocyst implantation and decidualization. Reproduction. 2007;134:635–43.
118. Lundkvist O, Nilsson BO. Ultrastructural studies of the temporal relationship between loss of zona pellucida and appearance of blastocyst-induced stromal changes during normal pregnancy in rats. Anat Embryol. 1984;170:45–9.
119. Kennedy TG, Doktorcik PE. Effects of analogues of prostaglandin E2 and F2 alpha on the decidual cell reaction in the rat. Prostaglandins. 1988;35:207–19.
120. Oettel M, Koch M, Kurischko A, Schubert K. Direct evidence for the involvement of prostaglandin F2 alpha in the first step of estrone-induced blastocyst implantation in the spayed rat. Steroids. 1979;33:1–8.
121. Granot I, Gnainsky Y, Dekel N. Endometrial inflammation and effect on implantation improvement and pregnancy outcome. Reproduction. 2012;144:661–8.
122. Kelly RW, King AE, Critchley HO. Cytokine control in human endometrium. Reproduction. 2001;121:3–19.
123. Ross JW, Malayer JR, Ritchey JW, Geisert RD. Characterization of the interleukin-1beta system during porcine trophoblastic elongation and early placental attachment. Biol Reprod. 2003;69:1251–9.
124. Boomsma CM, Kavelaars A, Eijkemans MJ, Amarouchi K, Teklenburg G, Gutknecht D, Fauser BJ, Heijnen CJ, Macklon NS. Cytokine profiling in endometrial secretions: a noninvasive window on endometrial receptivity. Reprod Biomed Online. 2009;18:85–94.
125. Simon C, Valbuena D, Krussel J, Bernal A, Murphy CR, Shaw T, Pellicer A, Polan ML. Interleukin-1 receptor antagonist prevents embryonic implantation by a direct effect on the endometrial epithelium. Fertil Steril. 1998;70:896–906.
126. Blitek A, Morawska E, Ziecik AJ. Regulation of expression and role of leukemia inhibitory factor and interleukin-6 in the uterus of early pregnant pigs. Theriogenology. 2012;78:951–64.
127. Modric T, Kowalski AA, Green ML, Simmen RC, Simmen FA. Pregnancy-dependent expression of leukaemia inhibitory factor (LIF), LIF receptor-beta and interleukin-6 (IL-6) messenger ribonucleic acids in the porcine female reproductive tract. Placenta. 2000;21:345–53.
128. Simon C, Piquette GN, Frances A, Polan ML. Localization of interleukin-1 type I receptor and interleukin-1 beta in human endometrium throughout the menstrual cycle. J Clin Endocrinol Metab. 1993;77:549–55.

129. Lass A, Weiser W, Munafo A, Loumaye E. Leukemia inhibitory factor in human reproduction. Fertil Steril. 2001;76:1091–6.
130. Bhatt H, Brunet LJ, Stewart CL. Uterine expression of leukemia inhibitory factor coincides with the onset of blastocyst implantation. ProcNatlAcad SciUS A. 1991;88:11408–12.
131. Stewart CL. The role of leukemia inhibitory factor (LIF) and other cytokines in regulating implantation in mammals. Ann N Y Acad Sci. 1994;734:157.
132. Cullinan EB, Abbondanzo SJ, Anderson PS, Pollard JW, Lessey BA, Stewart CL. Leukemia inhibitory factor (LIF) and LIF receptor expression in human endometrium suggests a potential autocrine/paracrine function in regulating embryo implantation. Proc Natl Acad Sci U S A. 1996;93:3115–20.
133. Nachtigall MJ, Kliman HJ, Feinberg RF, Olive DL, Engin O, Arici A. The effect of leukemia inhibitory factor (LIF) on trophoblast differentiation: a potential role in human implantation. J Clin Endocrinol Metab. 1996;81:801–6.
134. Hambartsoumian E. Endometrial leukemia inhibitory factor (LIF) as a possible cause of unexplained infertility and multiple failures of implantation. Am J Reprod Immunol. 1998;39:137–43.
135. Laird SM, Tuckerman EM, Dalton CF, Dunphy BC, Li TC, Zhang X. The production of leukaemia inhibitory factor by human endometrium: presence in uterine flushings and production by cells in culture. Hum Reprod. 1997;12:569–74.
136. Brinsden PR, Alam V, de Moustier B, Engrand P. Recombinant human leukemia inhibitory factor does not improve implantation and pregnancy outcomes after assisted reproductive techniques in women with recurrent unexplained implantation failure. Fertil Steril. 2009;91:1445–7.
137. Macklon NS, Geraedts JP, Fauser BC. Conception to ongoing pregnancy: the 'black box' of early pregnancy loss. Hum Reprod Update. 2002;8:333–43.
138. Fox C, Morin S, Jeong JW, Scott RT Jr, Lessey BA. Local and systemic factors and implantation: what is the evidence? Fertil Steril. 2016;105:873–84.
139. Kim BG, Yoo JY, Kim TH, Shin JH, Langenheim JF, Ferguson SD, Fazleabas AT, Young SL, Lessey BA, Jeong JW. Aberrant activation of signal transducer and activator of transcription-3 (STAT3) signaling in endometriosis. Hum Reprod. 2015;30:1069–78.
140. Evans-Hoeker E, Lessey BA, Jeong JW, Savaris RF, Palomino WA, Yuan L, Schammel DP, Young SL. Endometrial BCL6 overexpression in Eutopic endometrium of women with endometriosis. Reprod Sci. 2016;23:1234–41.
141. Tiberi L, Bonnefont J, van den Ameele J, Le Bon SD, Herpoel A, Bilheu A, Baron BW, Vanderhaeghen P. A BCL6/BCOR/SIRT1 complex triggers neurogenesis and suppresses medulloblastoma by repressing sonic hedgehog signaling. Cancer Cell. 2014;26:797–812.
142. Yoo JY, Kim TH, Fazleabas AT, Palomino WA, Ahn SH, Tayade C, Schammel DP, Young SL, Jeong JW, Lessey BAKRAS. Activation and over-expression of SIRT1/BCL6 contributes to the pathogenesis of endometriosis and progesterone resistance. Sci Rep. 2017;7:6765.
143. Maruyama T, Yoshimura Y. Molecular and cellular mechanisms for differentiation and regeneration of the uterine endometrium. Endocr J. 2008;55:795–810.
144. Walker SR, Nelson EA, Yeh JE, Pinello L, Yuan GC, Frank DA. STAT5 outcompetes STAT3 to regulate the expression of the oncogenic transcriptional modulator BCL6. Mol Cell Biol. 2013;33:2879–90.
145. Yoo JY, Jeong JW, Fazleabas AT, Tayade C, Young SL, Lessey BA. Protein inhibitor of activated STAT3 (PIAS3) is down-regulated in Eutopic endometrium of women with endometriosis. Biol Reprod. 2016;95(1):11.
146. Lim JJ, Lee DR, Song HS, Kim KS, Yoon TK, Gye MC, Kim MK. Heparin-binding epidermal growth factor (HB-EGF) may improve embryonic development and implantation by increasing vitronectin receptor (integrin alphanubeta3) expression in peri-implantation mouse embryos. J Assist Reprod Genet. 2006;23:111–9.
147. Yoo HJ, Barlow DH, Mardon HJ. Temporal and spatial regulation of expression of heparin-binding epidermal growth factor-like growth factor in the human endometrium: a possible role in blastocyst implantation. Dev Genet. 1997;21:102–8.

Chapter 2
Embryo and Endometrial Synchrony in Implantation Failure

Jason M. Franasiak and Richard T. Scott

Introduction

Normal embryo implantation requires synchronized interactions between the endometrium and the embryo. The concept of synchrony entails both of these components: the endometrium must be optimally receptive and it must be in that state at the same time that the embryo is ready to implant in order to attain optimal clinical outcomes. A loss of this synchrony—also termed *dyssynchrony* in the literature—occurs *either* when the endometrium is not optimally receptive *or* when the embryo is not developed to the point of optimal implantation capacity. When either of these scenarios occurs, dyssynchrony can cause implantation failure. Of great importance, this failure occurs in spite of the fact that the endometrium, given optimal timing, is capable of receiving an embryo and the embryo, given optimal developmental timing, is capable of implantation and progression to delivery of a healthy child. That is, dyssynchrony can cause implantation failure in the absence of true pathology—rather, this is a mishandling of physiology.

Much of the foundation of fundamental physiology of embryo implantation has been expertly reviewed elsewhere in this book—this chapter builds upon these concepts. Traditionally, dyssynchrony has been classified as true pathology. Faced with a poor outcome—failed implantation—it seems intuitive to attribute that failure to either an abnormality in the embryo or an impaired endometrium. Over the last 35 years, embryologist and endometrial physiologists have sought to isolate one factor or the other and identify the specific pathophysiologic changes resulting in failed implantation. In medicine and in science, we seek to employ Occam's razor,

J.M. Franasiak, MD, HCLD (✉) • R.T. Scott, MD, HCLD (✉)
Sidney Kimmel Medical College, Thomas Jefferson University Philadelphia, Philadelphia, PA, USA

IVI-RMA of New Jersey, Basking Ridge, NJ, USA
e-mail: jfranasiak@rmanj.com; rscott@rmanj.com

© Springer International Publishing AG 2018
J.M. Franasiak, R.T. Scott Jr. (eds.), *Recurrent Implantation Failure*,
https://doi.org/10.1007/978-3-319-71967-2_2

or *lex parsimoniae*—the law of parsimony, whenever possible. Indeed, many clinical disorders can ultimately be attributed to a single underlying pathologic abnormality with enough thought. However, while investigating implantation failures, one cannot anticipate that all failures will be attributed to a singular pathologic abnormality. Furthermore, while it is often presumed that implantation failure is due to some identifiable pathology, one must also consider the physiology of the circumstances—perhaps the failure is due to a misunderstanding of the physiology at work during embryo and endometrial development during assisted reproduction.

Pathology or Physiology

The scientists investigating failed implantation could largely be divided into two groups—the embryologists and the endometrial physiologists. The embryologists have traditionally focused on the morphologic and temporal aspects of embryo development. The retrospective review of large clinical experiences allowed investigators to determine criteria for optimal embryo morphology as well as temporal milestones for both early cleavage events and for the timing of blastulation, which commonly ranged from day 5–6 and rarely even day 7 of development [1, 2]. Meanwhile, the endometrial physiologists have focused on abnormal endometrial development by evaluating endometrial sonography, histologic milestones, specific cytokines, and markers of inflammation and, most recently, evaluating more comprehensively the endometrial transcriptome [3, 4].

We have learned a great deal about the specific pathologic abnormalities which may impair implantation. However, a large question remains: Is it possible for a completely normal embryo and a completely normal endometrium which are dyssynchronous leading to failed implantation? Might a circumstance exist when you have a normal endometrium and a normal embryo and these independently regulated entities, which must be temporally coordinated, are not in synch? The answer is yes, and this physiologic change cannot be ignored when attempting to optimize outcomes or when evaluating patients who have implantation failure.

This concept is clearly demonstrated by considering the difference between natural conceptions and those during cycles following controlled ovarian stimulation during assisted reproduction. During natural cycles and conception, embryonic development and the window of endometrial receptivity are controlled by the orderly development of the follicle under the regulation of the hypothalamic-pituitary-gonadal axis. A meaningful rise in progesterone occurs shortly after ovulation (Fig. 2.1a). This timing results in the oocyte being exposed to the spermatozoa at approximately the same time that secretory transformation begins in the endometrium. If both are normal, then development will be synchronous and implantation will be optimized.

In the case of controlled ovarian stimulation during an IVF cycle, this natural coordination is often lost. Due to stimulation parameters, the rise in progesterone

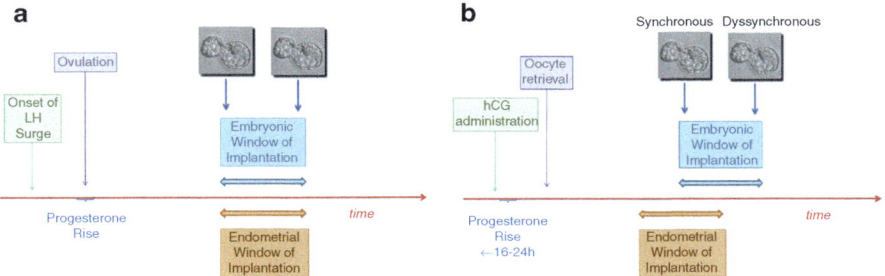

Fig. 2.1 Embryo and endometrial synchrony involves both the endometrium, whose window is determined by the progesterone stimulus, and the embryo, whose widow is relative to blastulation. During natural conception, a rise in progesterone follows the LH surge leading to the opening of the endometrial window of receptivity which overlaps with the window of embryonic blastulation and implantation (**a**). In the case of IVF, natural coordination can be lost. The rise in progesterone following ovulation trigger is faster and more robust, and the progesterone stimulus shifts the endometrial window of receptivity by 16–24 h. Additionally, blastulation may be delayed, particularly in older, low responders. These two factors, either alone or together, result in physiologic dyssynchrony which cannot be predicted prior to cycle start and may not necessarily be reproduced from cycle to cycle (**b**). Used with permission [5]

occurs earlier, and thus the hormonal signals which control the onset of secretory transformation occur earlier shifting the window of implantation. The result is that the endometrium is prepared for the embryo implantation event prior to the embryo reaching developmental maturity for optimal implantation—endometrial dyssynchrony (Fig. 2.1b).

The important difference between this physiologic phenomenon which leads to dyssynchrony and suboptimal implantation conditions and an underlying pathology is that the timing of the stimulus for secretory transformation varies from cycle to cycle. This results in the lack of reproducibility from cycle to cycle and dictates that this physiologic dyssynchrony is not something that can be screened for in advance. The practitioner and embryologist must coordinate in real time to optimize synchrony.

This concept of physiologic changes leading to dyssynchrony stands in contrast to true pathologic changes in the endometrium. The pathologic alterations in the rate of secretory transformation which has been hypothesized alter the timing of the window of receptivity, such as those studied with the endometrial receptivity array (ERA) test [6] among others, which seeks to characterize reproducible changes in the transcriptome which results in repeatedly altered windows of implantation—this effect is pathology in the cascade of events after the progesterone stimulus. While this is clearly important, receptivity pathology impacts only a relatively small percentage of the population. As noted, this alteration ought to be reproducible from cycle to cycle. In contrast, it could be hypothesized that all patients undergoing superovulation during IVF are at risk for embryonic-endometrial dyssynchrony based on timing when a critical level of progesterone is achieved as we will discuss further.

The Endometrium

The focus of the physiologic window of implantation in the uterus is progesterone. Progesterone represents the stimulus which, once a critical threshold is achieved, causes a well-timed and orderly secretory transformation. One can think of this threshold like a trigger which activates the natural timer with the window of receptivity opening several days later and then subsequently closing. Traditionally, there has been much emphasis placed on hormonal support. While this is required, the window of receptivity is more dependent on the timing of the onset of the stimulus than mid-luteal progesterone levels.

Traditionally, the window of endometrial receptivity had been thought of as being quite wide and forgiving, with implantations occurring in a 3–5-day window [7]. However, it is important to note that this concept was founded on data procured from the transfer of day 2 embryos from ovum donation cycles between days 16 and 24 of the cycle. Initially pregnancies were reported on days 17–19 with subsequent pregnancies reported from days 16–20. Subsequent studies have refined this window from what was *possible* to what is *optimal*—a very important distinction when discussing implantation failure with patients. The optimal window is in reality smaller than originally proposed with the highest rates occurring during a 2-day window [8]. In this study investigators utilized an ovum donation model with variation in the start of progesterone to control the window of implantation. Embryo transfers were performed following 2–6 days of progesterone. Pregnancies were achieved corresponding to days 17–20 with optimal days being 18–19. Rates began to fall by half on the late margin of the window. Indeed, delayed implantation on the far edge of the endometrial window may result in poor outcomes associated with abnormal placentation, reinforcing the difference between what is possible and optimal [9] (Fig. 2.2).

Given the apparent importance of the initial progesterone stimulus, it stands to reason that the natural question to follow would be: what is known about varied levels of progesterone and how these varied levels affect the secretory transformation which in turn leads to the optimal window of receptivity? Usadi et al., utilizing a controlled experimental design in which they varied progesterone dosing in healthy volunteers after controlled estrogen priming, showed that even very low levels of progesterone were able to cause differential expression of key genes known to be associated with the onset of secretory transformation leading to endometrial receptivity [10, 11]. These data and others, from the same investigators, suggest that even low serum levels of progesterone, perhaps level as low as 2.5 ng/mL, may initiate secretory transformation and ultimately control the window of time during which a reproductively competent embryo has the opportunity to implant.

In addition to the experimental and molecular evidence of a shift seen in response to the progesterone stimulus, there are several clinical studies in assisted reproduction showing that a premature rise in progesterone, and thus secretory transformation shift, causes an increase in failed implantations. Silverberg et al. measured serum progesterone on the day of ovulation trigger and noted that two breakpoints,

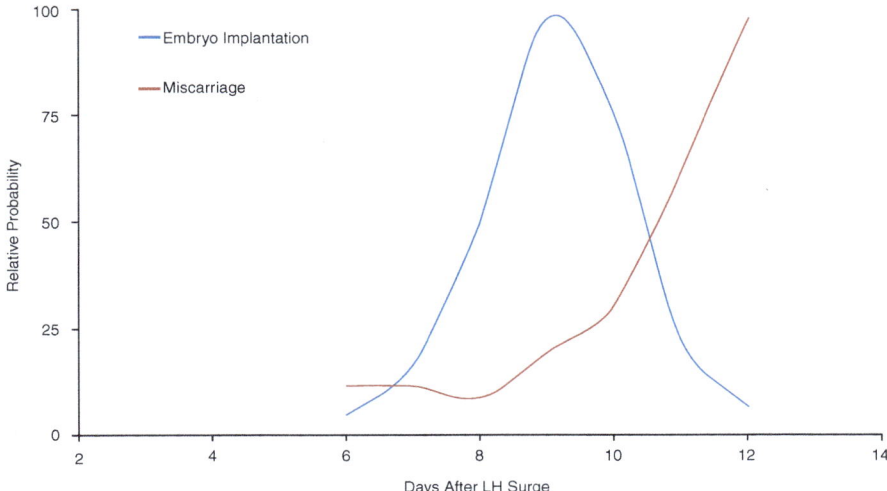

Fig. 2.2 The timing of implantation in naturally occurring pregnancies with increasing proportion of pregnancy loss with later implantation. The day of ovulation was defined as day 0. Modified from [9]

0.4 ng/mL and 0.9 ng/mL, were predictors of clinical pregnancy [3]. More recently, Bosch et al. evaluated serum progesterone levels on the day of hCG administration and found that patients with levels greater than 1.5 ng/mL had significantly lower ongoing pregnancy rates [4] (Fig. 2.3). Other investigators have shown similar detriment when there is premature progesterone elevation at levels of 1.5 ng/mL and 2 ng/mL [12].

It is important to interpret these data with caution. They do not necessarily mean that the endometrial secretory transformation begins at a progesterone level of 1.5 ng/mL. It is better to suggest that patients with that level of progesterone prior to the administration of the ovulation trigger are at increased risk of early-onset secretory transformation which would shift the window of implantation. It is important to note that those embryos which blastulate more slowly would then be at an even greater risk for being dyssynchronous with the endometrium—something we will discuss below.

As was mentioned before, it is important to note that in stimulated IVF cycles as compared to natural cycles, the progesterone rise is more rapid and robust following the ovulation stimulus. This is the result of the varied pharmacokinetics of hCG versus the natural LH surge. This can result in as much as a 16–24 h shift in the onset of the critical level of progesterone during stimulated cycles and would create a situation in which the endometrial window of receptivity is physiologically shifted in IVF. This window is of course all the more shifted if there is a premature rise in the progesterone prior to the administration of the ovulation trigger. This shift cannot be assessed prior to the cycle in question and is not reproducible from cycle to cycle—this must be actively managed in the current treatment cycle.

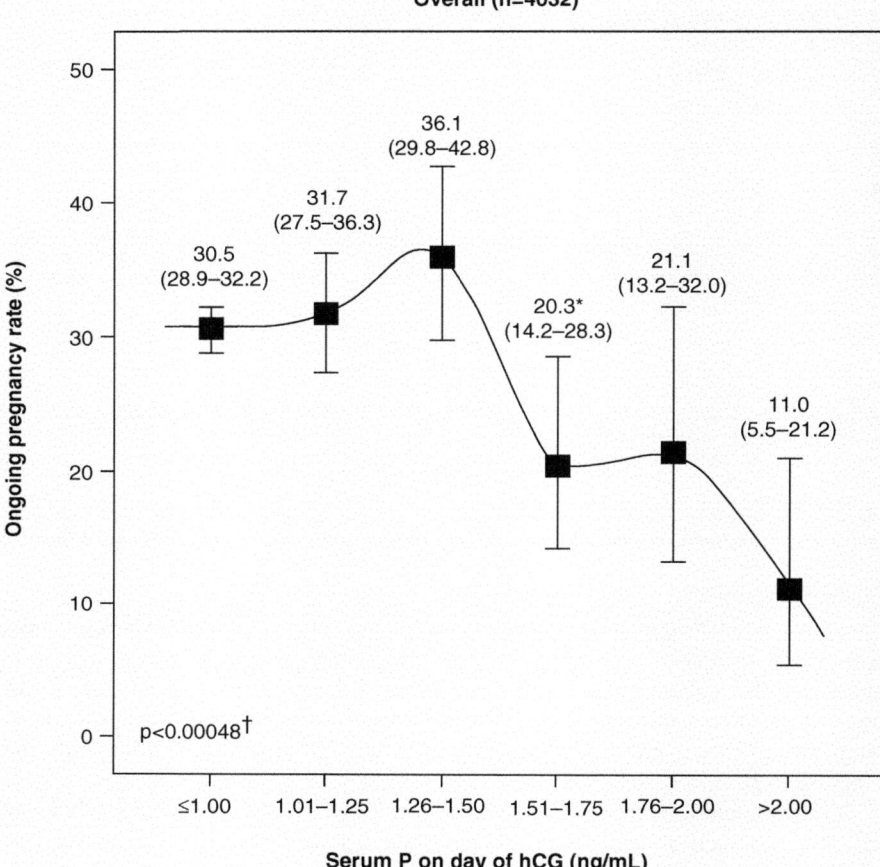

Fig. 2.3 Elevated serum progesterone levels on the day of hCG administration are associated with reduced ongoing pregnancy rates. In particular, serum progesterone levels of 1.5 ng/mL were associated with lower ongoing pregnancy rates following IVF/ICSI cycles. Used with permission from [4]

Furthermore, this focuses on only one half of the puzzle—the embryo's timing is also important.

The Embryo

Given that the time at which the embryo is ready to implant is the other half of the puzzle, it is important to look at what is known about variability in embryonic maturation. At the current time, the timing of blastulation is the best surrogate marker

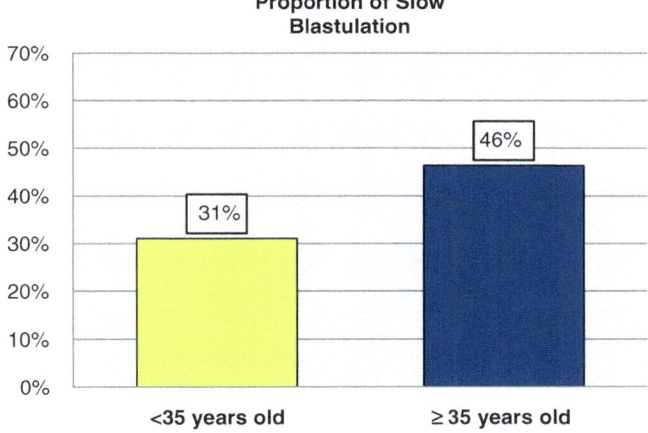

Fig. 2.4 Embryos in extended culture were assessed on day 5 utilizing Gardner's criteria for blastocyst grading. Those which were morula or B1 on the morning of day 5 were considered slowly blastulating. Patient over age 35 were at much higher risk for slowly blastulating embryos ($p < 0.0001$)

available in vitro. This physiology changes over time. It has been shown that blastulation rates differ given the woman's age. Shapiro et al. showed that patients under age 30 had much higher blastulation rates prior to day 6 than did patients 31–34 and 35–40 [13]. Forman et al. have shown that patients age 35 and above have a significantly higher proportion of embryos which have failed to blastulate by day 5 when compared to those patients under age 35 [14] (Fig. 2.4).

As for the clinical outcomes for these late blastulating embryos, similar to the shift in window seen with premature rises in progesterone in relation to the endometrium, the shift in the embryonic window confers a greater risk of implantation failure. Implantation rates of embryos which blastulate on day 6 versus day 5 were decreased by 15–18% [1, 2]. On first glance, one might suspect that this is due to some intrinsic deficit in the embryos. However, insightful studies have shown that cryopreservation of the late blastulating embryos and subsequent transfer in a synchronous programmed cycle allows for restoration of reproductive capacity [1, 14, 15]. This suggests that the decreased outcomes are due, in large part, to dyssynchrony and not to intrinsic deficits in embryonic reproductive competence.

Interestingly, these data also demonstrate why the impact of dyssynchrony may be greater in older women and contribute in part to the poorer outcomes in this population. The fact that the embryos from younger women complete blastulation earlier as compared to embryos in older patients may allow them to fall within the window of optimal endometrial receptivity even when the overall window is shifted 16–24 h earlier.

Management of Embryo and Endometrial Synchrony

Management of synchrony as it relates to these physiologic shifts requires monitoring and intervention in the current treatment cycle—the clinician is not able to anticipate it prior to initiation. Intuitively, it behooves the clinician to prevent dyssynchrony when possible. This may include changes in patient management during follicular stimulation, monitoring late follicular progesterone levels to determine if they exceed an "at-risk" threshold value, and observation of the timing of blastulation. Given the widespread availability of high-quality vitrification, it is possible to vitrify blastocysts and transfer them subsequently when embryo and endometrial synchrony may be assured.

Active management of the endometrium side of physiologic synchrony involves both a prevention and surveillance component. In order to prevent premature progesterone stimuli, it is necessary to keep progesterone levels low, below that stimulus level. Werner et al. have shown that the addition of an LH (or low-dose hCG) component to the ovarian stimulation regimen may help to prevent premature rises in progesterone [16]. Indeed, an LH-to-FSH ratio of 0.3–0.6 decreased the incidence of premature progesterone rise in all responders, both high and low (Fig. 2.5).

The second component to active management of the endometrial window is prevention of an embryo transfer in the event of a premature progesterone rise. This has traditionally been assessed based upon serum progesterone drawn on the day of ovulation trigger administration. Of note, an absolute level which would trigger a decision to cryopreserve embryos in a given cycle is not uniform. This level will be dependent upon the progesterone assay utilized by the laboratory in a given pro-

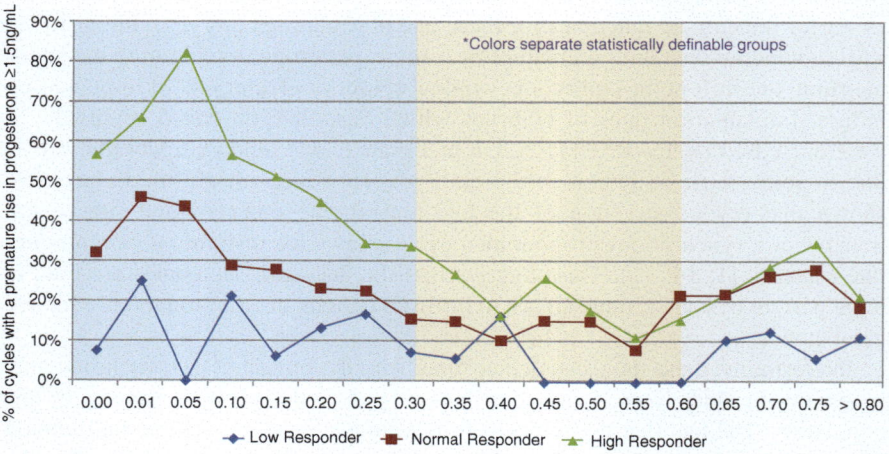

Fig. 2.5 The optimal ratio of exogenous LH-to-FSH to prevent a premature increase in progesterone according to response group (low, normal, and high). A ratio of 0.3–0.6 decreases the incidence or premature rise in all response groups. Used with permission [16]

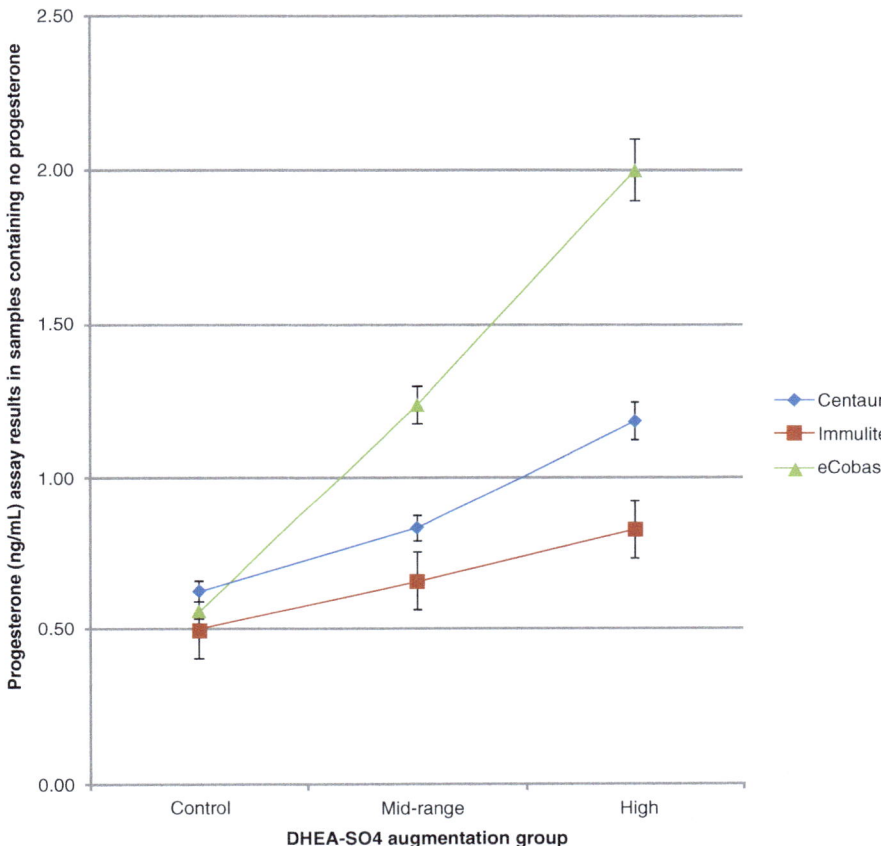

Fig. 2.6 Measurement of the manufacturer's DHEA-S controls showed a linear increase in the progesterone detected, ranging from 0.5 ng/mL without DHEA-S (control) in the blank control to as high as 2.0 ng/mL in the high control where DHEA-S was 722 μg/mL (High). This linear increase in progesterone was seen on all platforms despite the complete absence of progesterone in the sample being analyzed. *Mean* and *SE bars* shown. Used with permission [17]

gram and based on the clinical experiences which result at various cutoff values. Of note, it is important to determine if patients are on any medications which may interact with your progesterone assay and, as such, would alter clinical management. For example, DHEA has been shown to alter results of the progesterone assay to the extent that clinical decision would change [17] (Fig. 2.6).

Active management of the embryonic window at this point includes only a prevention arm as there is not a way to proactively affect blastulation rates. Prevention would involve extended culture of the embryos with an assessment of the embryos, commonly on day 5, to determine if they have begun to blastulate. There has been great focus on time-lapse imaging and prediction of blastulation. As present, the day of blastulation can be predicted to some extent by time-lapse monitoring but not as accurately as required for management of synchrony based upon the rate of cleavage [15]. If the embryo begins blastulating on day 5, it can be assumed that, when transferred to an endometrium that did not receive a premature progesterone stimulus, a synchronous transfer will occur. If the embryos have not yet blastulated, it might be an indication for cryopreservation and subsequent transfer in a synchronous cycle in order to preserve reproductive competence capabilities [1].

It is paramount once again to note that both these factors, the embryo and the endometrium, must be accounted for in this active management paradigm.

Summary

When discussing physiologic embryo and endometrial dyssynchrony, we focus on an embryo, when analyzed in isolation is reproductively competent, and an endometrium, when analyzed in isolation is capable of being receptive to an embryo. It is when the two are assessed together that dyssynchrony occurs, either due to premature progesterone stimulus on the endometrium or late blastulation of the embryo or both.

There are limitations which exist in implementation of this paradigm. From the embryonic component, more data and detailed assessment of the timing of blastulation are needed. In terms of the endometrial window, it has been refined from a broad period of approximately 5 days to a more optimal time frame of approximately 2–3 days. However, more data is needed to define and refine the outer limits of and the most optimal time within this window of endometrial receptivity.

While all this additional physiologic data on the embryo and endometrium may be of great scientific interest, it is possible that another solution may preclude its necessity on the clinical side. Indeed, cryopreservation of the embryo after blastulation, whether on day 5 or 6, followed by a synthetic programmed cycle with known progesterone start may ensure a much more precise alignment of these two windows and may be the paradigm in the future.

References

1. Shapiro BS, Daneshmand ST, Garner FC, Aguirre M, Ross R. Contrasting patterns in in vitro fertilization pregnancy rates among fresh autologous, fresh oocyte donor, and cryopreserved cycles with the use of day 5 or day 6 blastocysts may reflect differences in embryo-endometrium synchrony. Fertil Steril. 2008;89(1):20–6.
2. Barrenetxea G, López de Larruzea A, Ganzabal T, Jiménez R, Carbonero K, Mandiola M. Blastocyst culture after repeated failure of cleavage-stage embryo transfers: a comparison of day 5 and day 6 transfers. Fertil Steril. 2005;83(1):49–53.

3. Silverberg KM, Burns WN, Olive DL, Riehl RM, Schenken RS. Serum progesterone levels predict success of in vitro fertilization/embryo transfer in patients stimulated with leuprolide acetate and human menopausal gonadotropins. J Clin Endocrinol Metab. 1991;73(4):797–803.

4. Bosch E, Labarta E, Crespo J, Simon C, Remohi J, Jenkins J, et al. Circulating progesterone levels and ongoing pregnancy rates in controlled ovarian stimulation cycles for in vitro fertilization: analysis of over 4000 cycles. Hum Reprod. 2010;25:2092–100.

5. Franasiak JM, Ruiz-Alonso M, Scott RT, Simón C. Both slowly developing embryos and a variable pace of luteal endometrial progression may conspire to prevent normal birth in spite of a capable embryo. Fertil Steril. 2016;105(4):861–6.

6. Ruiz-Alonso M, Blesa D, Díaz-Gimeno P, Gómez E, Fernández-Sánchez M, Carranza F, et al. The endometrial receptivity array for diagnosis and personalized embryo transfer as a treatment for patients with repeated implantation failure. Fertil Steril. 2013;100(3):818–24.

7. Navot D, Scott RT, Droesch K, Veeck LL, Liu HC, Rosenwaks Z. The window of embryo transfer and the efficiency of human conception in vitro. Fertil Steril. 1991;55(1):114–8.

8. Prapas Y, Prapas N, Jones EE, Duleba AJ, Olive DL, Chatziparasidou A, et al. The window for embryo transfer in oocyte donation cycles depends on the duration of progesterone therapy. Hum Reprod Oxf Engl. 1998;13(3):720–3.

9. Wilcox AJ, Baird DD, Weinberg CR. Time of implantation of the conceptus and loss of pregnancy. N Engl J Med. 1999;340(23):1796–9.

10. Usadi RS, Groll JM, Lessey BA, Lininger RA, Zaino RJ, Fritz MA, et al. Endometrial development and function in experimentally induced luteal phase deficiency. J Clin Endocrinol Metab. 2008;93(10):4058–64.

11. Mesen TB, Young SL. Progesterone and the luteal phase: a requisite to reproduction. Obstet Gynecol Clin N Am. 2015;42(1):135–51.

12. Healy MW, Patounakis G, Connell MT, Devine K, DeCherney AH, Levy MJ, et al. Does a frozen embryo transfer ameliorate the effect of elevated progesterone seen in fresh transfer cycles? Fertil Steril. 2016;105(1):93–9.

13. Shapiro BS, Daneshmand ST, Garner FC, Aguirre M, Hudson C. Factors related to embryo-endometrium asynchrony in fresh IVF cycles increase in prevalence with maternal age. Fertil Steril. 2013;100(3):S287.

14. Forman EJ, Franasiak JM, Hong KH, Scott RT. Late expanding euploid embryos that are cryopreserved (CRYO) with subsequent synchronous transfer have high sustained implantation rates (SIR) similar to fresh normally blastulating euploid embryos. Fertil Steril. 2013;100(3):S99.

15. Franasiak J, Forman EJ, Hong KH, Werner MD, Upham KM, Scott RT Jr. Investigating the impact of the timing of blastulation on implantation: active management of embryo-endometrial synchrony increases implantation rates. Fertil Steril. 2013;100(3):S97.

16. Werner MD, Forman EJ, Hong KH, Franasiak JM, Molinaro TA, Scott RT. Defining the "sweet spot" for administered luteinizing hormone-to-follicle-stimulating hormone gonadotropin ratios during ovarian stimulation to protect against a clinically significant late follicular increase in progesterone: an analysis of 10,280 first in vitro fertilization cycles. Fertil Steril. 2014;102(5):1312–7.

17. Franasiak JM, Thomas S, Ng S, Fano M, Ruiz A, Scott RT, et al. Dehydroepiandrosterone (DHEA) supplementation results in supraphysiologic DHEA-S serum levels and progesterone assay interference that may impact clinical management in IVF. J Assist Reprod Genet. 2016;33(3):387–91.

Chapter 3
Spermatogenesis: Fertile Ground for Contributing to Recurrent Implantation Failure?

Sorena Keihani, Jeremy B. Myers, and James M. Hotaling

Abbreviations

ART	Assisted reproductive technology
ASRM	American Society for Reproductive Medicine
CGH	Comparative genomic hybridization
FISH	Fluorescent in situ hybridization
ICSI	Intracytoplasmic sperm injection
IMSI	Intracytoplasmic morphologically selected sperm injection
IVF	In vitro fertilization
PGS	Preimplantation genetic screening
RIF	Recurrent implantation failure
ROS	Reactive oxygen species
RPL	Recurrent pregnancy loss
SCD	Sperm chromatin dispersion
SCSA	Sperm chromatin structure assay
SDF	Sperm DNA fragmentation
TESA	Testicular sperm aspiration
TESE	Testicular sperm extraction
TUNEL	Terminal deoxy-nucleotide transferase-mediated dUTP nick end labeling

S. Keihani, MD • J.B. Myers, MD, FACS • J.M. Hotaling, MD, MS, FECSM (✉)
Center for Reconstructive Urology and Men's Health, Division of Urology,
University of Utah, Salt Lake City, UT, USA
e-mail: sorena.keihani@hsc.utah.edu; Jeremy.Myers@hsc.utah.edu; jim.hotaling
@gmail.com; Jim.Hotaling@hsc.utah.edu

© Springer International Publishing AG 2018
J.M. Franasiak, R.T. Scott Jr. (eds.), *Recurrent Implantation Failure*,
https://doi.org/10.1007/978-3-319-71967-2_3

Male Gamete Factor, Why it Matters?

Sperm, contributing one-half of the genomic material to the embryo, plays an incontrovertible role in initiating and maintaining a successful pregnancy. However, the evaluation of recurrent pregnancy loss (RPL) and recurrent implantation failure (RIF) is mostly focused on the female partner with little attention paid to male factors other than conventional semen parameters and paternal karyotype [1]. The underlying cause of RPL remains unexplained in greater than 50% of cases after natural conception [2], and only about 30% of assisted reproductive technology (ART) implantations are successful, with a large proportion failing for unknown reasons [3]. Thorough evaluation of male factor infertility in couples with RIF and RPL represents an understudied and potentially high-impact area of research.

A successful implantation after in vitro fertilization (IVF) or intracytoplasmic sperm injection (ICSI) relies on optimal sperm, oocyte, and endometrial quality. Recent evidence shows that paternal DNA fidelity influences all stages of early embryo development, with increased importance after the embryonic genome is activated [4]. Evidence from animal studies, as well as gestational trophoblastic diseases in humans, highlights the specific roles of the male gamete genome and epigenome. For example, paternal uniparental disomy (androgenote, i.e., embryo created by two male gametes) leads to placental overgrowth, little or no embryo development, and early fetal death, while maternal uniparental disomy (gynogenote) results in placental hypoplasia [5, 6]. These findings illuminate the critical role of sperm and imprinting factors in implantation, placental proliferation, and vascularization, as well as overall placental quality, which may affect the outcomes of conception.

There is a general agreement that conventional semen analyses fail to accurately discriminate between fertile and infertile men and lack the ability to predict reproductive outcomes after ART [7, 8]. Although some parameters, like morphology and motility, might correlate with sperm quality [9, 10], more recent evidence from RIF cases show high rates of DNA numerical and structural damage despite normozoospermic semen analyses [11, 12]. Hence, conventional semen parameters provide little, if any, information on sperm DNA quality and epigenetics. Thus, more sophisticated and complementary tests are needed for the evaluation of complex infertility cases such as couples with RIF.

Major Male Gamete Factors in Recurrent Implantation Failure

Sperm Chromosomal Aneuploidy

It is accepted that chromosomal abnormalities in parents can affect fertility and lead to recurrent miscarriage. American Society for Reproductive Medicine (ASRM) recommends peripheral karyotype analysis for both parents in couples struggling with RPL [2]. However, having a normal parental karyotype does not guarantee a euploid embryo. By investigating chromosomes in individual gametes, we can infer that sperm aneuploidies usually happen de novo in the presence of a normal parental karyotype [13]. Thus, it is crucial to directly study gametes to estimate aneuploidy risk during conception.

Different biological, clinical, and environmental factors may lead to chromosomal abnormalities by affecting meiosis during spermatogenesis. For example, paternal age, varicocele, radiation, toxins, smoking, alcohol consumption, and many medications can trigger higher rates of sperm aneuploidy [14]. Men with peripheral karyotypic abnormalities, severely abnormal semen analysis parameters, and those with nonobstructive azoospermia are at particularly high risk of having sperm aneuploidy [15]. Fluorescent in situ hybridization (FISH) is the gold standard to detect numerical and even some structural chromosomal abnormalities in sperm.

Interestingly, several studies have shown that rates of numerical chromosomal abnormalities are higher in sperm of patients experiencing RIF, and a large body of evidence now supports using FISH for screening of sperm in this subset of patients [15–17]. For example, Ramasamy et al. recommend that sperm FISH is indicated for men who, despite normal semen parameters, are faced with RPL or RIF [18]. This notion is partly based on findings that up to 45% of men with RPL and normal semen parameters can still have high sperm aneuploidy rates [19]. Although the 2012 ASRM committee opinion on RPL did not recommend routine use of FISH [2], the 2015 ASRM report for evaluation of the infertile male indicates that patients with RPL and RIF might benefit from screening for sperm aneuploidy [20]. This inconsistency may originate from limited data and uncertainty about the actual prognostic value of FISH regarding final pregnancy outcomes, as well as cost considerations [21].

Most FISH studies are traditionally focused on a number of "high-yield" chromosomes: namely, 13, 18, 21, X, and Y. The reason behind this is generally the higher prevalence of aneuploidies involving these chromosomes that will remain compatible with life [18]. A relevant and unanswered question is if this limited panel is sufficient for RIF and whether a more comprehensive panel would provide more information. For example, Neusser et al. disputed using the standard clinical FISH probe (i.e., 13, 18, 21, X, Y) and reported that in RPL, chromosomes 1, 2, 6, 15, 16, and 21 are more relevant targets for sperm aneuploidy screening, with chromosome 16 being the most promising diagnostic target [22]. This is somewhat intuitive, given that trisomy 16 is the most common trisomy identified in first trimester miscarriages, although it typically originates from the maternal germline [23].

In reality, current FISH chromosome sets were designed to detect clinically important viable aneuploidies. Thus, when the outcome of interest is shifted to recurrent miscarriage, it makes sense to target different chromosomes for diagnostic purposes. Ideally, all 23 chromosomes in sperm should be evaluated; however, the costs and technical issues hinder most centers from using this approach [24]. More sophisticated automated FISH analyzers are able to screen all chromosomes, but their availability is limited to some reference laboratories [25]. Newer and more costly techniques such as array-comparative genomic hybridization (aCGH), polymerase chain reaction (PCR), and, ultimately, whole-genome sequencing can be used to detect abnormalities in all chromosomes. However, the applicability of these methods in male infertility studies has been limited to date [16, 26, 27]. Considering that many chromosomal abnormalities occur concomitantly rather than in isolation, some would also advocate a qualitative approach using only a few selected FISH probes to identify "at-risk" patients [18, 28]. Proponents of this approach suggest including chromosome 21 and the sex chromosomes would be sufficient since most other autosomal aneuploidies have an accompanying sex chromosome abnormality [18, 28]. Regardless, the optimal screening panel in RIF patients remains unknown.

An important limitation of FISH (similar to most other genetic tests on sperm) is that the preparation process involves steps that eventually render the individual sperm unusable for ART [18]. For example, in ICSI, the final sperm used for fertilization cannot be the same sperm for which FISH information is available, as this sperm would be damaged in the FISH process. This hampers the role of sperm aneuploidy testing in directly correlating with implantation success. However, having the information obtained from FISH would help clinicians and patients to seek genetic counseling, use preimplantation genetic screening (PGS), and understand their chances of having a euploid embryo [17, 19].

Sperm DNA Damage/Sperm DNA Fragmentation (SDF)

As sperm cells contribute half of the nuclear DNA to the zygote, sperm DNA integrity is crucial for normal embryogenesis. Sperm DNA fragmentation (SDF) can be defined as "denatured or damaged sperm DNA that can not be repaired" [20], encompassing both single- and double-strand breaks. Sperm DNA damage encompasses a wider spectrum of abnormalities including strand breaks, base deletions or modifications, abnormal DNA cross-linkage, as well as defective DNA-protein cross-linking and protamine packaging [29]. Since not all studies discriminate between sperm DNA damage and SDF, these terms are used here interchangeably.

Sperm DNA damage can be present in spite of normal paternal karyotype, sperm FISH results, and semen parameters. In fact, low rates of SDF are a normal phenomenon seen in most fertile individuals [30]. Interestingly, there are now compelling evidence that sperm with DNA damage can successfully fertilize an egg and produce an embryo that may eventually fail or lead to an early miscarriage [31–35]. This might explain some cases of the so-called "unexplained" miscarriage of an embryo with normal karyotype, specifically when the paternal genome is activated during the later stages of embryonic development [12]. These facts make SDF a compelling subject to investigate in couples struggling with RPL and RIF.

Sperm have limited DNA repair mechanisms, rendering it vulnerable to a variety of factors causing DNA damage [36, 37]. Although a healthy oocyte can execute some limited sperm DNA repair, this is contingent on a high-quality oocyte that is typically found in younger, more fertile, women [38]. However, this may not always be the case in most ART candidates. Also, large amounts of DNA damage are not readily repairable even by a healthy strong oocyte [32]. Thus, it remains challenging to isolate the real impact of SDF and predict how much sperm DNA damage is safe in regards to pregnancy and implantation outcomes [38].

Multiple factors affecting nuclear and mitochondrial DNA are thought to cause SDF. Spermatogenesis is a complex process involving changes in nuclear proteins, dense chromatin packing, and chromosomal compaction. Defects in the sperm maturation process, as well as apoptosis pathways later in spermatogenesis, can lead to DNA damage [39]. However, reactive oxygen species (ROS) and post-testicular oxidative stress also play major roles in sperm DNA damage [39, 40]. A recent meta-analysis showed that male aging is associated with increased SDF rates, perhaps due to reduced replication fidelity and accumulation of de novo mutations in sperm progenitor cells [41]. Thus, both paternal and maternal age (due to decreased ability of oocytes to repair sperm DNA) can affect fertility by propagating sperm DNA damage. Both immature and damaged sperm escaping apoptosis produce large amounts of ROS. This oxidative stress can affect mature sperm during co-migration in seminiferous tubules, storage in the epididymis, and also after ejaculation [39]. Additional factors such as alcohol consumption, smoking, infections, medications, varicocele, and other diseases may also cause DNA damage via increased ROS production [42]. A list of potential environmental and clinical factors causing SDF is summarized in Fig. 3.1.

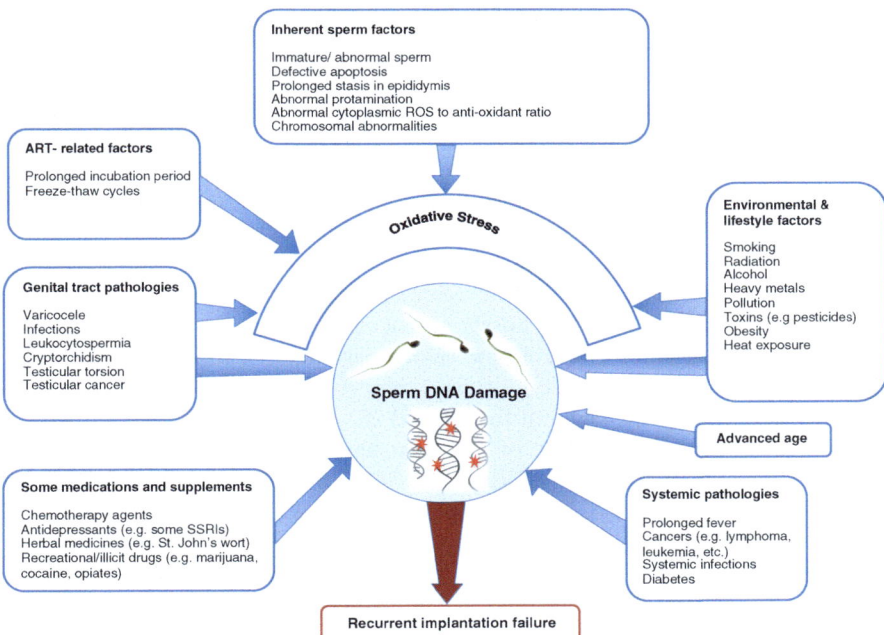

Fig. 3.1 Potential factors leading to sperm DNA damage or fragmentation. The figure depicts the factors that possibly can cause sperm DNA damage directly or via oxidative stress. Multiple pathways are possible for each of the factors listed. *ROS* reactive oxygen species, *ART* assisted reproductive technology, *SSRI* selective serotonin reuptake inhibitor

ROS are normally needed for a number of essential steps in sperm maturation. A correct balance between oxidative agents and antioxidants is thus essential for functions such as chromosomal compaction, capacitation, and acrosome activation [42]. An imbalance between ROS and antioxidants in the sperm environment can cause lipid peroxidation, which damages sperm membrane integrity and sperm motility [43]. Different methods are available to assess ROS levels in semen. However, in the absence of clinically meaningful cutoffs and definitions for abnormal ROS levels, these tests are of little use in clinic [44]. DNA damage is also mediated by caspases and endonucleases after exposure to non-physiologic concentrations of ROS [39]. Interestingly, overnight incubation and prolonged culture times during IVF is associated with higher SDF, possibly due to higher ROS generation and longer exposure of sperm to the ROS produced by immature sperm and other environmental factors [45, 46]. Hence, prior testing for SDF may also have some clinical significance for choosing the right ART protocol to minimize oxidative damage.

Different tests are available for detecting sperm DNA damage. Characteristics of the five most commonly used tests (terminal deoxy-nucleotide transferase-mediated dUTP nick end labeling [TUNEL], sperm chromatin structure assay [SCSA], sperm chromatin dispersion [SCD], Comet assay, and acridine orange assay) are summarized in Table 3.1. Other assays such as in situ nick translation assay (ISNT), aniline blue staining, toluidine blue, and chromomycin A3 (CMA3) are also available but less commonly used in the literature considering RIF and implantation outcomes. Additional information and comprehensive reviews on SDF tests are available elsewhere [47, 48].

Each test measures a different type of DNA damage and provides different information that is not necessarily correlated with the results of other SDF tests. Thus, it is important to keep in mind that these assays are not interchangeable. For example, Stahl et al. reported that the correlation between SCSA and TUNEL might actually be weaker than what was previously assumed [49]. Most SDF tests lack a standardized cutoff value, making comparison between different studies troublesome [50]. Currently, none of these modalities produce sperm useable for IVF/ICSI after SDF tests. Moreover, reliable clinical data regarding different SDF test results and the implantation outcomes are either missing or inconsistent.

Correlations between conventional semen parameters and sperm DNA damage are equivocal. Although some studies report associations with sperm concentration, morphology, and motility [35, 51–53], the results are not consistent [54–56]. Additionally, the type of SDF test used can impact this correlation. For example, a recent study reported that SCSA results are negatively correlated with sperm concentration and motility, while TUNEL results were independent of conventional semen parameters [49]. However, the key concept is that high SDF can be present despite normal bulk semen parameters [39, 54, 57]. Interestingly, Bareh et al. recently showed that even with normal sperm parameters, male partners of women with unexplained RPL had higher rates of sperm DNA damage [12]. Thus, SDF testing can provide clinically actionable information independent of bulk seminal parameters in patients under work-up for RPL and RIF [58].

Table 3.1 Characteristics of the methods commonly used for assessing sperm DNA damage/fragmentation

Assay	Principle	How results are expressed	Strengths	Limitations
TUNEL	Directly incorporates modified nucleotides at the site of damage	Percentage of sperm with DNA damage	Detects both single- and double-strand breaks	Requires fluorescence microscopy or flow cytometry (expensive)
			Better correlation with recurrent implantation failure in meta-analyses	Prolonged procedure
			High sensitivity	Variable protocols
			Reproducible when flow cytometry is used	Variable thresholds
SCSA	Measures differential susceptibility of DNA to denaturation according to level of DNA damage	Percentage of sperm with fragmented DNA	Measures large number of cells rapidly	Only detects single-strand breaks
			Highly standardized/reduced interlaboratory variation	Expensive
			Additional information on chromatin decondensation	Not readily available
			Better correlation with recurrent implantation failure in meta-analyses	
SCD (Halo assay)	Measures differential susceptibility of DNA to denaturation according to level of DNA damage and controlled protein depletion	Percentage of sperm with fragmented DNA	Simple and inexpensive	Only detects single-strand breaks
			Convenient technique	Low-contrasting images
			Low number of sperm needed	Interobserver subjectivity for interpretation of halos

(continued)

Assay	Principle	How results are expressed	Strengths	Limitations
Comet assay	Electrophoretic technique; selectively denatures partial DNA after alkaline or neutral lysis treatment to detect single- or double-strand breaks, respectively	Degree of DNA fragmentation in a single sperm is assessed by looking at halo measuring percentage of DNA in the tail of the comet, tail length, and intensity of staining	Inexpensive	Limited and inconsistent data on correlation with miscarriage after ART
			Suitable for small semen samples (~5000 sperm)	Non-standardized
			Can measure altered bases	Interlaboratory variation
			High sensitivity	Separate conditions (alkaline or neutral) are required for detecting double- and single-strand breaks
AO assay	Measures differential susceptibility of DNA to denaturation according to level of DNA damage and controlled protein depletion	Percentage of sperm with fragmented DNA	Inexpensive	Only detects single-strand breaks
				Limited and inconsistent data on correlation with miscarriage after ART
				Interobserver subjectivity
				Prolonged incubation times

TUNEL terminal deoxy-nucleotide transferase-mediated dUTP nick end labeling, *SCSA* sperm chromatin structure assay, *SCD* sperm chromatin dispersion, *AO assay* acridine orange assay, *ART* assisted reproductive technology

During the last decade, at least eight systematic reviews and meta-analyses were performed to assess the effects of SDF on different outcomes, including pregnancy rates, live birth rates, and pregnancy loss after natural pregnancy or ART [10, 50, 59–64]. The results are, however, inconsistent and hard to generalize. The results from four meta-analyses, which provided data on relationship between sperm DNA damage and miscarriage after IVF or ICSI, are summarized in Table 3.2. A 2008 meta-analysis by Zini et al. suggested that sperm DNA damage is predictive of miscarriage after IVF and ICSI [62]. They also reported that their findings were independent of the treatment method (IVF or ICSI), as well as the testing method (TUNEL or SCSA). A larger meta-analysis in 2012 showed an overall 2.16-fold increase in the risk of miscarriage with higher SDF compared to lower SDF; they also reported that significant results were obtained with TUNEL and SCSA but not with Comet and acridine orange assays [63].

In a more recent meta-analysis, Zhao et al. also reported a significantly increased miscarriage rate in patients with high sperm DNA damage; in the same study however, subgroup analysis for miscarriage was significant only for ICSI but not for IVF [10]. Also, similar to a study by Robinson et al., in a subgroup analysis based on SDF test type, the combined results (IVF and ICSI) were significant for TUNEL and SCSA, but not for the Comet assay and acridine orange combined [10]. These findings were not reproduced in a meta-analysis by Zhang et al., who reported nonsignificant results for effect of SDF on pregnancy loss after IVF or ICSI [64]. However, in 2015, Osman et al. performed a meta-analysis on the effect of SDF on live birth rate after ART and concluded that high SDF is associated with lower live birth rates after both IVF and ICSI, although the results were only marginally significant [50]. This was the first meta-analysis that assessed live birth rates as the outcome in relation to sperm DNA damage. High heterogeneity of the pooled data, using various assays and cutoffs in different studies, inadequate power for subgroup analyses, and variable inclusion and exclusion criteria are some of the obstacles in reaching a firm conclusion from these studies.

Despite the growing interest in DNA fragmentation and the large number of publications, especially during the last two decades, controversies are still ongoing on when and how DNA fragmentation tests should be used in current clinical practice, if at all [20, 65, 66]. Spurred by these inconsistencies, the most recent ASRM guideline for evaluation of infertile men refers to DNA integrity testing as "controversial" and does not recommend the routine use of SDF tests for male factor infertility work-up. However, the same report acknowledges that "the effect of abnormal sperm DNA fragmentation on the value of IUI or IVF and ICSI results may be clinically significant" [20]. Based on the current evidence, using SDF testing might be a viable option specifically in cases of RIF. The information provided allows for more informed decision-making and more realistic expectations. Patients with high SDF values might be good candidates for genetic counseling and consideration for alternative sperm selection methods (see below).

There is conflicting evidence regarding IVF vs. ICSI outcomes in cases of high sperm DNA damage. When considering live birth rates as an outcome, patients with

Table 3.2 Summary of meta-analyses assessing the association between sperm DNA damage and miscarriage rate

Reference	Number of included studies	Number of cycles/couples	OR (95% CI)[a] combined/IVF/ICSI	SDF assay	OR (95% CI)[a] based on assay	Comment
Zini et al. [62]	7 papers	1549 cycles	Combined: 2.48 (1.52–4.04)	TUNEL (n = 3)	SCSA: 1.77 (1.01–3.13)	OR with TUNEL was significantly higher than SCSA in meta-regression analysis
	1 IVF only	640 pregnancies	IVF: 2.17 (1.02–4.60)	SCSA (n = 4)	TUNEL: 7.04 (2.81–17.67)	
	2 ICSI only	122 miscarriages	ICSI: 2.73 (1.43–5.20)			
	4 both					
Robinson et al. [63]	16 papers	2962 couples	Combined: 2.16 (1.54–3.03)	TUNEL (n = 6)	SCSA: 1.47 (1.04–2.09)	Subgroup analysis on treatment type showed no significant difference in miscarriage (data not shown in the paper).
	1 IVF only	1252 pregnancies	IVF: not available	SCSA (n = 7)	TUNEL: 7.04 (3.94–6.32)	Analysis based on assay showed stronger association with TUNEL assay
	4 ICSI only	225 miscarriages	ICSI: not available	Comet (n = 2)	Comet: 1.43 (0.40–5.14)	
	10 both			AO (n = 1)	AO: 2.78 (0.59–13.11)	
	1 natural					
Zhao et al. [10]	14 papers	3106 cycles	Combined: 2.28 (1.55–3.35)	TUNEL (n = 7)	SCSA: 1.90 (1.01–3.59)	Modest publication bias reported for effect of SDF on miscarriage rate
	1 IVF only	2756 couples	IVF: 1.84 (0.98–3.46)	SCSA (n = 3)	TUNEL: 3.23 (1.67–6.27)	
	4 ICSI only	965 pregnancies	ICSI: 2.68 (1.40–5.14)	Comet (n = 2)	Comet + AO: 1.43 (0.82–2.50)	
	9 both	187 miscarriages		AO (n = 2)		
Zhang et al. [64]	8 papers	Not available	Combined: 0.54 (0.26–1.10)	TUNEL (n = 1)	SCSA: 0.79 (0.49–1.26)	The results were nonsignificant for different SCSA cutoff values (OR provided for DFI cutoff >27%)
	1 IVF only		IVF: 0.51 (0.19–1.34)	SCSA (n = 6)	TUNEL: 0.35 (0.10–1.17)	
	2 ICSI only		ICSI: 0.57 (0.20–1.64)	Comet (n = 1)	Comet: 0.50 (0.13–1.97)	
	5 both					

IVF in vitro fertilization, *ICSI* intracytoplasmic sperm injection, *OR* odds ratio, *CI* confidence interval, *TUNEL* terminal deoxy-nucleotide transferase-mediated dUTP nick end labeling, *SCSA* sperm chromatin structure assay, *SCD* sperm chromatin dispersion, *AO* acridine orange assay, *DFI* DNA fragmentation index
[a]OR (95% CI) corresponds to risk of miscarriage in patients with high DNA damage compared with those with low DNA damage based on treatment method (IVF, OR, and combined) or based on sperm DNA damage assay (SCSA, TUNEL, Comet, AO)

higher SDF appear to have poor results with IVF but not with ICSI [50, 67]. Data is limited in this regard, and the underlying reason behind this difference is largely unknown. As proposed by Lewis et al. [65], and also Bungum et al. [68], women undergoing ICSI may be younger and healthier compared to those undergoing IVF, so their oocytes might have a higher capacity for sperm DNA repair. Additionally, sperm used in IVF spend more time in culture media and has higher chances of oxidative damage due to proximity to immature sperm and other natural substances in the culture media overnight [65, 67]. Thus, choosing ICSI over IVF may lead to higher live birth rates for cases with high sperm DNA damage, since it bypasses many of the natural selection barriers. However, this might not be true when considering RPL and RIF as outcomes. It is arguable that natural sperm selection in IVF may deselect some sperm with high DNA damage. So if ICSI is used to bypass this step, despite higher fertilization rates achieved, a sperm with high DNA damage can still cause early pregnancy loss or yet unknown abnormalities in the embryo [50, 69]. This hypothesis can partly explain high rates of RIF encountered with both IVF and ICSI in those with high sperm DNA damage. Thus, current evidence does not indicate superiority of either IVF or ICSI when considering RPL and RIF. Also, the ramifications for offspring using sperm with significant DNA damage remain unknown.

The choice of SDF test for evaluation of RIF is also controversial. Theoretically SDF tests detecting double-strand DNA damage (e.g., TUNEL and alkaline Comet) should be more appropriate for predicting miscarriage since single-stranded DNA damages are usually of less significance and easier to repair by a healthy oocyte [39]. Data from current meta-analyses suggest that TUNEL and SCSA have better correlations with RIF. A DNA fragmentation index cutoff of 30% is commonly used for SCSA, and a threshold of 15–20% is used for TUNEL. However, the appropriate cutoff value to predict recurrent miscarriage after ART remains controversial and undetermined. Much of this stems from lack of standardized protocols with high interobserver and interlaboratory variations.

Sperm Epigenetics

A burgeoning area in infertility research is the role of epigenetics in male fecundity. Epigenetics includes noncoding changes in the genome that do not alter the basic DNA sequence. These alterations might occur via different mechanisms such as changes in methylation, histone modification, or via microRNAs [24, 70]. The sperm epigenetic profile might actually encompass a "historical record" of the spermatogenesis process and also provide information on a variety of environmental factors that can affect male fertility [24, 70].

During sperm maturation, 90–95% of histones are replaced by protamines (major nuclear sperm proteins). This protamination allows for a more efficient packaging of highly compacted chromatin and also protects the sperm from oxidative stress [71]. Any aberrations in this epigenetic process would render the sperm vulnerable to DNA damage and may have at least some diagnostic value for infertility work-up [70, 72]. DNA methylation is another important aspect of sperm epigenetics that plays a well-established role in imprinting disorders [70]. Interestingly, recent studies reported associations between differentially methylated areas in sperm DNA and fecundity in men [73, 74]. This underscores the diagnostic implications of sperm epigenetics. While the role of sperm epigenetics is currently confined to research and most of the diagnostic targets are not fully validated, this field holds tremendous promise for understanding RIF.

Potential Therapeutic Options and Interventions

High-level evidence is lacking for many of the behavioral, lifestyle, and nutritional interventions, as well as diagnostic and treatment options, in regard to RIF after ART. However, taking into account the known associations between many of the modifiable factors and sperm quality or overall fecundity, some general interventions or lifestyle modifications are recommended for male partners undergoing assessment for RIF (Table 3.3). It is noteworthy that any changes in sperm parameters probably need a 72-day period (a full spermatogenesis cycle) to come into full effect. Thus, any repeat testing or intervention, if indicated, should be performed with an appropriate time interval.

Alcohol: Heavy alcohol consumption is linked to systemic ROS generation and may negatively affect sperm parameters and create testicular pathology [75, 76]. Likewise, paternal alcohol consumption can specifically affect IVF outcomes and lead to lower rates of live birth and higher rates of miscarriage [77, 78]. Although the available studies are small and mostly include men with heavy alcohol consumption, male partners in couples with a history of RIF undergoing IVF or ICSI should avoid alcohol consumption or decrease its use significantly.

Smoking: Cigarette smoke contains various toxic agents including ROS and heavy metals and can cause direct and indirect damage to sperm. Smoking can negatively affect bulk semen parameters (e.g., count, motility, morphology, etc.) and also leads to double-strand DNA breaks and sperm DNA damage [42, 79]. Additionally, it can cause a variety of genetic, epigenetic, and molecular alterations affecting male fertility via poorly understood mechanisms [80, 81]. There is also a positive association between preconception (as well as during pregnancy and after birth) paternal smoking and certain childhood diseases including leukemia [82, 83]. Thus, smoking cessation is highly recommended for patients with RIF undergoing ART procedures.

Varicocele: About 15% of normal men have some degree of varicocele, and this figure reaches up to 40% in infertile males [105]. Varicocele is associated with oxidative stress and higher sperm DNA damage [90, 91]. There is now a consensus on surgical repair of varicoceles in infertile men, specifically when abnormal semen parameters are present [92, 105]. A meta-analysis in 2016 reported that treating varicocele increases pregnancy as well as live birth rates after ICSI [93]. Also,

Table 3.3 Modifiable factors causing sperm DNA damage or affecting ART outcomes

Modifiable factor	Negative impacts	Recommendation	Supporting references
Alcohol	Increases ROS generation; affects bulk semen parameters; creates testicular pathology; negatively impacts reproductive capability, pregnancy outcomes, and miscarriage rate	Avoid alcohol consumption or significantly decrease its use prior and during ART	La Vignera [75]
			Opuwari [76]
			Klonoff-Cohen [77]
			Nicolau [78]
Smoking	ROS-mediated and direct damage to sperm; negative effect on bulk semen parameters; strong association with high sperm DNA damage; increases risk of certain diseases (e.g., leukemia) in the offspring	Cessation of smoking	Sharma [79]
			Harlev [80]
		Avoid second-hand smoke	Esakky [81]
			Liu [82]
Testicular heat stress	Impairs spermatogenesis; increases sperm DNA damage	Avoid prolonged wet heat to groin area (sauna, hot tubs, Jacuzzi)	Rao [84]
			Rao [85]
			Garolla [86]
		Could consider to avoid wearing tightly fitted underwear, cycling with tight pants, and using laptop on closed legs. However, unconvincing data for these	Ahmad [87]
			Sheynkin [88]
			Southorn [89]
Varicocele	Associated with higher oxidative stress and sperm DNA damage; increases testicular heat stress; negative impact on bulk semen parameters	Screen and offer varicocelectomy to patients before ART	Pathak [90]
			Wang [91]
			Shauer [92]
			Esteves [93]
Abstinence time	Prolonged abstinence may lead to more oxidative sperm DNA damage	Consider shorter abstinence times (e.g., 1–2 days) before providing semen for ART	Agarwal [94]
			Mayorga-Torres [95]
			Gosalvez [96]
			Pons [97]
Environmental toxins *(Pesticides, heavy metals*, etc.)	Positive correlation with sperm DNA damage	Avoid pesticide exposure	Sengupta [98]
		Avoid occupational exposure to heavy metals and toxins if possible	Wright [42]
			Wirth [99]

(continued)

Table 3.3 (continued)

Modifiable factor	Negative impacts	Recommendation	Supporting references
Obesity and diet	High BMI might be associated with negative semen quality, fertility outcomes, and pregnancy loss after ART	Eat a healthy diet	Sermondade [100]
		Exercise regularly	Campbell [101]
		Maintain a healthy BMI	Barazani [102]
Medications *(antidepressants, calcium channel blockers, alpha-adrenergic blockers, anticonvulsants, antiretroviral)*	Some medications may alter semen quality or pregnancy outcomes	Avoid using drugs known to negatively impact sperm quality or use alternatives if possible	Brezina [103]
			Wright [42]
Recreational/illicit drugs	Negatively impact fertility, sperm function, and testicular structure	Avoid recreational drug use (e.g., marijuana, cocaine, opiates, anabolic steroids, etc.)	Fronczak [104]
			Barazani [102]

ART assisted reproductive technology, *ROS* reactive oxygen species, *BMI* body mass index

recent evidence from both observational studies and randomized controlled trials show that varicocelectomy before ART may decrease miscarriage rates and improve the pregnancy outcomes [106, 107], although controversial results are also reported [108]. Taken together, varicocelectomy is a feasible intervention before performing ART and may also benefit couples with RIF.

Testicular heat stress: Since spermatogenesis is a temperature-dependent process, occurring in lower than normal body temperatures, elevation in scrotal temperature could cause testicular heat stress or "thermal spermatotoxicity" and is associated with impaired spermatogenesis, increased immature sperm, increased ROS formation, autophagy, and higher SDF [87, 109]. For example, in a randomized clinical trial, Rao et al. showed that transient and frequent scrotal hyperthermia (by soaking in 43 °C water) causes severe but reversible changes in spermatogenesis [84, 85]. Tightly fitted underwear; moderate cycling; regular use of sauna, Jacuzzi, or hot tubs; as well as using laptop on closed legs all might increase scrotal temperature and potentially cause sperm DNA damage or decrease in sperm quality [42]. However the available evidence for most of these claims is limited. Male partners pursuing ART procedures may be advised to avoid these habits but must also be counseled that there is no conclusive evidence that anything other than exposure to wet heat is damaging [85, 110].

Shorter abstinence times: The World Health Organization (WHO) traditionally suggests 2–7 days of abstinence before providing a semen sample for analysis [111]. This is largely based on earlier studies reporting improved conventional semen parameters after this period. However, as previously discussed, conventional semen analysis does not take into account factors like ROS generation and sperm

DNA damage. More recent studies indicate that shorter abstinence is not associated with unfavorable sperm parameters, and in fact, with longer abstinence, rates of ROS and SDF are increased [94, 95]. On the other hand, a 1-day abstinence instead of the recommended 2–7 days leads to less sperm DNA damage and may be beneficial, especially for ART purposes [96, 97]. It is reasonable, although far from conclusive, to consider recommending shorter abstinence times to couples with RIF where the man has a high SDF.

Antibiotic treatment of leukocytospermia: Leukocytes in semen are a source for ROS generation and potentially higher sperm DNA damage [42, 112]. Although some reports suggest a negative impact of leukocytospermia on IVF and ICSI outcomes, many others do not show such a correlation [113, 114]. Thus, antibiotic treatment of leukocytospermia in the absence of infection currently lacks sufficient evidence in RIF cases. However, treatment of underlying infection might be helpful in resolving the leukocytospermia and potentially improving ART outcomes, although no specific study has yet assessed this claim. Moreover, appropriate leukocyte counting methods and cutoffs for clinically significant leukocytospermia remain controversial.

Other factors: Considering the potential detrimental effects of various environmental toxins, it is recommended that patients avoid occupational or environmental exposure to heavy metals, pesticides, bisphenol A (used in plastic packaging), and xenobiotics [42, 99]. Exposure to x-ray radiation should also be discouraged. A healthy diet and weight loss may be recommended as additional efforts to improve overall health and sperm quality [42, 102]. A thorough medication history, including supplements, herbal medicine, over-the-counter drugs, and also recreational drug use may also provide useful information. A number of medications such as some antidepressants, calcium channel blockers, opioids, and codeine may have detrimental effects on semen quality or fertility [42, 103].

Oral antioxidant therapy: As previously mentioned, oxidative stress is the main factor in SDF and can also damage the sperm membrane, causing fertility problems [40]. On the other hand, physiologic levels of ROS play an important role in sperm maturation. Therefore, using antioxidants may be considered a double-edged sword if consumed in excess. Semen naturally contains antioxidants such as vitamins E and C, selenium, zinc, folate, carnitine, and carotenoids [115, 116]. With rising interest in the role of ROS on semen parameters, several studies suggested that using antioxidants improves semen quality and sperm DNA damage. A Cochrane review in 2014 assessed the role of antioxidants for male subfertility and concluded that antioxidant supplementation might improve live birth and clinical pregnancy rates; however the evidence is of low quality [116]. In the same report, the authors analyzed results from two studies that specifically addressed the use of antioxidants in patients undergoing IVF or ICSI [117, 118]. Pooled data indicated antioxidants increase live birth rate after IVF or ICSI, when compared to placebo (OR 3.61, 95% CI: 1.27–10.29, from 2 randomized controlled trials, 90 men). However, the results were not statistically significant for clinical pregnancy (OR: 2.64, 95% CI: 0.94–7.41) [116]. Different antioxidant supplements such as vitamins C and E, carotene, selenium, glutathione, etc. are studied for improving SDF [42]. One of the aforementioned randomized trials used vitamin E (300 mg, twice a day for 3 months) [117], and the other one used Menevit (Bayer, Sydney, Australia; each capsule contains vitamin E 400 IU, vitamin C 100 mg, lycopene 6 mg, zinc 25 mg, selenium 26 microgram, folate 0.5 mg, garlic 1000 mg, palm oil [vehicle]), one capsule daily for 3 months prior to IVF cycle [118]. It remains difficult to make a strong recommendation based on this limited evidence; however a trial of oral antioxidant supplementation may be considered in RIF cases. The optimal antioxidant agent, dosing, and duration of treatment remains largely unknown. It is relevant to note that although evidence on adverse effects of antioxidants is of very low quality, miscarriage is included as a potential side effect [116].

Targeted sperm selection: For natural conception to occur, sperm go through a stringent physiologic screening process where only a few selected sperm reach the oocyte at the site of fertilization. Although our knowledge is limited on the physiologic selection of sperm in humans, it is intuitive that more "fit and fecund" sperm are selected in this process [119]. With advent of newer ART techniques, specifically ICSI, this natural process of sperm selection is bypassed. For example, sperm selection in ICSI has largely relied on gross morphology and motility characteristics [119]. By this circumvention, we are sometimes forcing an individual sperm, which would not otherwise pass the natural sperm selection challenge, to fertilize an egg. So it is highly likely that recurrent miscarriages could result if the selected sperm is not actually optimized for fertilization and early embryogenesis.

An ideal sperm selection method is noninvasive and quick, allows deselecting abnormal sperm and those with hidden DNA damage, selects for a "fit and fecund" male gamete, does not destroy the tested sperm or compromise its functional and structural integrity, and would eventually improve outcomes after ART. In the absence of such a "magic test" in the andrology armamentarium, a number of approaches are currently under development in hopes of choosing sperm with less DNA damage. However, evidence of their efficacy in improving RIF outcomes is very limited.

Conventional sperm sorting methods, namely, density gradient centrifugation (DGC), conventional sperm swim-up (CSW), and direct sperm swim-up (DSW), involve multiple washing and centrifugation steps that can lead to ROS generation and damage to sperm DNA [40, 120]. At the turn of the twentieth century, a new approach named "motile sperm organelle morphology examination" or MSOME was introduced that utilized real-time high magnification for sperm selection [121]. This allowed a modification to conventional ICSI by selecting a sperm with seemingly normal morphology and motility in a technique known as intracytoplasmic morphologically selected sperm injection (IMSI). Since then, controversies are ongoing on the potential benefits of IMSI over ICSI in different clinical situations. Although current evidence does not support superiority of IMSI for unselected patients [122], the data are more convincing for patients with previous ICSI failures or those with severe male infertility factors. For example, a recent meta-analysis reported a 70% decrease in miscarriage rate for IMSI, compared to ICSI, for this subpopulation of patients [123]. Therefore, until more sophisticated and reliable sperm selection techniques are more readily available, IMSI may be considered for cases with RIF and those with high SDF rates.

Some newer options are also available for sperm selection: birefringence, glass wool filtration, microfluidic-based sperm sorting, hyaluronic acid binding, magnetic-activated cell sorting, zeta potential, electrophoretic sperm isolation, and microelectrophoresis [124–130]. However, none of these methods are currently widely available, and none has shown convincing clinical value in improving pregnancy outcomes [58, 120]. More information on individual tests is available elsewhere [120, 130].

Testicular sperm extraction (TESE) and aspiration (TESA): Sperm directly retrieved from the testis are known to have less DNA fragmentation compared to the ejaculated sperm [58, 131, 132]. Recently, Esteves et al. performed a prospective cohort study on oligozoospermic men with high SDF and reported that DNA damage in sperm obtained by TESE/TESA was one-fifth of that in the ejaculated sperm; ICSI outcomes were also significantly better when the TESE/TESA sperm were used [131]. Interestingly, miscarriage rates were also significantly lower in the TESE/TESA group, compared to the ejaculated sperm group (OR: 0.29, 95% CI: 0.10–0.82) [131]. Importantly, some studies suggest that testicular sperm may actually have higher levels of sperm aneuploidy [18, 133]. For example, Moskovtsev et al. reported that although the TESE sperm had lower SDF compared to the ejaculated sperm, the rate of aneuploidy in chromosomes 13, 18, 21, X, and Y was in fact higher [134]. Taking these all together, using TESE/TESA may be a good option for some patients struggling with RIF, specifically those with higher rates of sperm DNA damage. Implementing preimplantation genetic screening to find aneuploidy, can serve as a complementary test with this approach so the potential benefits of TESE/TESA with ICSI would not be offset by increased rates of aneuploidy.

Preimplantation genetic screening (PGS): Generally, PGS can be recommended for most cases of RPL and RIF [135]. From a male factor perspective, PGS can be a beneficial and complementary test for patients with RIF, specifically when high rates of sperm DNA damage or sperm chromosomal aneuploidy are present. Interestingly, Rubio et al. reported that in patients with RPL, who had a sperm chromosomal abnormality detected by FISH, no miscarriages were found when PGS was implemented. So they suggested that detection of a sperm chromosomal abnormality would be a reliable indication for PGS [136]. Although costly, examination of the embryo using FISH, or more ideally aCGH, or newer sequencing techniques, aids in selecting healthier embryos for implantation and helps to avoid RIF in patients with known risk of low sperm quality.

Future Directions

With the rapid advent of newer technologies and tests for evaluating male factors, lack of well-designed studies and randomized controlled trials to assess clinical impact remains an important obstacle to applying them to clinical practice. For this reason, the first step would be standardization of available techniques and performance of high-quality studies to assess different pregnancy outcomes in well-defined and specific subpopulation of patients.

There is a growing need for a reliable noninvasive sperm-sorting test to select sperm with minimal DNA damage to improve outcomes after IVF or ICSI. In addition to the sperm selection methods named above, a number of other tests are also under investigation for future use. For example, Raman spectroscopy uses discrete laser scattering to assess the genetic material in live sperm and could potentially select for sperm with better molecular characteristics [120, 127]. "Omics" technology is also an emerging field dealing with intracellular interactions at different levels. Transcriptomics, proteomics, and metabolomics analyses on sperm are different areas of interest for infertility research, and the findings may have clinical implications in the future [119]. Sperm epigenetics is also an interesting and growing area for future infertility research. Epigenetic biomarkers are developing to help in better understanding of sperm fecundity, and also the effect of environmental exposures [24].

With the evidence we currently have in hand, testing for sperm chromosomal abnormalities is essential for couples with RIF. Although it remains difficult to predict the exact risk of unfavorable outcomes in presence of sperm DNA damage or aneuploidy diagnosed with current tests, the results can help clinicians and patients in a number of ways. It allows for a more informative discussion with patients and helps to offer additional options such as PGS and genetic counseling. For couples with high degrees of abnormal sperm genetic material, a detailed discussion about the risks and potential impacts of these findings on final ART outcomes enables the parents to make more educated, although difficult, decisions about their reproductive choices and allows them to also consider alternative options.

References

1. Puscheck EE, Jeyendran RS. The impact of male factor on recurrent pregnancy loss. Curr Opin Obstet Gynecol. 2007;19(3):222–8. https://doi.org/10.1097/GCO.0b013e32813e3ff0.
2. The Practice Committee of the American Society for Reproductive Medicine. Evaluation and treatment of recurrent pregnancy loss: a committee opinion. Fertil Steril. 2012;98(5):1103–11. https://doi.org/10.1016/j.fertnstert.2012.06.048.
3. Coughlan C, Ledger W, Wang Q, Liu F, Demirol A, Gurgan T, et al. Recurrent implantation failure: definition and management. Reprod Biomed Online. 2014;28(1):14–38. https://doi.org/10.1016/j.rbmo.2013.08.011.
4. Simon L, Murphy K, Shamsi MB, Liu L, Emery B, Aston KI, et al. Paternal influence of sperm DNA integrity on early embryonic development. Hum Reprod. 2014;29(11):2402–12. https://doi.org/10.1093/humrep/deu228.
5. McGrath J, Solter D. Completion of mouse embryogenesis requires both the maternal and paternal genomes. Cell. 1984;37(1):179–83.
6. Surani MA, Barton SC, Norris ML. Development of reconstituted mouse eggs suggests imprinting of the genome during gametogenesis. Nature. 1984;308(5959):548–50.
7. Guzick DS, Overstreet JW, Factor-Litvak P, Brazil CK, Nakajima ST, Coutifaris C, et al. Sperm morphology, motility, and concentration in fertile and infertile men. N Engl J Med. 2001;345(19):1388–93. https://doi.org/10.1056/NEJMoa003005.
8. Wang C, Swerdloff RS. Limitations of semen analysis as a test of male fertility and anticipated needs from newer tests. Fertil Steril. 2014;102(6):1502–7. https://doi.org/10.1016/j.fertnstert.2014.10.021.
9. Sun JG, Jurisicova A, Casper RF. Detection of deoxyribonucleic acid fragmentation in human sperm: correlation with fertilization in vitro. Biol Reprod. 1997;56(3):602–7.

10. Zhao J, Zhang Q, Wang Y, Li Y. Whether sperm deoxyribonucleic acid fragmentation has an effect on pregnancy and miscarriage after in vitro fertilization/intracytoplasmic sperm injection: a systematic review and meta-analysis. Fertil Steril. 2014;102(4):998–1005.e8. https://doi.org/10.1016/j.fertnstert.2014.06.033.
11. Ryu HM, Lin WW, Lamb DJ, Chuang W, Lipshultz LI, Bischoff FZ. Increased chromosome X, Y, and 18 nondisjunction in sperm from infertile patients that were identified as normal by strict morphology: implication for intracytoplasmic sperm injection. Fertil Steril. 2001;76(5):879–83.
12. Bareh GM, Jacoby E, Binkley P, Chang TC, Schenken RS, Robinson RD. Sperm deoxyribonucleic acid fragmentation assessment in normozoospermic male partners of couples with unexplained recurrent pregnancy loss: a prospective study. Fertil Steril. 2016;105(2):329–36. e1. https://doi.org/10.1016/j.fertnstert.2015.10.033.
13. Templado C, Uroz L, Estop A. New insights on the origin and relevance of aneuploidy in human spermatozoa. Mol Hum Reprod. 2013;19(10):634–43. https://doi.org/10.1093/molehr/gat039.
14. Chatziparasidou A, Christoforidis N, Samolada G, Nijs M. Sperm aneuploidy in infertile male patients: a systematic review of the literature. Andrologia. 2015;47(8):847–60. https://doi.org/10.1111/and.12362.
15. Carrell DT. The clinical implementation of sperm chromosome aneuploidy testing: pitfalls and promises. J Androl. 2008;29(2):124–33. https://doi.org/10.2164/jandrol.107.003699.
16. Caseiro AL, Regalo A, Pereira E, Esteves T, Fernandes F, Carvalho J. Implication of sperm chromosomal abnormalities in recurrent abortion and multiple implantation failure. Reprod Biomed Online. 2015;31(4):481–5. https://doi.org/10.1016/j.rbmo.2015.07.001.
17. Kohn TP, Kohn JR, Darilek S, Ramasamy R, Lipshultz L. Genetic counseling for men with recurrent pregnancy loss or recurrent implantation failure due to abnormal sperm chromosomal aneuploidy. J Assist Reprod Genet. 2016;33(5):571–6. https://doi.org/10.1007/s10815-016-0702-8.
18. Ramasamy R, Besada S, Lamb DJ. Fluorescent in situ hybridization of human sperm: diagnostics, indications, and therapeutic implications. Fertil Steril. 2014;102(6):1534–9. https://doi.org/10.1016/j.fertnstert.2014.09.013.
19. Ramasamy R, Scovell JM, Kovac JR, Cook PJ, Lamb DJ, Lipshultz LI. Fluorescence in situ hybridization detects increased sperm aneuploidy in men with recurrent pregnancy loss. Fertil Steril. 2015;103(4):906–9.e1. https://doi.org/10.1016/j.fertnstert.2015.01.029.
20. Practice Committee of the American Society for Reproductive Medicine. Diagnostic evaluation of the infertile male: a committee opinion. Fertil Steril. 2015;103(3):e18–25. https://doi.org/10.1016/j.fertnstert.2014.12.103.
21. Tempest HG, Martin RH. Cytogenetic risks in chromosomally normal infertile men. Curr Opin Obstet Gynecol. 2009;21(3):223–7. https://doi.org/10.1097/GCO.0b013e32832947c2.
22. Neusser M, Rogenhofer N, Durl S, Ochsenkuhn R, Trottmann M, Jurinovic V, et al. Increased chromosome 16 disomy rates in human spermatozoa and recurrent spontaneous abortions. Fertil Steril. 2015;104(5):1130–7.e1–10. https://doi.org/10.1016/j.fertnstert.2015.07.1160.
23. Lathi RB, Gray Hazard FK, Heerema-McKenney A, Taylor J, Chueh JT. First trimester miscarriage evaluation. Semin Reprod Med. 2011;29(6):463–9. https://doi.org/10.1055/s-0031-1293200.
24. Hotaling J, Carrell DT. Clinical genetic testing for male factor infertility: current applications and future directions. Andrology. 2014;2(3):339–50. https://doi.org/10.1111/j.2047-2927.2014.00200.x.
25. Carrell DT, Emery BR. Use of automated imaging and analysis technology for the detection of aneuploidy in human sperm. Fertil Steril. 2008;90(2):434–7. https://doi.org/10.1016/j.fertnstert.2007.06.095.
26. Patassini C, Garolla A, Bottacin A, Menegazzo M, Speltra E, Foresta C, et al. Molecular karyotyping of human single sperm by array-comparative genomic hybridization. PLoS One. 2013;8(4):e60922. https://doi.org/10.1371/journal.pone.0060922.
27. Pastuszak AW, Lamb DJ. The genetics of male fertility—from basic science to clinical evaluation. J Androl. 2012;33(6):1075–84. https://doi.org/10.2164/jandrol.112.017103.

28. Sarrate Z, Vidal F, Blanco J. Role of sperm fluorescent in situ hybridization studies in infertile patients: indications, study approach, and clinical relevance. Fertil Steril. 2010;93(6):1892–902. https://doi.org/10.1016/j.fertnstert.2008.12.139.
29. Aitken RJ, De Iuliis GN, McLachlan RI. Biological and clinical significance of DNA damage in the male germ line. Int J Androl. 2009;32(1):46–56. https://doi.org/10.1111/j.1365-2605.2008.00943.x.
30. Agarwal A, Said TM. Role of sperm chromatin abnormalities and DNA damage in male infertility. Hum Reprod Update. 2003;9(4):331–45.
31. Twigg JP, Irvine DS, Aitken RJ. Oxidative damage to DNA in human spermatozoa does not preclude pronucleus formation at intracytoplasmic sperm injection. Hum Reprod. 1998;13(7):1864–71.
32. Ahmadi A, Ng SC. Developmental capacity of damaged spermatozoa. Hum Reprod. 1999;14(9):2279–85.
33. Henkel R, Hajimohammad M, Stalf T, Hoogendijk C, Mehnert C, Menkveld R, et al. Influence of deoxyribonucleic acid damage on fertilization and pregnancy. Fertil Steril. 2004;81(4):965–72. https://doi.org/10.1016/j.fertnstert.2003.09.044.
34. Carrell DT, Liu L, Peterson CM, Jones KP, Hatasaka HH, Erickson L, et al. Sperm DNA fragmentation is increased in couples with unexplained recurrent pregnancy loss. Arch Androl. 2003;49(1):49–55.
35. Tomlinson MJ, Moffatt O, Manicardi GC, Bizzaro D, Afnan M, Sakkas D. Interrelationships between seminal parameters and sperm nuclear DNA damage before and after density gradient centrifugation: implications for assisted conception. Hum Reprod. 2001;16(10):2160–5.
36. Jansen J, Olsen AK, Wiger R, Naegeli H, de Boer P, van Der Hoeven F, et al. Nucleotide excision repair in rat male germ cells: low level of repair in intact cells contrasts with high dual incision activity in vitro. Nucleic Acids Res. 2001;29(8):1791–800.
37. Olsen AK, Duale N, Bjoras M, Larsen CT, Wiger R, Holme JA, et al. Limited repair of 8-hydroxy-7,8-dihydroguanine residues in human testicular cells. Nucleic Acids Res. 2003;31(4):1351–63.
38. Meseguer M, Santiso R, Garrido N, Garcia-Herrero S, Remohi J, Fernandez JL. Effect of sperm DNA fragmentation on pregnancy outcome depends on oocyte quality. Fertil Steril. 2011;95(1):124–8. https://doi.org/10.1016/j.fertnstert.2010.05.055.
39. Sakkas D, Alvarez JG. Sperm DNA fragmentation: mechanisms of origin, impact on reproductive outcome, and analysis. Fertil Steril. 2010;93(4):1027–36. https://doi.org/10.1016/j.fertnstert.2009.10.046.
40. Aitken RJ, Bronson R, Smith TB, De Iuliis GN. The source and significance of DNA damage in human spermatozoa; a commentary on diagnostic strategies and straw man fallacies. Mol Hum Reprod. 2013;19(8):475–85. https://doi.org/10.1093/molehr/gat025.
41. Johnson SL, Dunleavy J, Gemmell NJ, Nakagawa S. Consistent age-dependent declines in human semen quality: a systematic review and meta-analysis. Ageing Res Rev. 2015;19:22–33. https://doi.org/10.1016/j.arr.2014.10.007.
42. Wright C, Milne S, Leeson H. Sperm DNA damage caused by oxidative stress: modifiable clinical, lifestyle and nutritional factors in male infertility. Reprod Biomed Online. 2014;28(6):684–703. https://doi.org/10.1016/j.rbmo.2014.02.004.
43. Gomez E, Irvine DS, Aitken RJ. Evaluation of a spectrophotometric assay for the measurement of malondialdehyde and 4-hydroxyalkenals in human spermatozoa: relationships with semen quality and sperm function. Int J Androl. 1998;21(2):81–94.
44. Sikka SC, Hellstrom WJ. Current updates on laboratory techniques for the diagnosis of male reproductive failure. Asian J Androl. 2016;18(3):392–401. https://doi.org/10.4103/1008-682X.179161.
45. Muratori M, Maggi M, Spinelli S, Filimberti E, Forti G, Baldi E. Spontaneous DNA fragmentation in swim-up selected human spermatozoa during long term incubation. J Androl. 2003;24(2):253–62.

46. Cicare J, Caille A, Zumoffen C, Ghersevich S, Bahamondes L, Munuce MJ. In vitro incubation of human spermatozoa promotes reactive oxygen species generation and DNA fragmentation. Andrologia. 2015;47(8):861–6. https://doi.org/10.1111/and.12337.
47. Esteves SC, Sharma RK, Gosalvez J, Agarwal A. A translational medicine appraisal of specialized andrology testing in unexplained male infertility. Int Urol Nephrol. 2014;46(6):1037–52. https://doi.org/10.1007/s11255-014-0715-0.
48. Gosálvez J, López-Fernández C, Fernández JL, Esteves SC, Johnston SD. Unpacking the mysteries of sperm DNA fragmentation: ten frequently asked questions. J Reprod Biotech Fertil. 2015;4. https://doi.org/10.1177/2058915815594454.
49. Stahl PJ, Cogan C, Mehta A, Bolyakov A, Paduch DA, Goldstein M. Concordance among sperm deoxyribonucleic acid integrity assays and semen parameters. Fertil Steril. 2015;104(1):56–61.e1. https://doi.org/10.1016/j.fertnstert.2015.04.023.
50. Osman A, Alsomait H, Seshadri S, El-Toukhy T, Khalaf Y. The effect of sperm DNA fragmentation on live birth rate after IVF or ICSI: a systematic review and meta-analysis. Reprod Biomed Online. 2015;30(2):120–7. https://doi.org/10.1016/j.rbmo.2014.10.018.
51. Velez de la Calle JF, Muller A, Walschaerts M, Clavere JL, Jimenez C, Wittemer C, et al. Sperm deoxyribonucleic acid fragmentation as assessed by the sperm chromatin dispersion test in assisted reproductive technology programs: results of a large prospective multicenter study. Fertil Steril. 2008;90(5):1792–9. https://doi.org/10.1016/j.fertnstert.2007.09.021.
52. Evgeni E, Lymberopoulos G, Touloupidis S, Asimakopoulos B. Sperm nuclear DNA fragmentation and its association with semen quality in Greek men. Andrologia. 2015;47(10):1166–74. https://doi.org/10.1111/and.12398.
53. Omran HM, Bakhiet M, Dashti MG. DNA integrity is a critical molecular indicator for the assessment of male infertility. Mol Med Rep. 2013;7(5):1631–5. https://doi.org/10.3892/mmr.2013.1390.
54. Evgeni E, Charalabopoulos K, Asimakopoulos B. Human sperm DNA fragmentation and its correlation with conventional semen parameters. J Reprod Infertil. 2014;15(1):2–14.
55. Lin MH, Kuo-Kuang Lee R, Li SH, Lu CH, Sun FJ, Hwu YM. Sperm chromatin structure assay parameters are not related to fertilization rates, embryo quality, and pregnancy rates in in vitro fertilization and intracytoplasmic sperm injection, but might be related to spontaneous abortion rates. Fertil Steril. 2008;90(2):352–9. https://doi.org/10.1016/j.fertnstert.2007.06.018.
56. Karydis S, Asimakopoulos B, Papadopoulos N, Vakalopoulos I, Al-Hasani S, Nikoletos N. ICSI outcome is not associated with the incidence of spermatozoa with abnormal chromatin condensation. In Vivo. 2005;19(5):921–5.
57. Benchaib M, Lornage J, Mazoyer C, Lejeune H, Salle B, Francois Guerin J. Sperm deoxyribonucleic acid fragmentation as a prognostic indicator of assisted reproductive technology outcome. Fertil Steril. 2007;87(1):93–100. https://doi.org/10.1016/j.fertnstert.2006.05.057.
58. Agarwal A, Cho CL, Esteves SC. Should we evaluate and treat sperm DNA fragmentation? Curr Opin Obstet Gynecol. 2016;28(3):164–71. https://doi.org/10.1097/gco.0000000000000271.
59. Evenson D, Wixon R. Meta-analysis of sperm DNA fragmentation using the sperm chromatin structure assay. Reprod Biomed Online. 2006;12(4):466–72.
60. Collins JA, Barnhart KT, Schlegel PN. Do sperm DNA integrity tests predict pregnancy with in vitro fertilization? Fertil Steril. 2008;89(4):823–31. https://doi.org/10.1016/j.fertnstert.2007.04.055.
61. Zini A. Are sperm chromatin and DNA defects relevant in the clinic? Syst Biol Reprod Med. 2011;57(1–2):78–85. https://doi.org/10.3109/19396368.2010.515704.

62. Zini A, Boman JM, Belzile E, Ciampi A. Sperm DNA damage is associated with an increased risk of pregnancy loss after IVF and ICSI: systematic review and meta-analysis. Hum Reprod. 2008;23(12):2663–8. https://doi.org/10.1093/humrep/den321.
63. Robinson L, Gallos ID, Conner SJ, Rajkhowa M, Miller D, Lewis S, et al. The effect of sperm DNA fragmentation on miscarriage rates: a systematic review and meta-analysis. Hum Reprod. 2012;27(10):2908–17. https://doi.org/10.1093/humrep/des261.
64. Zhang Z, Zhu L, Jiang H, Chen H, Chen Y, Dai Y. Sperm DNA fragmentation index and pregnancy outcome after IVF or ICSI: a meta-analysis. J Assist Reprod Genet. 2015;32(1):17–26. https://doi.org/10.1007/s10815-014-0374-1.
65. Lewis SEM. The place of sperm DNA fragmentation testing in current day fertility management. Middle East Fertil Soc J. 2013;18(2):78–82. https://doi.org/10.1016/j.mefs.2013.01.010.
66. Barratt CLR, Mansell SA. Andrology is desperate for a new assay—let us make sure we get it right this time…. Middle East Fertil Soc J. 2013;18(2):82–3. https://doi.org/10.1016/j.mefs.2013.01.008.
67. Simon L, Proutski I, Stevenson M, Jennings D, McManus J, Lutton D, et al. Sperm DNA damage has a negative association with live-birth rates after IVF. Reprod Biomed Online. 2013;26(1):68–78. https://doi.org/10.1016/j.rbmo.2012.09.019.
68. Bungum M, Humaidan P, Axmon A, Spano M, Bungum L, Erenpreiss J, et al. Sperm DNA integrity assessment in prediction of assisted reproduction technology outcome. Hum Reprod. 2007;22(1):174–9. https://doi.org/10.1093/humrep/del326.
69. Oleszczuk K, Giwercman A, Bungum M. Sperm chromatin structure assay in prediction of in vitro fertilization outcome. Andrology. 2016;4(2):290–6. https://doi.org/10.1111/andr.12153.
70. Carrell DT. Epigenetics of the male gamete. Fertil Steril. 2012;97(2):267–74. https://doi.org/10.1016/j.fertnstert.2011.12.036.
71. Oliva R. Protamines and male infertility. Hum Reprod Update. 2006;12(4):417–35. https://doi.org/10.1093/humupd/dml009.
72. Aoki VW, Liu L, Jones KP, Hatasaka HH, Gibson M, Peterson CM, et al. Sperm protamine 1/protamine 2 ratios are related to in vitro fertilization pregnancy rates and predictive of fertilization ability. Fertil Steril. 2006;86(5):1408–15. https://doi.org/10.1016/j.fertnstert.2006.04.024.
73. Hammoud SS, Purwar J, Pflueger C, Cairns BR, Carrell DT. Alterations in sperm DNA methylation patterns at imprinted loci in two classes of infertility. Fertil Steril. 2010;94(5):1728–33. https://doi.org/10.1016/j.fertnstert.2009.09.010.
74. Jenkins TG, Aston KI, Meyer TD, Hotaling JM, Shamsi MB, Johnstone EB, et al. Decreased fecundity and sperm DNA methylation patterns. Fertil Steril. 2016;105(1):51–7.e1–3. https://doi.org/10.1016/j.fertnstert.2015.09.013.
75. La Vignera S, Condorelli RA, Balercia G, Vicari E, Calogero AE. Does alcohol have any effect on male reproductive function? A review of literature. Asian J Androl. 2013;15(2):221–5. https://doi.org/10.1038/aja.2012.118.
76. Opuwari CS, Henkel RR. An update on oxidative damage to spermatozoa and oocytes. Biomed Res Int. 2016;2016:9540142. https://doi.org/10.1155/2016/9540142.
77. Klonoff-Cohen H, Lam-Kruglick P, Gonzalez C. Effects of maternal and paternal alcohol consumption on the success rates of in vitro fertilization and gamete intrafallopian transfer. Fertil Steril. 2003;79(2):330–9.
78. Nicolau P, Miralpeix E, Sola I, Carreras R, Checa MA. Alcohol consumption and in vitro fertilization: a review of the literature. Gynecol Endocrinol. 2014;30(11):759–63. https://doi.org/10.3109/09513590.2014.938623.
79. Sharma R, Harlev A, Agarwal A, Esteves SC. Cigarette smoking and semen quality: a new meta-analysis examining the effect of the 2010 World Health Organization Laboratory methods for the examination of human semen. Eur Urol. 2016;70(4):635–45. https://doi.org/10.1016/j.eururo.2016.04.010.

80. Harlev A, Agarwal A, Gunes SO, Shetty A, du Plessis SS. Smoking and male infertility: an evidence-based review. World J Mens Health. 2015;33(3):143–60. https://doi.org/10.5534/wjmh.2015.33.3.143.
81. Esakky P, Moley KH. Paternal smoking and germ cell death: a mechanistic link to the effects of cigarette smoke on spermatogenesis and possible long-term sequelae in offspring. Mol Cell Endocrinol. 2016;435:85–93. https://doi.org/10.1016/j.mce.2016.07.015.
82. Liu R, Zhang L, McHale CM, Hammond SK. Paternal smoking and risk of childhood acute lymphoblastic leukemia: systematic review and meta-analysis. J Oncol. 2011;2011:854584. https://doi.org/10.1155/2011/854584.
83. Milne E, Greenop KR, Scott RJ, Bailey HD, Attia J, Dalla-Pozza L, et al. Parental prenatal smoking and risk of childhood acute lymphoblastic leukemia. Am J Epidemiol. 2012;175(1):43–53. https://doi.org/10.1093/aje/kwr275.
84. Rao M, Zhao XL, Yang J, Hu SF, Lei H, Xia W, et al. Effect of transient scrotal hyperthermia on sperm parameters, seminal plasma biochemical markers, and oxidative stress in men. Asian J Androl. 2015;17(4):668–75. https://doi.org/10.4103/1008-682X.146967.
85. Rao M, Xia W, Yang J, Hu LX, Hu SF, Lei H, et al. Transient scrotal hyperthermia affects human sperm DNA integrity, sperm apoptosis, and sperm protein expression. Andrology. 2016;4(6):1054–63. https://doi.org/10.1111/andr.12228.
86. Garolla A, Torino M, Sartini B, Cosci I, Patassini C, Carraro U, et al. Seminal and molecular evidence that sauna exposure affects human spermatogenesis. Hum Reprod. 2013;28(4):877–85. https://doi.org/10.1093/humrep/det020.
87. Ahmad G, Moinard N, Esquerre-Lamare C, Mieusset R, Bujan L. Mild induced testicular and epididymal hyperthermia alters sperm chromatin integrity in men. Fertil Steril. 2012;97(3):546–53. https://doi.org/10.1016/j.fertnstert.2011.12.025.
88. Sheynkin Y, Welliver R, Winer A, Hajimirzaee F, Ahn H, Lee K. Protection from scrotal hyperthermia in laptop computer users. Fertil Steril. 2011;95(2):647–51. https://doi.org/10.1016/j.fertnstert.2010.10.013.
89. Southorn T. Great balls of fire and the vicious cycle: a study of the effects of cycling on male fertility. J Fam Plann Reprod Health Care. 2002;28(4):211–3.
90. Pathak P, Chandrashekar A, Hakky TS, Pastuszak AW. Varicocele management in the era of in vitro fertilization/intracytoplasmic sperm injection. Asian J Androl. 2016;18(3):343–8. https://doi.org/10.4103/1008-682X.178482.
91. Wang YJ, Zhang RQ, Lin YJ, Zhang RG, Zhang WL. Relationship between varicocele and sperm DNA damage and the effect of varicocele repair: a meta-analysis. Reprod Biomed Online. 2012;25(3):307–14. https://doi.org/10.1016/j.rbmo.2012.05.002.
92. Schauer I, Madersbacher S, Jost R, Hubner WA, Imhof M. The impact of varicocelectomy on sperm parameters: a meta-analysis. J Urol. 2012;187(5):1540–7. https://doi.org/10.1016/j.juro.2011.12.084.
93. Esteves SC, Roque M, Agarwal A. Outcome of assisted reproductive technology in men with treated and untreated varicocele: systematic review and meta-analysis. Asian J Androl. 2016;18(2):254–8. https://doi.org/10.4103/1008-682X.163269.
94. Agarwal A, Gupta S, Du Plessis S, Sharma R, Esteves SC, Cirenza C, et al. Abstinence time and its impact on basic and advanced semen parameters. Urology. 2016;94:102–10. https://doi.org/10.1016/j.urology.2016.03.059.
95. Mayorga-Torres BJ, Camargo M, Agarwal A, du Plessis SS, Cadavid AP, Cardona Maya WD. Influence of ejaculation frequency on seminal parameters. Reprod Biol Endocrinol. 2015;13:47. https://doi.org/10.1186/s12958-015-0045-9.
96. Gosalvez J, Gonzalez-Martinez M, Lopez-Fernandez C, Fernandez JL, Sanchez-Martin P. Shorter abstinence decreases sperm deoxyribonucleic acid fragmentation in ejaculate. Fertil Steril. 2011;96(5):1083–6. https://doi.org/10.1016/j.fertnstert.2011.08.027.

97. Pons I, Cercas R, Villas C, Brana C, Fernandez-Shaw S. One abstinence day decreases sperm DNA fragmentation in 90% of selected patients. J Assist Reprod Genet. 2013;30(9):1211–8. https://doi.org/10.1007/s10815-013-0089-8.

98. Sengupta P, Banerjee R. Environmental toxins: alarming impacts of pesticides on male fertility. Hum Exp Toxicol. 2014;33(10):1017–39. https://doi.org/10.1177/0960327113515504.

99. Wirth JJ, Mijal RS. Adverse effects of low level heavy metal exposure on male reproductive function. Syst Biol Reprod Med. 2010;56(2):147–67. https://doi.org/10.3109/19396360903582216.

100. Sermondade N, Faure C, Fezeu L, Shayeb AG, Bonde JP, Jensen TK, et al. BMI in relation to sperm count: an updated systematic review and collaborative meta-analysis. Hum Reprod Update. 2013;19(3):221–31. https://doi.org/10.1093/humupd/dms050.

101. Campbell JM, Lane M, Owens JA, Bakos HW. Paternal obesity negatively affects male fertility and assisted reproduction outcomes: a systematic review and meta-analysis. Reprod Biomed Online. 2015;31(5):593–604. https://doi.org/10.1016/j.rbmo.2015.07.012.

102. Barazani Y, Katz BF, Nagler HM, Stember DS. Lifestyle, environment, and male reproductive health. Urol Clin North Am. 2014;41(1):55–66. https://doi.org/10.1016/j.ucl.2013.08.017.

103. Brezina PR, Yunus FN, Zhao Y. Effects of pharmaceutical medications on male fertility. J Reprod Infertil. 2012;13(1):3–11.

104. Fronczak CM, Kim ED, Barqawi AB. The insults of illicit drug use on male fertility. J Androl. 2012;33(4):515–28. https://doi.org/10.2164/jandrol.110.011874.

105. Male Infertility Best Practice Policy Committee of the American Urological Association; Practice Committee of the American Society for Reproductive Medicine. Report on varicocele and infertility. Fertil Steril. 2004;82(Suppl 1):S142–5. https://doi.org/10.1016/j.fertnstert.2004.05.057.

106. Esteves SC, Oliveira FV, Bertolla RP. Clinical outcome of intracytoplasmic sperm injection in infertile men with treated and untreated clinical varicocele. J Urol. 2010;184(4):1442–6. https://doi.org/10.1016/j.juro.2010.06.004.

107. Mansour Ghanaie M, Asgari SA, Dadrass N, Allahkhah A, Iran-Pour E, Safarinejad MR. Effects of varicocele repair on spontaneous first trimester miscarriage: a randomized clinical trial. Urol J. 2012;9(2):505–13.

108. Pasqualotto FF, Braga DP, Figueira RC, Setti AS, Iaconelli A Jr, Borges E Jr. Varicocelectomy does not impact pregnancy outcomes following intracytoplasmic sperm injection procedures. J Androl. 2012;33(2):239–43. https://doi.org/10.2164/jandrol.110.011932.

109. Durairajanayagam D, Agarwal A, Ong C. Causes, effects and molecular mechanisms of testicular heat stress. Reprod Biomed Online. 2015;30(1):14–27. https://doi.org/10.1016/j.rbmo.2014.09.018.

110. Jung A, Schuppe HC. Influence of genital heat stress on semen quality in humans. Andrologia. 2007;39(6):203–15. https://doi.org/10.1111/j.1439-0272.2007.00794.x.

111. World Health Organization. WHO laboratory manual for the examination and processing of human semen. 5th ed. Geneva: World Health Organization; 2010.

112. Agarwal A, Mulgund A, Alshahrani S, Assidi M, Abuzenadah AM, Sharma R, et al. Reactive oxygen species and sperm DNA damage in infertile men presenting with low level leukocytospermia. Reprod Biol Endocrinol. 2014;12:126. https://doi.org/10.1186/1477-7827-12-126.

113. Ricci G, Granzotto M, Luppi S, Giolo E, Martinelli M, Zito G, et al. Effect of seminal leukocytes on in vitro fertilization and intracytoplasmic sperm injection outcomes. Fertil Steril. 2015;104(1):87–93. https://doi.org/10.1016/j.fertnstert.2015.04.007.

114. Cavagna M, Oliveira JB, Petersen CG, Mauri AL, Silva LF, Massaro FC, et al. The influence of leukocytospermia on the outcomes of assisted reproductive technology. Reprod Biol Endocrinol. 2012;10:44. https://doi.org/10.1186/1477-7827-10-44.

115. Talevi R, Barbato V, Fiorentino I, Braun S, Longobardi S, Gualtieri R. Protective effects of in vitro treatment with zinc, d-aspartate and coenzyme q10 on human sperm motility,

lipid peroxidation and DNA fragmentation. Reprod Biol Endocrinol. 2013;11:81. https://doi. org/10.1186/1477-7827-11-81.

116. Showell MG, Mackenzie-Proctor R, Brown J, Yazdani A, Stankiewicz MT, Hart RJ. Antioxidants for male subfertility. Cochrane Database Syst Rev. 2014;12:CD007411. https://doi.org/10.1002/14651858.CD007411.pub3.

117. Kessopoulou E, Powers HJ, Sharma KK, Pearson MJ, Russell JM, Cooke ID, et al. A double-blind randomized placebo cross-over controlled trial using the antioxidant vitamin E to treat reactive oxygen species associated male infertility. Fertil Steril. 1995;64(4):825–31.

118. Tremellen K, Miari G, Froiland D, Thompson J. A randomised control trial examining the effect of an antioxidant (Menevit) on pregnancy outcome during IVF-ICSI treatment. Aust N Z J Obstet Gynaecol. 2007;47(3):216–21. https://doi.org/10.1111/j.1479-828X.2007.00723.x.

119. Sakkas D, Ramalingam M, Garrido N, Barratt CL. Sperm selection in natural conception: what can we learn from mother nature to improve assisted reproduction outcomes? Hum Reprod Update. 2015;21(6):711–26. https://doi.org/10.1093/humupd/dmv042.

120. Rappa KL, Rodriguez HF, Hakkarainen GC, Anchan RM, Mutter GL, Asghar W. Sperm processing for advanced reproductive technologies: where are we today? Biotechnol Adv. 2016;34(5):578–87. https://doi.org/10.1016/j.biotechadv.2016.01.007.

121. Bartoov B, Berkovitz A, Eltes F. Selection of spermatozoa with normal nuclei to improve the pregnancy rate with intracytoplasmic sperm injection. N Engl J Med. 2001;345(14):1067–8. https://doi.org/10.1056/NEJM200110043451416.

122. La Sala GB, Nicoli A, Fornaciari E, Falbo A, Rondini I, Morini D, et al. Intracytoplasmic morphologically selected sperm injection versus conventional intracytoplasmic sperm injection: a randomized controlled trial. Reprod Biol Endocrinol. 2015;13:97. https://doi. org/10.1186/s12958-015-0096-y.

123. Setti AS, Braga DP, Figueira RC, Iaconelli A Jr, Borges E. Intracytoplasmic morphologically selected sperm injection results in improved clinical outcomes in couples with previous ICSI failures or male factor infertility: a meta-analysis. Eur J Obstet Gynecol Reprod Biol. 2014;183:96–103. https://doi.org/10.1016/j.ejogrb.2014.10.008.

124. Sakkas D, Manicardi GC, Tomlinson M, Mandrioli M, Bizzaro D, Bianchi PG, et al. The use of two density gradient centrifugation techniques and the swim-up method to separate spermatozoa with chromatin and nuclear DNA anomalies. Hum Reprod. 2000;15(5):1112–6.

125. Degheidy T, Abdelfattah H, Seif A, Albuz FK, Gazi S, Abbas S. Magnetic activated cell sorting: an effective method for reduction of sperm DNA fragmentation in varicocele men prior to assisted reproductive techniques. Andrologia. 2015;47(8):892–6. https://doi.org/10.1111/ and.12343.

126. Magli MC, Crippa A, Muzii L, Boudjema E, Capoti A, Scaravelli G, et al. Head birefringence properties are associated with acrosome reaction, sperm motility and morphology. Reprod Biomed Online. 2012;24(3):352–9. https://doi.org/10.1016/j.rbmo.2011.12.013.

127. Samuel R, Badamjav O, Murphy KE, Patel DP, Son J, Gale BK, et al. Microfluidics: the future of microdissection TESE? Syst Biol Reprod Med. 2016;62(3):161–70. https://doi.org/ 10.3109/19396368.2016.1159748.

128. Ainsworth C, Nixon B, Aitken RJ. Development of a novel electrophoretic system for the isolation of human spermatozoa. Hum Reprod. 2005;20(8):2261–70. https://doi.org/10.1093/ humrep/dei024.

129. Simon L, Murphy K, Aston KI, Emery BR, Hotaling JM, Carrell DT. Micro-electrophoresis: a noninvasive method of sperm selection based on membrane charge. Fertil Steril. 2015;103(2):361–6.e3. https://doi.org/10.1016/j.fertnstert.2014.10.047.

130. Said TM, Land JA. Effects of advanced selection methods on sperm quality and ART outcome: a systematic review. Hum Reprod Update. 2011;17(6):719–33. https://doi.org/10.1093/ humupd/dmr032.

131. Esteves SC, Sanchez-Martin F, Sanchez-Martin P, Schneider DT, Gosalvez J. Comparison of reproductive outcome in oligozoospermic men with high sperm DNA fragmentation under-

going intracytoplasmic sperm injection with ejaculated and testicular sperm. Fertil Steril. 2015;104(6):1398–405. https://doi.org/10.1016/j.fertnstert.2015.08.028.
132. Greco E, Scarselli F, Iacobelli M, Rienzi L, Ubaldi F, Ferrero S, et al. Efficient treatment of infertility due to sperm DNA damage by ICSI with testicular spermatozoa. Hum Reprod. 2005;20(1):226–30. https://doi.org/10.1093/humrep/deh590.
133. Huang WJ, Lamb DJ, Kim ED, de Lara J, Lin WW, Lipshultz LI, et al. Germ-cell nondisjunction in testes biopsies of men with idiopathic infertility. Am J Hum Genet. 1999;64(6):1638–45. https://doi.org/10.1086/302402.
134. Moskovtsev SI, Alladin N, Lo KC, Jarvi K, Mullen JB, Librach CL. A comparison of ejaculated and testicular spermatozoa aneuploidy rates in patients with high sperm DNA damage. Syst Biol Reprod Med. 2012;58(3):142–8. https://doi.org/10.3109/19396368.2012.667504.
135. Ly KD, Agarwal A, Nagy ZP. Preimplantation genetic screening: does it help or hinder IVF treatment and what is the role of the embryo? J Assist Reprod Genet. 2011;28(9):833–49. https://doi.org/10.1007/s10815-011-9608-7.
136. Rubio C, Buendia P, Rodrigo L, Mercader A, Mateu E, Peinado V, et al. Prognostic factors for preimplantation genetic screening in repeated pregnancy loss. Reprod Biomed Online. 2009;18(5):687–93.

Chapter 4
Embryonic Factors Associated with Recurrent Implantation Failure

Daniel J. Kaser and Catherine Racowsky

Abbreviations

AC	Abnormal cleavage
AH	Assisted hatching
CPR	Clinical pregnancy rate
FISH	Fluorescence in situ hybridization
HPI	Hours post-insemination
ICM	Inner cell mass
IR	Implantation rate
LBR	Live birth rate
NGS	Next-generation sequencing
PGT-A	Preimplantation genetic testing for aneuploidy
TE	Trophectoderm
TLI	Time-lapse imaging
RC	Reverse cleavage
RCT	Randomized controlled trial
RIF	Recurrent implantation failure
ZP	Zona pellucida

D.J. Kaser, MD
Sidney Kimmel Medical College, Thomas Jefferson University Philadelphia, Philadelphia, PA, USA

IVI-RMA of New Jersey, Basking Ridge, NJ, USA
e-mail: dkaser@rmanj.com

C. Racowsky, PhD, HCLD (✉)
Department of Obstetrics and Gynecology, Brigham and Women's Hospital, Harvard Medical School, Boston, MA, USA
e-mail: CRACOWSKY@PARTNERS.ORG

© Springer International Publishing AG 2018
J.M. Franasiak, R.T. Scott Jr. (eds.), *Recurrent Implantation Failure*,
https://doi.org/10.1007/978-3-319-71967-2_4

Cleavage Stage Embryos

Developmental Rate and Abnormal Kinetics in the Cleavage Stage Embryo

The human preimplantation embryo develops along a predictable timeline, as first demonstrated by Edwards et al. [1] (Fig. 4.1). Accordingly, developmental rate and morphologic appearance traditionally have been the two main considerations for noninvasive selection of embryos for transfer. Both the Society for Assisted Reproductive Technology [2] and the Alpha Scientists in Reproductive Medicine/ESHRE Special Interest Group of Embryology [3] have recently described cleavage stage scoring systems in detail. Such scoring, whether performed once on the day of transfer (i.e., single parameter) or serially to generate a cumulative score (i.e., combined parameter), considers cell number, fragmentation, symmetry, and other features such as cytoplasmic granularity, multinucleation, and loss of membrane definition at the cleavage stage.

Two measurements of developmental rate, in particular, have been associated with implantation potential following day 3 transfer—early cleavage (division to the two-cell stage by 26–28-h post-insemination (HPI)) and total cell number at 64–68 HPI [4, 5]. In a prospective cohort study, Sakkas et al. [6] demonstrated that early cleavage was predictive of implantation (early cleavage 58/219, 25.5% vs. no early cleavage 43/290, 14.8%; $P = 0.01$). This finding has been corroborated by several other groups [7, 8]. Regarding total cell number, numerous studies have shown a direct correlation between cell number and implantation potential at the cleavage stage [9–11]. Racowsky et al. [5] clarified the optimal cell number at the day 3 evaluation and showed in a retrospective analysis of 1823 embryos with known implantation fate that embryos containing eight cells at 64–68 HPI had the highest implantation potential, followed by embryos with greater than eight cells,

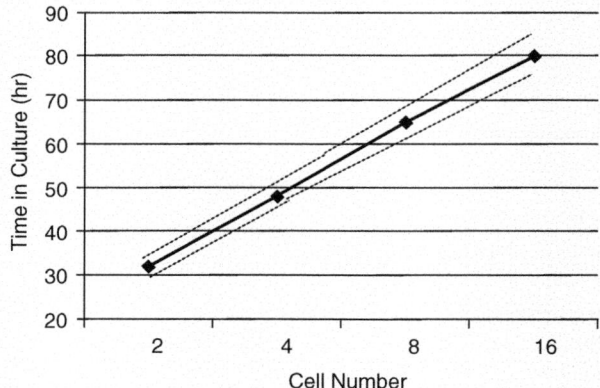

Fig. 4.1 Normal developmental kinetics of the human cleavage stage embryo. Solid line represents mean time in hours; dashed lines represent the 95% confidence intervals. Reprinted with permission from Edwards et al. Am J Obstet Gynecol 1981;141:408–16

which in turn had higher implantation rates (IR) than those with seven or fewer cells. Of note, neither early cleavage nor blastomere number has been specifically evaluated in the RIF population.

With the advent of time-lapse imaging (TLI) systems, in which images are acquired at frequent, preset time intervals (every 5–20 min), the nature of cleavage kinetics has been further characterized. While many of these time-based parameters have been shown to predict blastocyst formation, fewer have a clear association with implantation (reviewed by Kaser and Racowsky [12]). TLI parameters that have been demonstrated to predict implantation potential include the duration of the first cytokinesis; the time to the two-cell, three-cell, and five-cell stages; and the duration of the two-cell and three-cell stages [13–16]. These time-based assessments have been incorporated into hierarchal ranking systems as an adjunct to selection by conventional morphology alone [17]; however, no one selection algorithm has emerged as dominant. Indeed, the clinical utility of TLI has been called into question by the four randomized controlled trials (RCTs) performed to date. Three of these failed to demonstrate an improvement in clinical pregnancy rates (CPR) when TLI was used for embryo selection [18–20], and the one showing a significant improvement in IR [21] involved several biases in favor of the TLI group associated with differences between the culture systems used for the control and study groups [22]. Adjunctive use of TLI has not been studied in the RIF population, and it remains to be seen whether this selection strategy will be beneficial in this unique group of patients.

Morphologic Features Associated with Implantation at the Cleavage Stage

Several morphologic features of the human preimplantation embryo have been shown to correlate with implantation at the cleavage stage, including fragmentation [5, 23, 24], blastomere symmetry [5, 25], multinucleation at the four-cell stage [26–28], poor membrane definition/early compaction [29, 30], and zona pellucida (ZP) thickness [31–33]. A comprehensive review of each of these features, along with their relative contributions to the likelihood of implantation following day 3 transfer, was written by Skiadas and Racowsky [34]. The only morphologic parameter that has been studied specifically in the RIF population is ZP thickness, as described below.

Laboratory Interventions to Improve Implantation Potential at the Cleavage Stage

Time-Lapse Imaging for Detection of Abnormal Cleavage Patterns, Abnormal Phenotypes, and Multinucleated Embryos

While TLI has not been shown in prospective studies to improve CPR when used in hierarchal scoring algorithms, it is capable of detecting abnormal kinetic and morphologic parameters that conventional morphology cannot. Ultimately, where TLI may confer an advantage over conventional morphology is not in the measurement of certain intervals or cell durations but rather in the identification of abnormal cleavage (AC) and reverse cleavage (RC) patterns. AC is defined as the division of one cell into three, rather than two, daughter cells; RC is defined as blastomere fusion (i.e., two daughter cells fusing to form one cell). Both of these cleavage patterns have been shown to be highly predictive of implantation failure. Athayde Wirka et al. [35] reported that embryos exhibiting AC have lower IR than those that cleave normally (1/27, 3.7% vs. 19/105, 18.0%; $P = 0.05$); similarly, embryos with RC also have decreased implantation potential (0/22, 0% vs. 29/131, 22.1%; $P = 0.01$) [36]. The incidence of AC and RC has not been described in the RIF population, and studies evaluating the deselection of embryos based solely on these parameters have not been undertaken.

Similar to these abnormal cleavage patterns, TLI is also able to detect abnormal morphologic features that cannot be seen with static observations. Two that deserve mention are abnormal syngamy and abnormal first cytokinesis. In a retrospective analysis of embryos with known implantation fate, Athayde Wirka et al. [35] showed that embryos exhibiting abnormal syngamy, defined as disordered pronuclei movement within the cytoplasm accompanied by delayed dispersion of the nuclear envelopes at the time of pronuclei fading, had a non-statistically significant decrease in implantation (0/14, 0% vs. 19/106, 17.9%; $P = 0.08$). Similarly, those with an abnormal first cytokinesis, defined as the presence of oolemma ruffling and pseudo-furrow formation prior to the first mitotic division, likewise may have decreased implantation potential (2/32, 6.2% vs. 15/91, 16.5%; $P = 0.1$). The impact of these phenotypes has not been evaluated prospectively or in the RIF population.

It should also be noted that multinucleation, while observable with conventional morphology, may be more readily detected with the use of TLI, particularly when bright-field imaging is used. Goodman et al. [19] demonstrated the utility of TLI in the detection of multinucleation in a randomized controlled trial (RCT) of embryo selection with or without adjunctive TLI-based annotation. When embryos were cultured in a TLI system but selected for transfer based on conventional morphology alone, only 76/1080 (7.0%) were called multinucleated at the four-cell stage; in contrast, when the TLI videos of these same embryos were reviewed retrospectively, an additional 305 embryos were found to exhibit multinucleation (381/1080, 35.3%). In a multivariate analysis, multinucleation was independently and inversely associated with implantation potential (OR 0.51; 95% CI 0.30–0.86; $P = 0.01$) [19]. Deselection of multinucleated embryos has never been specifically evaluated in RIF patients.

Assisted Hatching for Treatment of the Thick Zona Pellucida

The ZP is a tetravalent glycoprotein coat surrounding the mammalian oocyte that is responsible for sperm binding, the initiation of the acrosome reaction, and prevention of polyspermy. In vivo the ZP is likewise important for protecting the preimplantation embryo as it traverses along the oviduct and into the uterus. Escapement of the embryo from the ZP (i.e., hatching), via both mechanical and chemical efforts, is a prerequisite for interaction between the trophectoderm and the uterine epithelium. Indeed, embryos that fail to hatch are not able to implant [37].

Accordingly, many studies have attempted to correlate certain morphologic features of the ZP, including thickness, hardness, and variation, with implantation potential [31–33]. Both a thinner ZP and one in which there is more varied thickness have been associated with higher IR [38].

These observations led to the development of assisted hatching (AH), which is a catchall term for several different micromanipulation techniques aimed to artificially thin or breach the ZP. AH can be performed by partial zona dissection with a glass microneedle [39], zona drilling with acidified Tyrode's solution [37], infrared laser photoablation [40], or the use of a piezoelectric pulse [41]. While studies exist comparing the clinical efficacy of these techniques, there is no definitive evidence that one method is superior to another [42].

The first RCT of AH reported higher IR following zona drilling of "poor prognosis" embryos, defined as those with a thickness >15 μm, a low blastomere number, and high degree of fragmentation [43]. Subsequent studies revealed conflicting results: some noted higher IR with AH [44, 45], while others showed no difference [46, 47], and still other showed harm [48, 49]. This heterogeneity is also apparent in trials that specifically evaluated the role of AH among patients with a history of RIF. Valojerdi et al. [50] randomized 796 RIF patients to transfer of a day 2 embryo with a breached or intact ZP; there was no difference in CPR or IR in the treatment and control group. In contrast, Stein et al. [51] randomized 154 RIF patients to partial zona dissection or no intervention and observed a significantly higher CPR following hatching among a subgroup of patients greater than age 38 years (23.9% in the study group vs. 7% in the control group; $P < 0.05$).

A Cochrane systematic review and meta-analysis analyzed 31 RCTs on the effect of AH on CPR (2933 patients in the AH group vs. 2795 patients in the control group) and noted a slightly higher CPR in the treatment group (OR 1.13; 95% CI 1.01–1.27) [42]. Notably, there was considerable study heterogeneity in this analysis ($I^2 = 49\%$), indicating that differences in study design, patient characteristics, operator experience, and hatching method may render it problematic to generate summary statistics from these trials [52]. Subgroup analysis of patients undergoing their first IVF/ICSI cycle failed to show a benefit of AH (six RCTs; $n = 650$; OR 0.77; 95% CI 0.54–1.10), while those who had failed at least one prior cycle had a modest improvement in CPR following AH (nine RCTs; $n = 1365$; OR 1.42; 95% CI 1.11–1.81). Only two of these nine studies independently demonstrated a higher CPR with AH ([53, 54]; Fig. 4.2), but the overall effect estimate excluded one, suggesting that the intervention may be beneficial in patients with a prior failed cycle. Among the studies that included live birth rate (LBR) as an outcome, there was no difference between the control and AH groups when all cycles were considered (nine RCTs; $n = 1921$; OR 1.03; 95% CI 0.85–1.25) or after subanalyses restricted to only first cycles (one RCT; $n = 20$; OR 0.24; 95% CI 0.03–2.03) or repeat cycles (one RCT; $n = 150$; OR 1.4; 95% CI 0.62–3.13).

Thus, in summary, the requirement that an embryo hatches from the ZP in order to implant raises the possibility that AH may be beneficial for RIF patients. Available

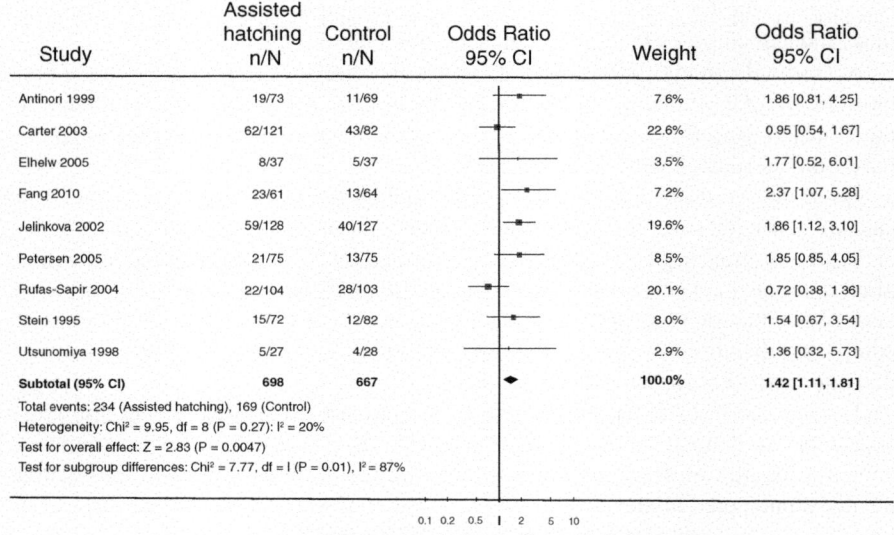

Study	Assisted hatching n/N	Control n/N	Odds Ratio 95% CI	Weight	Odds Ratio 95% CI
Antinori 1999	19/73	11/69		7.6%	1.86 [0.81, 4.25]
Carter 2003	62/121	43/82		22.6%	0.95 [0.54, 1.67]
Elhelw 2005	8/37	5/37		3.5%	1.77 [0.52, 6.01]
Fang 2010	23/61	13/64		7.2%	2.37 [1.07, 5.28]
Jelinkova 2002	59/128	40/127		19.6%	1.86 [1.12, 3.10]
Petersen 2005	21/75	13/75		8.5%	1.85 [0.85, 4.05]
Rufas-Sapir 2004	22/104	28/103		20.1%	0.72 [0.38, 1.36]
Stein 1995	15/72	12/82		8.0%	1.54 [0.67, 3.54]
Utsunomiya 1998	5/27	4/28		2.9%	1.36 [0.32, 5.73]
Subtotal (95% CI)	**698**	**667**		**100.0%**	**1.42 [1.11, 1.81]**

Total events: 234 (Assisted hatching), 169 (Control)
Heterogeneity: Chi² = 9.95, df = 8 (P = 0.27): I² = 20%
Test for overall effect: Z = 2.83 (P = 0.0047)
Test for subgroup differences: Chi² = 7.77, df = I (P = 0.01), I² = 87%

0.1 0.2 0.5 I 2 5 10
Favors control   Favors hatching

Fig. 4.2 Forest plot of clinical pregnancy rates comparing assisted hatching to no assisted hatching among patients with at least one prior failed cycle. Reprinted with permission from Carney et al. Cochrane Database Syst Rev. 2012;12:CD001894

evidence indicates that for patients with a history of at least one prior failed cycle, AH may, indeed, improve the CPR. However, there is no evidence that AH improves the LBR, regardless of treatment history.

Co-culture of Embryos

Prior to the introduction of complex culture media, extended culture of human embryos to the blastocyst stage required a feeder layer of cells in order to overcome cleavage stage block (reviewed by Ménézo et al. [55]). Co-culture, or simultaneous culture of embryos with a variety of somatic cell types, including trophoblast tissue, oviductal or uterine epithelial cells, or even primate cell lines such as green monkey kidney Vero cells, proved to support in vitro development of embryos beyond the cleavage stage. In initial studies of unselected patient populations, co-culture systems appeared to improve embryo quality and perhaps IR when compared to simple media (meta-analysis by Kattal et al. [56]). Importantly, none of the included 17 RCTs in this meta-analysis compared co-culture to complex media, and the reported improvement in IR following co-culture was only 3.0% in those studies ($n = 6$) that had complete data for analysis. For patients with a history of RIF, nonrandomized studies and those comparing co-culture systems to simple media likewise suggest a modest improvement in CPR with co-culture [57, 58]. Again, the comparator in these studies was simple, not complex, media. In the only RCT of co-culture vs.

complex media (G-Series, Vitrolife) among patients with RIF (defined as having failed at least three prior transfers), there was no improvement in IR (23.1% vs. 19.8%, not significant) [59]. Accordingly, available evidence is insufficient to recommend the use of co-culture systems, even in the RIF population.

Extended Culture of Embryos to the Blastocyst Stage

In contrast to the limited evidence to support the use of co-culture, extended culture to day 5 or day 6 with subsequent blastocyst transfer has been shown to improve IR both in the general infertility population and in RIF patients. In a recent Cochrane database meta-analysis of cleavage stage vs. blastocyst transfer, the CPR and LBR following fresh transfer were higher in the blastocyst group (CPR 27 RCTs; $n = 4031$; OR 1.30; 95% CI 1.14–1.47; $I^2 = 56\%$) (LBR 13 RCTs; $n = 1630$; OR 1.48; 95% CI 1.2–1.82; $I^2 = 45\%$) [60]. While there were more patients in the blastocyst group who had their embryo transfer canceled due to poor development (17 RCTs; $n = 2577$; OR 2.50; 95% CI 1.76–3.55; $I^2 = 36\%$) and also more patients in the blastocyst group who had no supernumerary embryos available for cryopreservation (14 RCTs; $n = 2292$; OR 0.48; 95% CI 0.40–0.57; $I^2 = 84\%$), there were no differences in the cumulative pregnancy rate following fresh and frozen-thawed transfer after one retrieval (five RCTs; $n = 632$; OR 0.89; 95% CI 0.64–1.22; $I^2 = 71\%$).

In the RIF population specifically, blastocyst transfer likewise seems to be beneficial. In a prospective cohort study of 276 patients who had failed at least two prior cleavage stage transfers, a day 5 or day 6 transfer was associated with higher rates of implantation (25.4% vs. 12.4%; $P < 0.05$) and clinical pregnancy (34.1% vs. 22.4%; $P < 0.05$) per cycle as compared to a day 2 transfer [61]. Levitas et al. [62] randomized 54 patients who had failed at least three prior cycles to a cleavage stage transfer on day 2 or day 3 or blastocyst transfer on day 5, day 6, or day 7. The IR was higher in the blastocyst group (21.2% vs. 6.0%; $P < 0.01$).

Thus, blastocyst transfer is associated with higher IR per transfer in the general infertility and RIF population, likely due to improved embryo selection and possibly better embryo-endometrial synchrony.

Blastocyst Stage Embryos

Developmental Rate and Abnormal Kinetics in the Blastocyst

Embryo quality at the blastocyst stage is scored at 116–120 HPI on day 5 and approximately 140 HPI on day 6 according to the developmental stage (degree of cavitation and expansion), along with quality of the inner cell mass (ICM) and trophectoderm (TE) [63]. Blastocysts with a greater degree of expansion have higher IR, as first evidenced by Gardner et al. [64] in a retrospective analysis of double blastocyst transfer. In this study, the IR following transfer of full, expanded, or hatching blastocysts was 72.8% (99/136), compared to 28.1% (9/32) for early blastocysts ($P < 0.001$). This correlation between blastocyst stage and implantation potential has been reproduced in several other studies [5, 65–67].

Indeed, the timing of blastocyst formation may be a critical determinant of IR in fresh transfers (see Chap. 2 for complete discussion). Briefly, two retrospective studies suggested that embryos that reach the full blastocyst stage on day 5 of culture have higher implantation potential than morphologically similar embryos that complete blastulation on day 6 [68, 69]. In the Shapiro et al. study [68], blastocysts transferred on day 5 had a nearly twofold increased rate of implantation (36.3% vs. 19.0%; $P < 0.001$). In the Barrenetxea et al. study [69], day 5 transfer of a cavitating embryo was likewise associated with a higher IR than day 6 transfer of an equivalent stage embryo (23.3% vs. 4.9%; $P = 0.001$). Thus, delayed blastulation seems to be detrimental in fresh transfers, likely due, at least in part, to a shift in embryo-endometrial synchrony. Time-lapse studies have likewise demonstrated that the time to the start of cavitation and the time to blastocyst expansion are correlated with implantation [19, 70].

Interestingly, transfer of embryos with delayed blastulation in a subsequent frozen cycle may rescue the pregnancy rate. Shapiro et al. [71] demonstrated that the CPR for day 5 fresh blastocyst transfer was higher than that of day 6 fresh blastocyst transfer (51.0 vs. 33.3%; $P < 0.001$); however, there was no difference following frozen embryo transfer according to the day of cryopreservation (day 5 63.6% vs. day 6 58.9%; not significant). Other retrospective studies have confirmed this finding [72, 73]. These studies indicate that autologous day 6 blastocysts transferred in frozen cycles have significantly higher IR than morphologically equivalent embryos transferred in fresh cycles. This observation raises the possibility of elective cryopreservation of all embryos, or at least those with delayed blastulation as described below, as a possible intervention to improve pregnancy rates following extended culture.

Morphologic Features of the Blastocyst Associated with Implantation

In addition to the developmental stage, the Gardner and Schoolcraft system of blastocyst scoring assigns a grade to the ICM and TE, based on the number, size, and cohesiveness of its cells. In both fresh and frozen embryo transfers, the TE quality seems to be the most important morphologic parameter at this stage. Ahlstrom et al. [74] reported that while ICM quality was predictive of live birth in univariate analyses following fresh single blastocyst transfer, after adjusting for potential confounders (including female age, number of prior failed cycles, total gonadotropin dose, and number of good-quality embryos), the ICM grade no longer was associated with live birth. TE grade, in contrast, was significantly associated with live birth in multivariate analyses (A, n = 234, 49.9% [Referent]; B, n = 128, 33.9% [OR 0.51; 95% CI 0.39–0.68]; C, n = 2, 8.0% [OR 0.17, 95% CI 0.04–0.73]). Hill et al. [67] confirmed these findings in an analysis of 694 single blastocyst transfers: LBRs were 57%, 40%, and 25% for TE grades A, B, and C, respectively ($P < 0.001$). Similar to the Ahlstrom et al. [74] study, ICM quality was not associated with live birth in multivariate analysis. These studies established the importance of TE grade on clinical outcome following fresh autologous transfer at the blastocyst stage. Likewise, in an analysis of more than 1000 vitrified/warmed cycles, TE grade was significantly associated with ongoing pregnancy, while ICM was not [75]. The relative importance of ICM and TE grades has not been evaluated specifically in the RIF population.

Laboratory Interventions to Improve Implantation Potential at the Blastocyst Stage

Freeze-All Strategy

With improved cryosurvival following vitrification, pregnancy rates following frozen embryo transfer have approached, if not surpassed, fresh transfers. Accordingly, the segmentation of IVF cycles into two phases (such that controlled ovarian stimulation, oocyte retrieval, and freeze all are performed during one menstrual cycle, followed by a so-called "deferred" frozen transfer in a subsequent menstrual cycle) has become increasingly popular ([76]; reviewed by Kaser and Racowsky [77]). There have been four RCTs that allocated patients to elective cryopreservation of all embryos or fresh transfer [78–81]. All of these studies demonstrated an improvement in pregnancy rates with the freeze-all strategy, although, of note, one study has since been withdrawn [78]. Two of the remaining three studies [79, 81] reported statistically significant results. The stage of embryo development (pronucleate vs. blastocyst) at the time of freeze all does not seem to affect the rates of implantation, clinical pregnancy, or cumulative pregnancy [82].

Whether or not these data are applicable to the RIF population remains to be seen. There is only one retrospective cohort study that evaluates the role of freeze-all cycles in RIF patients [83]. Patients who had failed at least one prior blastocyst transfer were given the choice of another fresh blastocyst transfer (n = 163) or freeze all at the pronucleate stage with subsequent warming, extended culture, and blastocyst transfer (n = 106). In multivariate analyses, elective cryopreservation was associated with a higher LBR after the first transfer (OR 3.8; 95% CI 2.1–7.2; $P < 0.0001$); notably, cumulative pregnancy rates were also higher (OR 1.9; 95% CI 1.1–3.3; $P = 0.03$). Taken together, these findings suggest that cycle segmentation may be beneficial for RIF patients. There are no prospective studies evaluating the role of fresh vs. freeze-all cycles in this patient population.

Vitrification of Blastocysts Undergoing Delayed Expansion

Embryos that ultimately blastulate typically vary in both morphological quality and the timing for compaction, blastulation, and expansion (Fig. 4.3). As discussed above, embryos that blastulate on day 6 have lower IR than those that blastulate on day 5 when transferred in a fresh cycle. While such embryos were initially considered to be of lesser intrinsic quality, it is now apparent that the observed lower rates of implantation likely result from a shift in synchrony between the embryo and the endometrium, as frozen transfer of delayed embryos results in pregnancy rates

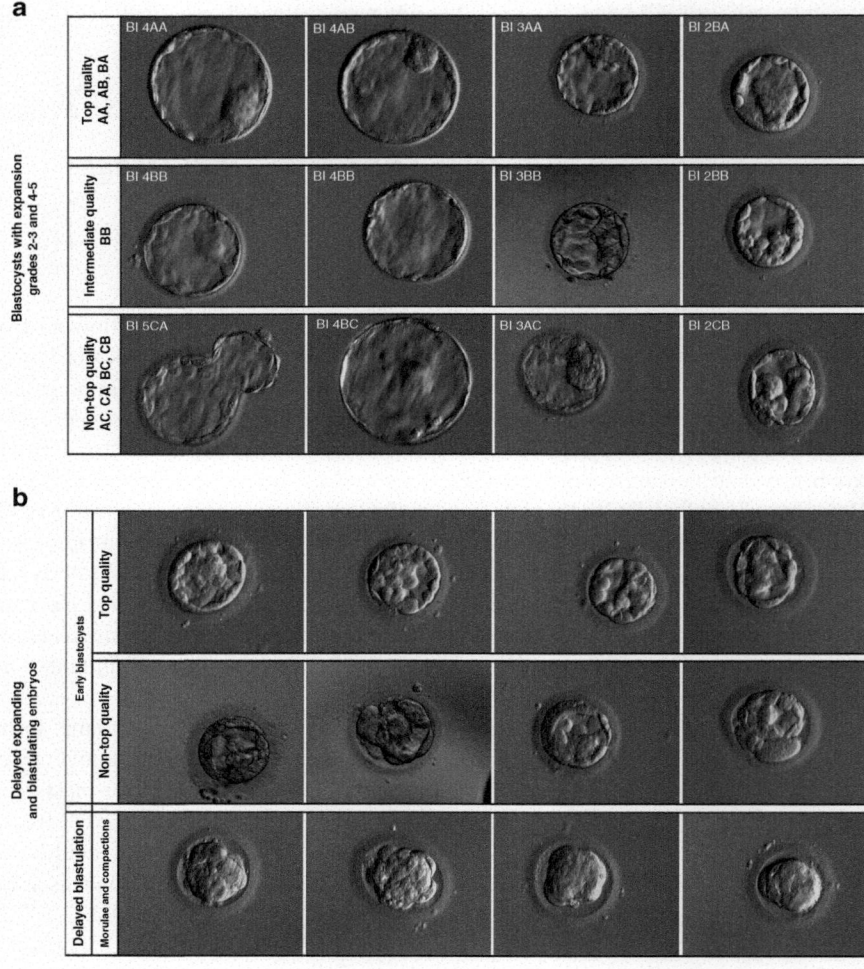

Fig. 4.3 Bright-field images of embryos on day 5 with varying degrees of cavitation and expansion. (**a**) Blastocysts with expansion grades 2–3 and 4–5. (**b**) Delayed expanding and blastulating embryos. Reprinted with permission from Wirleitner et al. Hum Reprod 2016;31:1685–95

equivalent to fresh transfer of embryos with timely blastulation (see Chap. 2 for complete discussion).

Accordingly, one laboratory intervention that may prove beneficial is to defer fresh transfer of embryos with delayed blastulation and/or expansion and transfer them in a subsequent warmed cycle. Wirleitner et al. [84] offered evidence in support of this practice in a large retrospective cohort study of autologous patients, in which IR following fresh (n = 1010) vs. vitrified/warmed blastocyst transfer (n = 1270) were compared according to their developmental stage in the same cohort of patients. Two important points were evident from this study: (1) while embryos with Gardner expansion grades of 4 or 5 had similar IR in fresh and frozen transfers (29.8% vs. 27.4%, $P > 0.05$), those earlier in development with expansion grades of 2 or 3 had significantly higher IR if transferred in a warmed cycle (45.0% vs. 24.8%; $P < 0.001$); and (2) early blastocysts, morulae, and compacting cleavage stage embryos had a very low likelihood of implanting in a fresh transfer (3.1–8.0%), but if cultured longer and vitrified on day 6, IR were significantly higher (21.9–24.7%; $P < 0.001$). Thus, the authors concluded that prolonged culture and vitrification of non-top-quality blastocysts, and also those with delayed cavitation or blastulation, may improve IR, at least in fresh autologous IVF cycles in which the endometrium may be advanced relative to embryonic development. This strategy has, indeed, been shown to be beneficial in patients with at least one prior failed blastocyst transfer, highlighting the special importance of embryo-endometrial synchrony for patients with a history of implantation failure [83].

Other Emerging Treatment Options

There are several other laboratory interventions available that may have applications to improve outcomes in RIF patients, including the following:

(a) Preimplantation genetic testing for aneuploidy

Preimplantation genetic testing for aneuploidy (PGT-A) allows the deselection of embryos with an abnormal chromosomal complement. While class 1 data support the utility of this technology in improving sustained implantation and live birth rates in the general infertility population [85], data are lacking for RIF patients specifically. There have been several important limitations to the few studies of PGT-A in RIF patients: all have been retrospective and have lacked appropriate non-PGT control groups; all have involved biopsy at the cleavage stage which is known to be detrimental to implantation potential [86]; and all have used outdated technologies such as fluorescence in situ hybridization (FISH) [87, 88]. There are no prospective studies of PGT-A in patients with a history of RIF.

As the paradigm for embryo biopsy continues to evolve (from day 3 biopsy with fresh blastocyst transfer to day 5 or day 6 biopsy with cryopreservation and deferred transfer), along with the platforms for genetic analysis (from FISH to array comparative genomic hybridization, quantitative PCR, and now next-generation sequencing, NGS), it will be important to assess the role of PGT-A in specific populations, such as those with RIF. Indeed, NGS may yield insight into why certain embryos fail to implant, as the technology is capable of detecting not only whole chromosomal aneuploidies but also segmental aneuploidies and mosaicism (see Chap. 5 for complete discussion). The clinical relevance of such microduplications and deletions has recently been described in a non-selection study of targeted NGS in which embryos were biopsied and transferred without knowledge of the assay results: interestingly, embryos containing segmental aneuploidies were nearly half as likely to result in live birth (13/39, 33.3% vs. 141/229, 61.6%; $P = 0.001$) [89]. The incidence of these types of mitotic errors in the RIF population as compared to the general infertility population has not been defined.

(b) Metabolic screening of culture media and peripheral blood
Metabolic assays of both spent culture media and also peripheral blood of patients with RIF also have been undertaken to determine if there are signatures associated with implantation. In an analysis of spent media from post-compaction embryos, Gardner et al. [90] noted that glucose consumption was significantly higher in those that implanted, consistent with a preferential shift toward glycolysis at the blastocyst stage. Alterations in certain metabolites involved in lipid and arginine metabolism (e.g., adipic acid and urea) have been shown to be upregulated in peripheral blood samples of patients with RIF, compared to other infertile controls matched on age and BMI [91].

(c) Mitochondrial DNA copy number measurements
Another indirect measure of metabolic activity is mitochondrial DNA copy number, which has been studied retrospectively in 280 patients undergoing euploid embryo transfer with known implantation status [92]. When normalized to nuclear DNA content, the amount of mitochondrial DNA is inversely proportional to the implantation potential of an embryo; that is, euploid embryos with less mitochondrial DNA had higher rates of implantation. A prospective validation of this assay is currently ongoing.

Whether these techniques will ultimately prove useful in the RIF population remains to be seen.

Conclusions

RIF is a challenging clinical situation, the underlying causes of which often involve abnormal embryonic factors. While there are strategies in the ART laboratory that target these abnormalities, with the exception of assisted hatching and blastocyst transfer, only low- to moderate-quality evidence is available to support most of these strategies in this specific patient population. Laboratory interventions that may overcome currently identified embryonic factors involved in RIF include:

– Assisted hatching
– Time-lapse imaging to deselect embryos with abnormal cleavage kinetics and phenotypes (abnormal and reverse cleavage, abnormal syngamy and first cytokinesis, and multinucleation)

- Extended culture with day 5 transfer of expanded blastocysts and vitrification of those undergoing delayed expansion
- IVF cycle segmentation with freeze-all and deferred cryopreserved embryo transfer
- Preimplantation genetic testing for detection of whole chromosomal and segmental aneuploidies and mosaicism
- Metabolic assessment through analysis of spent culture media, peripheral blood and/or measurement of mitochondrial DNA copy number in embryos

References

1. Edwards RG, Purdy JM, Steptoe PC, Walters DE. The growth of human preimplantation of embryos. Am J Obstet Gynecol. 1981;141:408–16.
2. Racowsky C, Vernon M, Mayer J, Ball GD, Behr B, Pomeroy KO, et al. Standardization of grading embryo morphology. Fertil Steril. 2010;94:1152–3.
3. Alpha Scientists in Reproductive Medicine and ESHRE Special Interest Group of Embryology. The Istanbul consensus workshop on embryo assessment: proceedings of an expert meeting. Hum Reprod. 2011;22:632–46.
4. Sakkas D, Shoukir Y, Chardonnens D, Bianchi PG, Campana A. Early cleavage of human embryos to the two-cell stage after intracytoplasmic sperm injection as an indicator of embryo viability. Hum Reprod. 1998;13:182–7.
5. Racowsky C, Combelles CMH, Nureddin A, Pan Y, Finna A, Miles L, et al. Day 3 and day 5 morphological predictors of embryo viability. Reprod Biomed Online. 2003;6:76–84.
6. Sakkas D, Percival G, D'Arcy Y, Sharif K, Afnan M. Assessment of early cleaving in vitro fertilized human embyos at the 2-cell stage before transfer improves embryo selection. Fertil Steril. 2001;76:1150–6.
7. Lundin K, Bergh C, Hardarson T. Early embryo cleavage is a strong indicator of embryo quality in human IVF. Hum Reprod. 2001;16:2652–7.
8. Giorgetti C, Hans E, Terriou P, Salzmann J, Barry B, Chabert-Orsini V, et al. Early cleavage: an additional predictor of high implantation rate following elective single embryo transfer. Reprod Biomed Online. 2007;14:85–91.
9. Puissant F, Van Rysselberge M, Barlow P, Deweze J, Leroy F. Embryo scoring as a prognostic tool in IVF treatment. Hum Reprod. 1987;2:705–8.
10. Steer C, Mills C, Tan S, Campbell S, Edwards RG. The cumulative embryo score: a predictive embryo scoring technique to select the optimal number of embryos to transfer in an in-vitro fertilization and embryo transfer program. Hum Reprod. 1992;7:117–9.
11. Carrillo AJ, Lane B, Pridman DD, Risch PP, Pool TB, Silverman IH, et al. Improved clinical outcomes for in vitro fertilization with delay of embryo transfer from 48 to 72 h after oocyte retrieval: use of glucose- and phosphate-free media. Fertil Steril. 1998;69:329–34.
12. Kaser DJ, Racowsky C. Clinical outcomes following selection of human preimplantation embryos with time-lapse monitoring: a systematic review. Hum Reprod Update. 2014;20:617–31.
13. Meseguer M, Herrero J, Tejera A, Hilligsoe KM, Ramsing NB, Remohi J. The use of morphokinetics as a predictor of embryo implantation. Hum Reprod. 2011;26:2658–71.
14. Rubio I, Kuhlmann R, Agerholm I, Kirk J, Herrero J, Escriba MJ, et al. Limited implantation success of direct-cleaved human zygotes: a time-lapse study. Fertil Steril. 2012;98:1458–63.
15. Kirkegaard K, Kesmodel US, Hindkjaer JJ, Ingerslev HJ. Time-lapse parameters as predictors of blastocyst development and pregnancy outcome in embryos from good prognosis patients: a prospective cohort study. Hum Reprod. 2013;28:2643–51.

16. Chen AA, Tan L, Suraj V, Reijo Pera R, Shen S. Biomarkers identified with time-lapse imaging: discovery, validation, and practical application. Fertil Steril. 2013;99:1035–43.
17. Meseguer M, Rubio I, Cruz M, Basile N, Marcos J, Requena A. Embryo incubation and selection in a time-lapse monitoring system improves pregnancy outcome compared with a standard incubator: a retrospective cohort study. Fertil Steril. 2012;98:1481–9.
18. Kahraman S, Cetinkaya M, Pirkevi C, Yelke H, Kumtepe Y. Comparison of blastocyst development and cycle outcome in patients with eSET using either conventional or time lapse incubators. A prospective study of good prognosis patients. J Reprod Stem Cell Biotechnol. 2013;3:55–61.
19. Goodman LR, Goldberg J, Falcone T, Austin C, Desai N. Does the addition of time-lapse morphokinetics in the selection of embryos for transfer improve pregnancy rates? A randomized controlled trial. Fertil Steril. 2016;105:275–85.
20. Kaser DJ, Bormann CL, Missmer SA, Farland LV, Ginsburg ES, Racowsky C. Eeva™ pregnancy pilot study: a randomized controlled trial of single embryo transfer on day 3 or day 5 with or without time-lapse imaging selection. Fertil Steril. 2016;106:e312.
21. Rubio I, Galan A, Larreategui Z, Ayerdi F, Bellver J, Herrero J, et al. Clinical validation of embryo culture and selection by morphokinetic analysis: a randomized, controlled trial of the EmbryoScope. Fertil Steril. 2014;102:1287–94.
22. Racowsky C, Kovacs P, Martins WP. A critical appraisal of time-lapse imaging for embryo selection: where are we and where do we need to go? J Assist Reprod Genet. 2015;32:1025–30.
23. Ziebe S, Petersen K, Lindenberg S, Andersen AG, Gabrielsen A, Andersen AN. Embryo morphology or cleavage stage: how to select the best embryos for transfer after in-vitro fertilization. Hum Reprod. 1997;12:1545–9.
24. Alikani M, Calderon G, Tomkin G, Garrisi J, Kokot M, Cohen J. Cleavage anomalies in early human embryos and survival after prolonged culture in-vitro. Hum Reprod. 2000;15:2634–43.
25. Hardarson T, Hanson C, Sjogren A, Lundin K. Human embryos with unevenly sized blastomeres have lower pregnancy and implantation rates: indications for aneuploidy and multinucleation. Hum Reprod. 2001;16:313–8.
26. Kligman I, Benadiva C, Alikani M, Munne S. The presence of multinucleated blastomeres in human embryos is correlated with chromosomal abnormalities. Hum Reprod. 1996;11:1492–8.
27. Jackson K, Ginsburg E, Hornstein M, Rein MS, Clarke RN. Multinucleation in normally fertilized embryos is associated with an accelerated ovulation induction response and lower implantation and pregnancy rates in in vitro fertilization-transfer cycles. Fertil Steril. 1998;70:60–6.
28. Saldeen P, Sundstrom P. Nuclear status of four-cell preembryos predicts implantation potential in in vitro fertilization treatment cycles. Fertil Steril. 2005;84:584–9.
29. Tao J, Tamis R, Fink K, Williams B, Nelson-White T, Craig R. The neglected morula/compact stage embryo transfer. Hum Reprod. 2002;17:1513–8.
30. Skiadas C, Jackson K, Racowsky C. Early compaction on day 3 may be associated with increased implantation potential. Fertil Steril. 2006;86:1386–91.
31. Schiewe MC, Araujo E Jr, Asch RH, Balmaceda JP. Enzymatic characterization of zona pellucida hardening in human eggs and embryos. J Assist Reprod Genet. 1995;12:2–7.
32. Palmstierna M, Murkes D, Csemiczky G, Andersson O, Wramsby H. Zona pellucida thickness variation and occurrence of visible mononucleated blastomeres in pre-embryos are associated with a high pregnancy rate in IVF treatment. J Assist Reprod Genet. 1998;15:70–5.
33. Gabrielsen A, Bhatnager PR, Petersen K, Lindenberg S. Influence of zona thickness of human embryos on clinical pregnancy outcome following in vitro fertilization treatment. J Assist Reprod Genet. 2000;17:323–8.
34. Skiadas CC, Racowsky C. Developmental rate, cumulative scoring, and embryo viability. In: Elder K, Cohen J, editors. Human preimplantation embryo selection. London: Informa Healthcare; 2007. p. 101–21.
35. Athayde Wirka K, Chen AA, Conaghan J, Ivani K, Gvakharia M, Behr B, et al. Atypical embryo phenotypes identified by time-lapse microscopy: high prevalence and association with embryo development. Fertil Steril. 2014;101:1637–48.

36. Liu Y, Chapple V, Roberts P, Matson P. Prevalence, consequence, and significance of reverse cleavage by human embryos viewed with the use of the Embryoscope time-lapse video system. Fertil Steril. 2014;102:1295–300.
37. Gordon JW, Dapunt U. Restoration of normal implantation rates in mouse embryos with a hatching impairment by use of a new method of assisted hatching. Fertil Steril. 1993;59:1302–7.
38. Cohen J, Wiemer KE, Wright G. Prognostic value of morphologic characteristics of cryopreserved embryos: a study using videocinematography. Fertil Steril. 1988;49:827–34.
39. Malter HE, Cohen J. Partial zona dissection of the human oocyte: a nontraumatic method using micromanipulation to assist zona pellucida penetration. Fertil Steril. 1989;51:139–48.
40. Obruca A, Strohmer H, Sakkas D, Menezo Y, Kogosowski A, Barak Y, et al. Use of lasers in assisted fertilization and hatching. Hum Reprod. 1994;9:1723–6.
41. Nakayama T, Fujiwara H, Tastumi K, Fujita K, Higuchi T, Mori T. A new assisted hatching technique using a piezo-micromanipulator. Fertil Steril. 1998;69:784–8.
42. Carney SK, Das S, Blake D, Farquhar C, Seif MM, Nelson L. Assisted hatching on assisted conception in vitro fertilisation (IVF) and intracytoplasmic sperm injection (ICSI). Cochrane Database Syst Rev. 2012;12:CD001894.
43. Cohen J, Alikani M, Trowbridge J, Rosenwaks Z. Implantation enhancement by selective assisted hatching using zona drilling of human embryos with poor prognosis. Hum Reprod. 1992;7:685–91.
44. Nagy ZP, Rienzi L, Iacobelli M, Morgia F, Ubaldi F, Schimberni M, et al. Laser-assisted hatching and removal of degenerated blastomere(s) of frozen-thawed embryo improves pregnancy rate. Fertil Steril. 1999;72:S4.
45. Balaban B, Urman B, Yakin K, Isiklar A. Laser assisted hatching increases pregnancy and implantation rates in cryopreserved embryos that were allowed to cleave in-vitro after thawing: a prospective randomised study. Hum Reprod. 2006;21:2136–40.
46. Carter J, Graham J, Han T, Davis A, Richter K, Widra E. Preliminary results of a prospective randomized study to assess the value of laser assisted hatching before cleavage stage embryo transfer among good-prognosis in vitro fertilization (IVF) patients. Fertil Steril. 2003;80:S94.
47. Sagoskin AW, Levy MJ, Tucker MJ, Richter KS, Widra EA. Laser assisted hatching in good prognosis patients undergoing in vitro fertilisation embryo transfer: a randomised control trial. Fertil Steril. 2007;87:283–7.
48. Primi M-P, Senn A, Montag M, Van der Ven H, Mandelbaum J, Veiga A, et al. A European multicentre prospective randomized study to assess the use of assisted hatching with a diode laser and the benefit of immunosuppressive/antibiotic treatment in different patient populations. Hum Reprod. 2004;19:2325–33.
49. Valojerdi MR, Eftekhari-Yazdi P, Karimian L, Hassani F, Movaghar B. Effect of laser zona thinning on vitrified-warmed embryo transfer at the cleavage stage: a prospective, randomized study. Reprod Biomed Online. 2010;20:234–42.
50. Valojerdi MR, Eftekhari-Yazdi P, Karimian L, Ashtiani SK. Effect of laser zona pellucida opening on clinical outcome of assisted reproduction technology in patients with advanced female age, recurrent implantation failure, or frozen-thawed embryos. Fertil Steril. 2008;90:84–91.
51. Stein A, Rufas O, Amit S, Avrech O, Pinkas H, Ovadia J, et al. Assisted hatching by partial zona dissection of human pre-embryos in patients with recurrent implantation failure after in vitro fertilization. Fertil Steril. 1995;63:838–41.
52. Simon A, Laufer N. Assessment and treatment of repeated implantation failure. J Assist Reprod Genet. 2012;29:1227–39.
53. Jelinkova L, Pavelkova J, Strehler E, Paulus W, Zivny J, Sterzik K. Improved implantation rate after chemical removal of the zona pellucida. Fertil Steril. 2003;79:1299–303.
54. Fang C, Li T, Miao BY, Zhuang GL, Zhou C. Mechanically expanding the zona pellucida of human frozen thawed embryos: a new method of assisted hatching. Fertil Steril. 2010;94:1302–7.
55. Ménézo YJR, Servy E, Veiga A, Hazout A, Elder A. Culture systems: embryo co-culture. In: Smith G, Swain JE, Pool TB, editors. Embryo culture: methods and protocols. New York: Springer; 2012. p. 231–42.

56. Kattal N, Cohen J, Barmat LI. Role of coculture in human in vitro fertilization: a meta-analysis. Fertil Steril. 2008;90:1069–76.
57. Spandorfer SD, Pascal P, Parks J, Clark R, Veeck L, Davis OK, et al. Autologous endometrial coculture in patients with IVF failure: outcome of the first 1,030 cases. J Reprod Med. 2004;49:463–7.
58. Eyheremendy V, Raffo FG, Papayannis M, Barnes J, Granados C, Blaquier J. Beneficial effect of autologous endometrial cell co-culture in patients with repeated implantation failure. Fertil Steril. 2010;93:769–73.
59. Benkhalifa M, Demirol A, Sari T, Balashova E, Tsouroupaki M, Giakoumakis Y, et al. Autologous embryo-cumulus cells co-culture and blastocyst transfer in repeated implantation failures: a collaborative prospective randomized study. Zygote. 2012;7:1–8.
60. Glujovsky D, Blake D, Farquhar C, Bardach A. Cleavage stage versus blastocyst stage embryo transfer in assisted reproductive technology. Cochrane Database Syst Rev. 2016;6:CD002118.
61. Guerif F, Bidault R, Gasnier O, Couet ML, Gervereau O, Lansac J, et al. Efficacy of blastocyst transfer after implantation failure. Reprod Biomed Online. 2004;9:630–6.
62. Levitas E, Lunenfeld E, Har-Vardi I, Albotiano S, Sonin Y, Hackmon-Ram R, et al. Blastocyst-stage embryo transfer in patients who failed to conceive in three or more day 2-3 embryo transfer cycles: a prospective, randomized study. Fertil Steril. 2004;81:567–71.
63. Gardner DK, Schoolcraft WB. In vitro culture of human blastocyst. In: Jansen R, Mortimer D, editors. Towards reproductive certainty: infertility and genetics beyond 1999. Carnforth: Parthenon; 1999. p. 378–88.
64. Gardner DK, Surrey E, Minjarez D, Leitz A, Stevens J, Schoolcraft WB. Single blastocyst transfer: a prospective randomized trial. Fertil Steril. 2004;8:551–5.
65. Guerif F, Le Gouge A, Giraudeau B, Poindrom J, Bidault R, Gasnier O, et al. Limited value of morphological assessment at days 1 and 2 to predict blastocyst development: a prospective study based on 4,042 embryos. Hum Reprod. 2007;22:1973–81.
66. Van den Abbeel E, Balaban B, Ziebe S, Lundin K, Cuesta MJ, Klein BM, et al. Association between blastocyst morphology and outcome of single-blastocyst transfer. Reprod Biomed Online. 2013;27:353–61.
67. Hill MJ, Richter KS, Heitmann RJ, Grahm JR, Tucker MJ, DeCherney AH, et al. Trophectoderm grade predicts outcomes of single-blastocyst transfers. Fertil Steril. 2013;99:1283–9.
68. Shapiro BS, Richter KS, Harris DC, Daneshmand ST. A comparison of day 5 and day 6 blastocyst transfers. Fertil Steril. 2001;75:1126–30.
69. Barrenetxea G, López de Larruzea A, Ganzabal T, Jiménez R, Carbonero K, Mandiola M. Blastocyst culture after repeated failure of cleavage-stage embryo transfers: a comparison of day 5 and day 6 transfers. Fertil Steril. 2005;83:49–53.
70. Campbell A, Fishel S, Bowman N, Duffy S, Sedler M, Thornton S. Retrospective analysis of outcomes after IVF using an aneuploidy risk model derived from time-lapse imaging without PGS. Reprod Biomed Online. 2013;27:140–6.
71. Shapiro BS, Daneshmand ST, Garner FC, Aguirre M, Ross R. Contrasting patterns in in vitro fertilization pregnancy rates among fresh autologous, fresh oocyte donor, and cryopreserved cycles with the use of day 5 or day 6 blastocysts may reflect differences in embryo-endometrium synchrony. Fertil Steril. 2008;89:20–6.
72. Richter KS, Shipley SK, McVearry I, Tucker MJ, Widra EA. Cryopreserved embryo transfers suggest that endometrial receptivity may contribute to reduced success rates of later developing embryos. Fertil Steril. 2006;86:862–6.
73. Shapiro BS, Daneshmand ST, Restrepo H, Garner FC, Aguirre M, Hudson C. Matched-cohort comparison of single-embryo transfers in fresh and frozen-thawed embryo transfer cycles. Fertil Steril. 2013;99:389–92.
74. Ahlstrom A, Westin C, Reismer E, Wikland M, Hardarson T. Trophectoderm morphology: an important parameter for predicting live birth after single blastocyst transfer. Hum Reprod. 2011;26:3289–96.
75. Honnma H, Baba T, Sasaki M, Hashiba Y, Ohno H, Fukunaga T, et al. Trophectoderm morphology significantly affects the rates of ongoing pregnancy and miscarriage in frozen-thawed single-blastocyst transfer cycle in vitro fertilization. Fertil Steril. 2012;98:361–7.

76. Devroey P, Polyzos NP, Blockeel C. An OHSS-free clinic by segmentation of IVF treatment. Hum Reprod. 2011;26:2593–7.
77. Kaser DJ, Racowsky C. Should we eliminate fresh embryo transfer from ART. In: Schlegel PN, et al., editors. Biennial review of infertility, vol. 3. New York: Springer; 2013. p. 203–14.
78. Aflatoonian A, Oskouian H, Ahmadi S, Oskouian L. Can fresh embryo transfers be replaced by cryopreserved-thawed embryo transfers in assisted reproductive cycles? A randomized controlled trial. J Assist Reprod Genet. 2010;27:357–63.
79. Shapiro BS, Daneshmand ST, Garner FC, et al. Evidence of impaired endometrial receptivity after ovarian stimulation for in vitro fertilization: a prospective randomized trial comparing fresh and frozen- thawed embryo transfer in normal responders. Fertil Steril. 2011a;96:344–8.
80. Shapiro BS, Daneshmand ST, Garner FC, Aguirre M, Hudson C, Thomas S. Evidence of impaired endometrial receptivity after ovarian stimulation for in vitro fertilization: a prospective randomized trial comparing fresh and frozen-thawed embryo transfers in high responders. Fertil Steril. 2011b;96:516–8.
81. Chen ZJ, Shi Y, Sun Y, Zhang B, Liang X, Cao Y, et al. Fresh versus frozen embryos for infertility in the polycystic ovary syndrome. N Engl J Med. 2016;375:523–33.
82. Shapiro BS, Daneshmand ST, Garner FC, Aguirre M, Hudson C. Freeze-all at the blastocyst or bipronuclear stage: a randomized controlled trial. Fertil Steril. 2015;104:1138–44.
83. Shapiro BS, Daneshmand ST, Garner FC, Aguirre M, Hudson C. Freeze-all can be a superior therapy to another fresh cycle in patients with prior fresh blastocyst implantation failure. Reprod Biomed Online. 2014;29:286–90.
84. Wirleitner B, Schuff M, Stecher A, Murtinger M, Vanderzwalmen P. Pregnancy and birth outcomes following fresh or vitrified embryo transfer according to blastocyst morphology and expansion stage, and culturing strategy for delayed development. Hum Reprod. 2016;31:1685–95.
85. Scott RT Jr, Uphapm KM, Forman EJ, Hong KH, Scott KL, Taylor D, et al. Blastocyst biopsy with comprehensive chromosomal screening and fresh embryo transfer significantly increases in vitro fertilization implantation and delivery rates: a randomized controlled trial. Fertil Steril. 2013a;100:697–703.
86. Scott RT Jr, Upham KM, Forman EJ, Zhao T, Treff NR. Cleavage-stage biopsy significantly impairs human embryonic implantation potential while blastocyst biopsy does not: a randomized and paired clinical trial. Fertil Steril. 2013b;100:624–30.
87. Platteau P, Staessen C, Michiels A, Van Steirteghem A, Liebaers I, Devroey P. Which patients with recurrent implantation failure after IVF benefit from PGD for aneuploidy screening? Reprod Biomed Online. 2006;12:334–9.
88. Pagidas K, Ying Y, Keefe D. Predictive value of preimplantation genetic diagnosis for aneuploidy screening in repeated IVF-ET cycles among women with recurrent implantation failure. J Assist Reprod Genet. 2008;25:103–6.
89. Werner MD, Goodrich D, Tao X, Zhan Y, Franasiak JM, Juneau CR, et al. NGS provides accurate predictions of segmental aneuploidy and prognosticates reduced reproductive potential of the human blastocyst. Fertil Steril. 2016;106:e68.
90. Gardner DK, Wale PL, Collins R, Lane M. Glucose consumption of single post-compaction human embryos is predictive of embryo sex and live birth outcome. Hum Reprod. 2011;26:1981–6.
91. RoyChoudhury S, Singh A, Gupta NJ, Srivastava S, Joshi MV, Chakravarty B, et al. Repeated implantation failure versus repeated implantation success: discrimination at a metabolomic level. Hum Reprod. 2016;31:1265–74.
92. Diez-Juan A, Rubio C, Marin C, Martinez S, Al-Asmar N, Riboldi M, et al. Mitochondrial DNA content as a viability score in human euploid embryos: less is better. Fertil Steril. 2015;104:534–41.

Chapter 5
The Genetics of Pregnancy Failure

Eric J. Forman, Nathan Treff, and Rebekah S. Zimmerman

Having a normal genetic composition is a necessary, but not sufficient, requirement for an embryo to implant and progress to a healthy delivery. By testing products of conception, it has been known for decades that whole chromosome aneuploidy, primarily trisomy, is the leading cause of failure of clinically recognized pregnancies. Clarifying the role of aneuploidy and other genetic abnormalities in the failure of embryos to implant has been more elusive but was assumed to be an important factor based on the strong association of advancing reproductive age and infertility. The development and rapid utilization of assisted reproductive technologies (ART) have provided invaluable insight into the genetic causes of failed embryonic implantation. The application of robust genetic testing platforms—from microarrays to real-time polymerase chain reaction (PCR) to next-generation sequencing (NGS)—to test the genetic status of gametes and preimplantation embryos has improved our understanding of the genetic contribution to an ongoing conceptus. Recent advances have focused on the impact of segmental imbalances and mosaicism on implantation and progression to normal deliveries. Future ART research will focus on other genetic causes that influence the ability of a euploid embryo to implant.

E.J. Forman, MD, HCLD (✉)
Reproductive Endocrinology and Infertility, Columbia University, New York, NY, USA
e-mail: eforman@rmanj.com

N. Treff, PhD
Rutgers University School of Medicine, Newark, NJ, USA

Genomic Prediction, Newark, NJ, USA

R.S. Zimmerman, PhD, FACMG
Icahn School of Medicine at Mount Sinai, New York, NY, USA
e-mail: rzimmerman@feclabs.org

© Springer International Publishing AG 2018   77
J.M. Franasiak, R.T. Scott Jr. (eds.), *Recurrent Implantation Failure*,
https://doi.org/10.1007/978-3-319-71967-2_5

The Role of Genetics in Early Pregnancy Failure

Cytogenetic Findings in POCs

Approximately 20% of clinically detected pregnancies result in a loss, with over 50% of losses being attributed to a whole chromosome abnormality. An early study reported in 1975 used Giemsa staining (G-banding) to analyze the karyotypes of nearly 1500 miscarriage specimens and found that over 61% of samples had an abnormal karyotype, which included monosomies, trisomies, double trisomies, triploidy, and tetraploidy [1]. As this study and many subsequent studies showed, trisomies are overwhelmingly responsible for first trimester pregnancy loss, most commonly trisomy 16 and trisomy 22. Monosomies and polyploidy account for the majority of the remaining abnormalities. Turner syndrome (45,X) is the most common monosomy finding in first trimester miscarriages. Although Turner syndrome is a viable aneuploidy, nearly 99% of 45,X fetuses spontaneously abort [2].

While G-banding is able to identify the majority of abnormalities, the method is not able to detect maternal cell contamination (MCC), which could cause a false-negative result in the case of an apparently normal female (46,XX) miscarriage. More recently, several studies have been published examining the utilization of newer molecular technologies to diagnose products of conception [3–6]. Microarrays using comparative genomic hybridization (CGH) and single nucleotide polymorphisms (SNPs) and NGS generate higher-resolution data, allowing for increases in reportable results and diagnostic yield. Similar to earlier findings, across all four studies (Table 5.1), approximately 50% of products of conception had at least one whole chromosome abnormality detected. Of the remaining samples, 40–48.4% were left with a normal diagnosis, 2.3–7.5% were triploid, and <0.5% were tetraploid. Now with the ability to detect partial chromosomal abnormalities, the studies reported that 1.3–5.3% had at least one segmental aneuploidy detected (in the absence of a translocation history in a parent). Mosaicism was reported at a very low frequency (0.67%) in the 1975 study, but not in the noted molecular studies.

Chromosome Rearrangement History

Chromosome rearrangements, including balanced translocations, inversions, and Robertsonian translocations, are often implicated in the etiology of recurrent pregnancy loss [7–9]. In the general population, approximately 1 in 500 individuals is likely to carry an apparently balanced chromosome rearrangement [10, 11]. Carriers of a balanced rearrangement typically are asymptomatic but present with fertility issues generally in the form of recurrent pregnancy loss due to the risk of a fetus inheriting an unbalanced derivative of the rearrangement. Thus, the recurrent

Table 5.1 Genetic characterization of products of conception

	Boue (1975)	Levy (2014)	Maslow (2015)	Shen (2016)	Sahoo (2016)
No. of samples	1498	2392	62	436	8118[a]
Platform	G-banding	SNP microarray (ILMN)	SNP microarray	aCGH (ILMN) and NGS (WGS on PGM)	SNP microarray (81.6%), array CGH (BAC and oligo) (18.4%)
Fresh or paraffin POC?	Fresh	Fresh	Paraffin	Fresh	Fresh and FFPE
Result rate	NR	99.9% (2389/2392)	71% (44/62)	100%	91.1% (7396/8118)
Resolution of segmental aneuploidy		>10 Mb	5 Mb (1–5 Mb clinically relevant)	~4 Mb to 111 Mb	>2.4 Mb (BAC aCGH), 112 kb (oligo aCGH), 20 kb (SNP array)
Genetics					
Maternal cell contamination	NR	22% (528/2392)	24% (15/62)	NR	NR
Normal	38.5% (577/1498)	40.6% (755/1861)	43% (19/44)	48.4% (211/436)	44.3% (3272/7396)
Aneuploid	42.5% (636/1498)	50.8% (945/1861)	54.5% (24/44)	43.1% (188/436)	42.9% (3176/7396)
Partial aneuploidy (no hx of translocation)	NR	1.3% (24/1861)[b]	NR	5.3% (23/436)	1.7% (127/7396)
Triploid	12.2% (183/1498)	6.1% (114/1861)	2.3% (1/44)	3.2% (14/436)	7.5% (554/7396)[c]
Tetraploidy	3.8% (57/1498)	0.2% (4/1861)	NR	NR	0.03% (2/7396)
Uniparental disomy (UPD)	NR	0.16% (3/1861)	NR	NR	0.5% (37/7396)
Mosaicism	0.67% (10/1498)	NR	NR	NR	NR

NR not reported, *ILMN* illumina
[a]Includes 99 non-POC samples
[b]Includes marker and isodicentric chromosomes
[c]FISH used on fresh, non-SNP array cases

pregnancy loss population likely has a higher incidence of chromosome rearrangements, and a recurrent pregnancy loss work-up usually includes obtaining a karyotype on the patient and partner, and if a rearrangement is found, miscarriage can be avoided by using preimplantation genetic diagnosis to select for balanced or normal embryos [12]. Robertsonian translocations are the products of the fusion of two acrocentric chromosomes (13, 14, 15, 21, and 22) and are found at an increased frequency in patients with recurrent pregnancy loss [13, 14].

Single Gene Disorders and Recurrent Pregnancy Loss

While relatively rare in comparison to aneuploidy in pregnancy, there are several single gene disorders (SGD) that are associated with recurrent pregnancy loss or fetal demise.

Some autosomal recessive disorders that present with multiple congenital anomalies can have lethal presentations in utero. Smith-Lemli-Opitz (SLO) is caused by deficiency in an important component of cholesterol metabolism, 7-dehydrocholesterol (7-DHC). Mutations in the *DHCR7* gene, which encodes 7-DHC, cause SLO, and approximately 1 in 30 to 1 in 70 individuals in the general population are thought to be carriers of a single mutation in *DHCR7*. Congenital disorder of glycosylation type Ia (CDG-Ia) is caused by mutations in the *PMM2* gene and has a carrier frequency of approximately 1 in 70 European Caucasians.

Interestingly, the reported carrier frequencies of these disorders are much higher than expected if calculated using the disease incidence. For example, SLO incidence in Canadian and European populations ranges from 1/60,000 to 1/20,000, which would suggest that the carrier frequency in these populations is approximately 1/120 to 1/70, respectively. However, laboratories performing carrier screening for SLO are finding the carrier frequency closer to 1/40 to 1/50 [15]. Keeping in mind that most labs screen for only common mutations, this suggests that the carrier frequency could be even higher and that either the disease is significantly variable and underreported or there is a significant amount of fetal demise associated with the disorder. The W151X mutation in *DHCR7*, when homozygous, has been reported in first trimester miscarriages [16]. The same can apply to CDG—the R141H mutation in *PMM2* is also thought to be lethal when homozygous [17], and to date, no homozygotes have been reported [18]. Both of these mutations can be screened for on most expanded carrier screening panels, and this testing could be considered during a recurrent pregnancy loss work-up.

There are also genes involved in chromosome segregation that, when mutated, can be implicated in pregnancy loss. *SYCP3* is a gene primarily involved in homologous chromosome pairing and recombination. Loss of SYCP3 in mice is associated with male infertility and decreased fertility in females. In humans, the T657C variant in SYCP3 has been very strongly associated with recurrent pregnancy loss [19].

Complete (CM) and partial (PM) hydatidiform molar pregnancies are typically isolated events for a patient; however, some patients have been found to have recurrent molar pregnancies. CM most often arise from the inheritance of all 46 paternal chromosomes and no maternal chromosomes. PM have a different pathology and are typically due to triploidy (69,XXX or 69,XXY). Mutations in either NLRP7 or KHDC3L are associated with recessive inheritance of recurrent molar pregnancies [20].

It is well known that some losses can be attributed to mutations or polymorphisms in coagulation pathway genes, such as Factor V, prothrombin, and Factor II. A recent meta-analysis was performed and found 37 genes that have strong associations with pregnancy loss due to hyperactive immune response, thrombophilia, abnormal placental function, and disruption in the regulation of metabolism [21].

The Role of Genetics in Implantation

Whereas the genetic contribution to pregnancy failure has been well established by studying miscarriage specimens, understanding the role of the genetics in the pre-implantation embryo's ability to successfully implant has been more elusive. Though challenged in recent years by animal and preliminary human studies proposing the presence of oogonial stem cells [22], the established dogma of human oocyte physiology remains that women are born with their lifetime endowment of approximately 1–2 million follicles and oocytes. While the menopause and the complete exhaustion of the follicle pool herald an absolute barrier to successful pregnancy, there is a well-established age-related decline in fertility, likely related to the decline in oocyte quantity and quality. The gradual decline in oocyte quantity, which accelerates after age 37, has been documented by studying tissue specimens at the time of oophorectomy [23].

Although some markers, such as an elevated serum follicle-stimulating hormone (FSH) levels on day 3 of the menstrual cycle, have been correlated with a reduced chance for a viable pregnancy, there is no definitive assay for oocyte quality. A good-quality oocyte can be considered one of the sufficient qualities to complete meiosis, achieve cytoplasmic and nuclear maturity to allow for normal fertilization after activation by viable spermatozoa, and then develop into an embryo capable of implantation and progression to a normal viable neonate. Several lines of evidence support the proposition that oocyte quality declines with increasing age and that this decline accelerates in the late 30s and even more rapidly in the early 40s. In historical populations that predated contraception and family planning, there was a clear decline in fertility rate with increasing maternal age [24]. While compelling, this association does not prove that the aging oocyte, and likely chromosomal aneuploidy, fully explains this decline in fecundity. Several other possible explanations exist, including a decline in sperm quality and function, decreased coital activity, increased risk of uterine abnormalities such as leiomyomas and synechiae, and increased risk of other medical comorbidities.

One model that could correct for several of these variables is women seeking to conceive with timed intrauterine insemination using thawed sperm from fertile donors. This population includes presumably fertile women requiring the use of donor sperm because they are single, are lesbian, or have a partner with azoospermia. The CECOS study evaluated 2193 married French women who underwent donor sperm and timed insemination because their husbands were azoospermic [25]. This study found a significant decline in the chance for pregnancy, with 73% of women under age 31 conceiving within 12 cycles, compared with 54% over age 35 ($P < 0.001$). The decline would likely be even sharper if women over age 40 were analyzed separately. This diminution in live birth rate most likely reflects an increase in the chance of mature oocytes being released that are not of sufficient quality to implant and progress to delivery. Other studies suggest that the decline in fecundity is primarily related to an age-related decline in oocyte quality, independent of quantity. One study from Ottawa found that women using timed donor insemination had a similar chance of conceiving whether they had low or high antral follicle counts, a marker of ovarian reserve [26]. In women attempting to conceive, a low AMH level—another reliable marker of ovarian reserve—does not appear to be predictive of natural fertility [27], indicating that the decline in oocyte quality is mostly related to advanced reproductive age rather than simply depletion of the follicular pool.

While the aging oocyte is less likely to result in a viable offspring, there are several potential causes for this including genetic (increased risk of aneuploidy, mosaicism, de novo segmental imbalances or mutations, epigenetic changes), cytoplasmic (increase in mitochondrial dysfunction, perhaps due to accumulation of reactive oxygen species from dysfunctional recycling of organelles/autophagy), or reduced ability of the uterus to facilitate implantation of a viable embryo. The advent of ART and its clinical application has shed light on these factors, confirming the pivotal role of genetics in embryonic competence.

Even before there was the ability to reliably assess the chromosomal status of preimplantation embryos, the relationship between increased maternal age and decreased rates of successful implantation became apparent. The first successful application of in vitro fertilization performed by the late Sir Robert Edwards (Nobel Laureate 2010) and Patrick Steptoe was in a 29-year-old woman, at the peak of her fertility, who had tubal factor infertility. The early practitioners of IVF attempted to compensate for diminished oocyte and embryo quality by stimulating multiple follicles to mature with the use of exogenous gonadotropins extracted from human menopausal urine. Since the average embryo was not capable of progressing to delivery, multiple embryos would routinely be transferred to the uterus. Even still, pregnancy rates in women of advanced reproductive age remained dismal, and miscarriage rates increased with increasing age. Schieve et al. found that miscarriage rates after IVF increased from 10.1% among women in their 20s to 39.3% for women older than 43 [28]. Similar to the prior spontaneous abortion literature, the most common cause of clinical miscarriage after ART appears to be aneuploidy, accounting for more than half of the losses in most reviews of products of conception after ART [33, 29–33]. The rate of aneuploid losses after ART does not appear to differ from natural conceptions, though one review reported a higher risk from intracytoplasmic sperm injection (ICSI) as compared to conventional insemination to achieve assisted fertilization [34]. Similar to natural conceptions, autosomal trisomy accounts for most of the aneuploid miscarriages after ART [35].

The introduction of donor oocyte programs further proved the primary role of the aging oocyte's contribution to the age-related decline in fertility. When transferred to the uterus of women of advanced reproductive age, even into the late 40s, embryos created from oocytes donated by women typically in their 20s resulted in successful implantations at rates commensurate with the oocyte donor rather than the recipient age [36]. Thus, it appears unlikely that there is an intrinsic decline in uterine receptivity with increasing maternal age, at least through the mid-40s. Unlike the well-established increase in miscarriage risk with increasing age, pregnancies conceived after oocyte donation had a 13.1% miscarriage risk that did not significantly vary with the age of the recipient. Similarly, delivery rates from egg donation remained high independent of paternal age, mitigating the causative role of sperm in the age-related decline in fertility [37]. The risk of de novo autosomal dominant mutations, however, appears to increase with increasing paternal age [38], a finding thought to relate to exposure of the paternal genome to reactive oxygen species over time.

Still, while the decline in oocyte quality with age is now well established, the ability to reliably test the genetics of preimplantation embryos was required to determine the relative contribution of genetics to implantation failure.

Preimplantation Genetic Screening (PGS): First Generation, Limited by Suboptimal Biopsy and Testing Methodology

Given the decreased implantation rates from transferred embryos in older women and the higher risk of aneuploid miscarriages, it seemed reasonable that testing embryos and selecting against aneuploid embryos would enhance IVF success rates. The first attempt at this strategy, given the technology available at the time, relied on biopsy of a single blastomere at the cleavage stage (day 3) of embryo development with subsequent fixation for fluorescence in situ hybridization (FISH) analysis [39]. While intriguing, there were several limitations of this approach. To facilitate biopsy of a single blastomere, embryos had to be placed in a magnesium-calcium-free media that could impact their further development into competent blastocysts. Next removal of one or two out of an embryo with typically six to ten cells was required, representing a substantial portion of the embryo that could impact its developmental competence. Furthermore, the accuracy of FISH, though proven in other clinical settings such as after chorionic villus sampling, was not reliably validated on single blastomeres since there is not a gold standard to retest the same blastomere. Finally, only the chromosomes most often found in clinically recognized abnormal pregnancies (including 13, 16, 18, 21, X, Y) were probed for. It is now known that errors can occur on any chromosome and, therefore, some embryos may have been misdiagnosed as normal. In addition, a reanalysis of embryos predicted to be abnormal by FISH found that 58% were euploid when analyzed by a more robust microarray platform at the blastocyst stage [40], indicating a high false-positive rate.

Retrospective, nonrandomized studies of the application of FISH-based preimplantation genetic screening (PGS) appeared to show benefit, especially for women of advanced reproductive age. However, several randomized trials failed to show benefit, and some even showed a detrimental effect. A meta-analysis reviewed nine randomized trials, five limited to women of advanced reproductive age, and concluded that FISH-based PGS resulted in a lower chance for delivery after IVF (26% vs. 18% per cycle) [41]. The most significant trial was led by Mastenbroek et al. and effectively dealt the death knell to FISH use in clinical ART [42]. In this trial of 408 women who underwent 836 total IVF cycles, those randomized to PGS had a lower live birth rate (24% vs. 35%). A later trial by the group at Instituto Valenciano de Infertilidad (IVI) used day three biopsy and nine chromosome FISH (13, 15, 17, 16, 18, 21, 22, X, Y) and found benefit in women of advanced reproductive age, but not in those with recurrent implantation failure (≥3 IVF failures) [43]. By the time this trial was published, the field had already advanced to employ a different biopsy technique and more robust genetic screening technologies.

Preimplantation Genetic Screening: Second Generation, Improved Biopsy, and Comprehensive Testing Platforms

While FISH-based PGS was unable to improve IVF success, it did not invalidate the general principle that selecting chromosomally normal embryos could improve the chance of live birth after IVF. Efforts then focused on using more sophisticated methodologies including SNP microarrays, array CGH, real-time PCR, and then NGS, to better diagnose embryos with aneuploidy by using a new method of PGS, called comprehensive chromosome screening (CCS), to detect the copy number status of all 22 autosomes and the sex chromosomes.

Many CCS platforms begin with whole genome amplification (WGA), which can be performed with any number of commercially available kits such as REPLI-g, GenomiPhi, GenomePlex, SurePlex, or MALBAC. The basic concept is random amplification of the genome such that the resulting product represents the relative quantity and genotypes present in the original sample. Of course, none of the methods of WGA provide a perfect representation, and thus downstream methods of analysis with highly parallel testing of the genome, such as SNP array or array CGH, have been applied in order to help overcome WGA inaccuracies. NGS has also been developed as a downstream analysis method that along with molecular barcoding has helped reduce the costs associated with CCS.

Preclinical studies showed that these technologies could reliably detect chromosome imbalance in samples from cell lines and then from embryos. Given the experience with FISH, the SNP array platform was validated with a "nonselection" trial in which embryos were biopsied and transferred with the clinicians not being privy to the PGS prediction [44]. The biopsies were then analyzed and the result correlated with the clinical outcome of the transferred embryo (using DNA fingerprinting in the case of multiple embryo transfer). The result clearly demonstrated that euploid embryos had a higher chance of implanting successfully than unselected and aneuploid embryos (41.4% vs. 28.2% vs. 4%, $P < 0.001$). The low false-positive rate was low enough to justify discarding abnormal embryos in an effort to enhance outcomes with the selective transfer of euploid embryos. The predictive value of euploid blastocyst implanting was significantly higher than a euploid day 3 cleavage stage embryo (48.2% vs. 29.2%, $P < 0.01$).

A paired randomized trial from the same group was performed to assess the safety of embryo biopsy at the cleavage vs. blastocyst stage. A double embryo transfer was performed in 116 women with one embryo undergoing biopsy and one not biopsied. The biopsy was used to later perform DNA fingerprinting to confirm which embryo is implanted in the case of a singleton delivery. The removal of a single cell on day 3 of development resulted in a significant 39% decrease in implantation potential, whereas removal of approximately five cells from the outer trophectoderm layer of the blastocyst did not significantly impair the chance of the embryo implanting and progressing to delivery [45]. Clinical studies of embryo biopsy for PGD evaluation of a monogenic disorder (beta-thalassemia) found that significantly more blastomere biopsies did not yield a result (25%) compared with trophectoderm biopsy (4%) [46] and the embryos undergoing trophectoderm biopsy were more likely to implant. Polar body biopsy has been proposed as a less invasive form of biopsy [47] since the polar bodies are naturally extruded during oocyte maturation and fertilization. When applied to preimplantation screening for aneuploidy using the SNP arrays, however, analysis of both polar bodies was found to disagree with the subsequent embryo biopsy 30% of the time and was less predictive of implantation potential [48]. Since premature separation of sister chromatids has been shown to be the predominant cause of meiotic errors in the oocyte, an embryo originating from an oocyte with reciprocal errors in the polar bodies often is actually euploid [49, 50]. Thus, it appears that trophectoderm biopsy at the blastocyst stage is the optimal stage for preimplantation analysis [51].

Given the high predictive values of these tests, the next step was to demonstrate clinical benefit in a randomized controlled trial. A trial comparing transfer of a single untested blastocyst vs. a biopsied euploid blastocyst by array CGH demonstrated improved success in a relatively young (<35 years old) patient population [52], with ongoing pregnancy rates of 41.7% vs. 69.1% ($P = 0.009$). Another study compared the transfer of two untested vs. two euploid blastocysts as determined by a validated real-time PCR assay [53]. This randomized trial also showed significant improvement in delivery rates with 84.7% of cycles delivering after transfer of euploid embryos compared with 67.5% of cycles transferring untested embryos [54]. Finally, the Blastocyst Euploid Selective Transfer (BEST) trial demonstrated that in women with normal ovarian reserve up to age 42, transferring one euploid blastocyst was not inferior to transferring two untested blastocysts (60.7% vs. 65.1% ongoing pregnancy rate to 24 weeks gestation) but had a much lower risk of multiples (0% vs. 53.4%) [55]. A follow-up study determined that those women randomized to transfer of a single euploid blastocyst had a much lower risk of having a baby with low birth weight and preterm delivery or requiring NICU admission [56]. A meta-analysis [57] and systematic review [58] both conclude that trophectoderm biopsy and comprehensive chromosome screening to select euploid blastocysts for transfer result in improved outcomes, particularly in good-prognosis patients with normal ovarian reserve.

The increased utilization of PGS clinically has provided a large body of data providing insight into the origins and prevalence of aneuploidy in preimplantation embryos. Retrospective analysis of outcomes using array CGH to screen for aneuploidy found that transferring euploid embryos corrected for the expected age-related decline in IVF pregnancy rates, at least up until age 42 [59]. An analysis of 247 blastomere biopsies from cleavage stage embryos using microarray and parental genotyping confirmed that the origin of aneuploidy can mostly be traced to errors in maternal meiosis [60].

A large clinical experience of the real-time, quantitative PCR CCS platform by Franasiak et al. evaluated 15,169 consecutive trophectoderm biopsies from blastocysts and found that the rate of aneuploidy remained stable in the low 30% range in the early 30s age group, rising rapidly in the late 30s and reaching 75% by age 42 [61]. The majority of errors in women in their 30s involved a single chromosome error, with the proportion of monosomies and trisomies being roughly equivalent. However, the incidence of multiple chromosome errors increased with age, and more than two-thirds of affected embryos in women over age 43 had more than one abnormal chromosome. In addition, the relative proportion of trisomies increased with advancing maternal age. Another study using the same dataset found an increase in the incidence of abnormalities involving chromosomes that are known to be found in clinically recognized pregnancies resulting in miscarriage [62].

While the array-based and PCR platforms demonstrated benefit in prospective trials, there are limitations. An analysis of 2354 clinically recognized pregnancies achieved after the transfer of euploid embryo testing with PCR found that there was a 0.13% error rate with resulting aneuploid pregnancies [63]. Follow-up testing revealed some of these pregnancies exhibited mosaicism, which is a known limitation of PGS since a prediction of the whole embryo has to be made from a small biopsy. A similar evaluation of pregnancies achieved after aCGH PGS found an error rate of 1.5% in clinical pregnancies [64].

Improvements in massive parallel sequencing technology allowed for the development of NGS at lower cost with the ability to barcode embryos and run dozens of samples on one sequencing chip [65]. A nonselection study of a targeted NGS approach again demonstrated high predictive values with euploid embryos implanting ~58% of the time and none of the predicted aneuploid embryos implanting. The development of NGS also led to the identification of segmental aneuploidy and mosaicism, i.e., a predicted mix of normal and abnormal cells. A nonselection trial for segmental aneuploidy demonstrated a significantly lower implantation rate for embryos harboring a >5 Mb deletion or duplication. Clinical studies have also shown lower chance of ongoing pregnancy from predicted mosaic range embryos and a higher risk of miscarriage [66].

Clinical CCS studies have also demonstrated reduced miscarriage rates. For example, Forman et al. found a significant decrease in clinical pregnancies resulting in a miscarriage when embryos were first screened by CCS (10.5%) compared to untested embryos (24.8%), Sher et al. found a significant reduction from 12% to 4% when incorporating CCS [67], and Keltz et al. found an 11% miscarriage rate in CCS tested embryos compared to 26% in untested embryos [68].

Interestingly, there remains a subset of cases where miscarriage occurred despite the transfer of a chromosomally normal embryo. While there are many possible explanations for this observation, there may be additional genetic causes other than whole chromosome uniform aneuploidy to consider. For example, mosaicism may contribute to some extent. Mosaicism originates from mitotic nondisjunction errors resulting in an embryo with cell lines with differing chromosomal makeup. Some evidence suggests that embryos predicted to be mosaic from a trophectoderm biopsy may possess reduced reproductive potential.

In addition, segmental aneuploidy may also represent a genetic factor that reduces reproductive potential. Many CCS methods have demonstrated the ability to detect segmental aneuploidy associated with inheritance of unbalanced chromosomes from carriers of a balanced translocation. These same methods may be capable of detecting de novo segmental imbalances. Preliminary data suggests that the majority of de novo segmental aneuploidies are of mitotic origin, making it important to demonstrate the ability to detect mosaic range segmental imbalances in a trophectoderm biopsy.

While these factors are among the most obvious targets for selection of competent embryos, there remains an enormous amount of uncharacterized molecular biology. For example, the preimplantation stage of embryo development represents the most dynamic period of time with respect to epigenetic modification of the embryonic genome. Characterizing the methylome during preimplantation development will undoubtedly improve our understanding of normal embryogenesis and potentially lead to new biomarkers of reproductive potential.

Conclusion

The evidence is clear that genetics plays an essential role in the ability of a fertilized embryo to progress to delivery of a healthy newborn. Decades worth of data studying products of conception from clinical miscarriages proved that chromosomal aneuploidy is the single largest factor contributing to the failure of established pregnancies to progress to delivery. Historical data also demonstrated that the aging oocyte is the major cause of the age-related decline in fertility, in large part due to the rapid increase in aneuploidy. The development of ART has provided valuable insight, conclusively demonstrating that aneuploidy increases dramatically with age. By using a safe biopsy technique, embryos can be selected for transfer that are chromosomally normal, resulting in a higher chance of delivery and lower risk of miscarriage and ongoing aneuploid gestation. Still, these testing platforms are not perfect, and there are other causes of failed implantation beyond whole chromosome aneuploidy. In addition, there are no proven interventions to reduce the prevalence of age-related aneuploidy in oocytes and embryos. Future developments will likely focus on improved methods of embryo selection to optimize the outcomes with transfer of genetically normal, competent embryos.

References

1. Boue J, Bou A, Lazar P. Retrospective and prospective epidemiological studies of 1500 karyotyped spontaneous human abortions. Teratology. 1975;12(1):11–26.
2. Nussbaum RL, McInnes RR, Willard HF, Thompson MW, Hamosh A. Thompson & Thompson genetics in medicine. 7th ed. Philadelphia: Saunders/Elsevier; 2007. p. xi, 585pp.
3. Shen J, Wu W, Gao C, Ochin H, Qu D, Xie J, et al. Chromosomal copy number analysis on chorionic villus samples from early spontaneous miscarriages by high throughput genetic technology. Mol Cytogenet. 2016;9:7.

4. Maslow BS, Budinetz T, Sueldo C, Anspach E, Engmann L, Benadiva C, et al. Single-nucleotide polymorphism-microarray ploidy analysis of paraffin-embedded products of conception in recurrent pregnancy loss evaluations. Obstet Gynecol. 2015;126(1):175–81.
5. Sahoo T, Dzidic N, Strecker MN, Commander S, Travis MK, Doherty C, et al. Comprehensive genetic analysis of pregnancy loss by chromosomal microarrays: outcomes, benefits, and challenges. Genet Med. 2017;19:83.
6. Levy B, Sigurjonsson S, Pettersen B, Maisenbacher MK, Hall MP, Demko Z, et al. Genomic imbalance in products of conception: single-nucleotide polymorphism chromosomal microarray analysis. Obstet Gynecol. 2014;124(2 Pt 1):202–9.
7. Neri G, Serra A, Campana M, Tedeschi B. Reproductive risks for translocation carriers: cytogenetic study and analysis of pregnancy outcome in 58 families. Am J Med Genet. 1983;16(4):535–61.
8. Campana M, Serra A, Neri G. Role of chromosome aberrations in recurrent abortion: a study of 269 balanced translocations. Am J Med Genet. 1986;24(2):341–56.
9. De Braekeleer M, Dao TN. Cytogenetic studies in couples experiencing repeated pregnancy losses. Hum Reprod. 1990;5(5):519–28.
10. Jacobs PA, Browne C, Gregson N, Joyce C, White H. Estimates of the frequency of chromosome abnormalities detectable in unselected newborns using moderate levels of banding. J Med Genet. 1992;29(2):103–8.
11. Maeda T, Ohno M, Matsunobu A, Yoshihara K, Yabe N. A cytogenetic survey of 14,835 consecutive liveborns. Jinrui Idengaku Zasshi. 1991;36(1):117–29.
12. Treff NR, Northrop LE, Kasabwala K, Su J, Levy B, Scott RT Jr. Single nucleotide polymorphism microarray-based concurrent screening of 24 chromosome aneuploidy and unbalanced translocations in preimplantation human embryos. Fertil Steril. 2010;95(5):1606–12.e1-2.
13. Therman E, Susman B, Denniston C. The nonrandom participation of human acrocentric chromosomes in Robertsonian translocations. Ann Hum Genet. 1989;53(Pt 1):49–65.
14. Fryns JP, Van Buggenhout G. Structural chromosome rearrangements in couples with recurrent fetal wastage. Eur J Obstet Gynecol Reprod Biol. 1998;81(2):171–6.
15. Lazarin GA, Haque I, Evans EA, Goldberg JD. Smith-Lemli-Opitz syndrome carrier frequency and estimates of in utero mortality rates. Prenat Diagn. 2017;37:350.
16. Loffler J, Trojovsky A, Casati B, Kroisel PM, Utermann G. Homozygosity for the W151X stop mutation in the delta7-sterol reductase gene (DHCR7) causing a lethal form of Smith-Lemli-Opitz syndrome: retrospective molecular diagnosis. Am J Med Genet. 2000;95(2):174–7.
17. Schollen E, Kjaergaard S, Legius E, Schwartz M, Matthijs G. Lack of Hardy-Weinberg equilibrium for the most prevalent PMM2 mutation in CDG-Ia (congenital disorders of glycosylation type Ia). Eur J Hum Genet. 2000;8(5):367–71.
18. Lek M, Karczewski KJ, Minikel EV, Samocha KE, Banks E, Fennell T, et al. Analysis of protein-coding genetic variation in 60,706 humans. Nature. 2016;536(7616):285–91.
19. Sazegari A, Kalantar SM, Pashaiefar H, Mohtaram S, Honarvar N, Feizollahi Z, et al. The T657C polymorphism on the SYCP3 gene is associated with recurrent pregnancy loss. J Assist Reprod Genet. 2014;31(10):1377–81.
20. Eagles N, Sebire NJ, Short D, Savage PM, Seckl MJ, Fisher RA. Risk of recurrent molar pregnancies following complete and partial hydatidiform moles. Hum Reprod. 2015;30(9):2055–63.
21. Shi X, Xie X, Jia Y, Li S. Maternal genetic polymorphisms and unexplained recurrent miscarriage: a systematic review and meta-analysis. Clin Genet. 2017;91:265.
22. Woods DC, Tilly JL. Isolation, characterization and propagation of mitotically active germ cells from adult mouse and human ovaries. Nat Protoc. 2013;8(5):966–88.
23. Block E. Quantitative morphological investigations of the follicular system in women; variations at different ages. Acta Anat. 1952;14(1-2):108–23.
24. Menken J, Trussell J, Larsen U. Age and infertility. Science. 1986;233(4771):1389–94.
25. Schwartz D, Mayaux MJ. Female fecundity as a function of age: results of artificial insemination in 2193 nulliparous women with azoospermic husbands. Federation CECOS. N Engl J Med. 1982;306(7):404–6.

26. Ripley M, Lanes A, Leveille MC, Shmorgun D. Does ovarian reserve predict egg quality in unstimulated therapeutic donor insemination cycles? Fertil Steril. 2015;103(5):1170–5.e2.
27. Streuli I, de Mouzon J, Paccolat C, Chapron C, Petignat P, Irion OP, et al. AMH concentration is not related to effective time to pregnancy in women who conceive naturally. Reprod Biomed Online. 2014;28(2):216–24.
28. Schieve LA, Tatham L, Peterson HB, Toner J, Jeng G. Spontaneous abortion among pregnancies conceived using assisted reproductive technology in the United States. Obstet Gynecol. 2003;101(5 Pt 1):959–67.
29. Causio F, Fischetto R, Sarcina E, Geusa S, Tartagni M. Chromosome analysis of spontaneous abortions after in vitro fertilization (IVF) and intracytoplasmic sperm injection (ICSI). Eur J Obstet Gynecol Reprod Biol. 2002;105(1):44–8.
30. Kim JW, Lee WS, Yoon TK, Seok HH, Cho JH, Kim YS, et al. Chromosomal abnormalities in spontaneous abortion after assisted reproductive treatment. BMC Med Genet. 2010;11:153.
31. Bingol B, Abike F, Gedikbasi A, Tapisiz OL, Gunenc Z. Comparison of chromosomal abnormality rates in ICSI for non-male factor and spontaneous conception. J Assist Reprod Genet. 2012;29(1):25–30.
32. Nayak S, Pavone ME, Milad M, Kazer R. Aneuploidy rates in failed pregnancies following assisted reproductive technology. J Women's Health. 2011;20(8):1239–43.
33. Werner M, Reh A, Grifo J, Perle MA. Characteristics of chromosomal abnormalities diagnosed after spontaneous abortions in an infertile population. J Assist Reprod Genet. 2012;29(8):817–20.
34. Lathi RB, Milki AA. Rate of aneuploidy in miscarriages following in vitro fertilization and intracytoplasmic sperm injection. Fertil Steril. 2004;81(5):1270–2.
35. Nasseri A, Mukherjee T, Grifo JA, Noyes N, Krey L, Copperman AB. Elevated day 3 serum follicle stimulating hormone and/or estradiol may predict fetal aneuploidy. Fertil Steril. 1999;71(4):715–8.
36. Navot D, Drews MR, Bergh PA, Guzman I, Karstaedt A, Scott RT Jr, et al. Age-related decline in female fertility is not due to diminished capacity of the uterus to sustain embryo implantation. Fertil Steril. 1994;61(1):97–101.
37. Sagi-Dain L, Sagi S, Dirnfeld M. The effect of paternal age on oocyte donation outcomes. Obstet Gynecol Surv. 2016;71(5):301–6.
38. Dubov T, Toledano-Alhadef H, Bokstein F, Constantini S, Ben-Shachar S. The effect of parental age on the presence of de novo mutations - lessons from neurofibromatosis type I. Mol Genet Genomic Med. 2016;4(4):480–6.
39. Munne S, Lee A, Rosenwaks Z, Grifo J, Cohen J. Diagnosis of major chromosome aneuploidies in human preimplantation embryos. Hum Reprod. 1993;8(12):2185–91.
40. Northrop LE, Treff NR, Levy B, Scott RT Jr. SNP microarray-based 24 chromosome aneuploidy screening demonstrates that cleavage-stage FISH poorly predicts aneuploidy in embryos that develop to morphologically normal blastocysts. Mol Hum Reprod. 2010;16(8):590–600.
41. Mastenbroek S, Twisk M, van der Veen F, Repping S. Preimplantation genetic screening: a systematic review and meta-analysis of RCTs. Hum Reprod Update. 2011;17(4):454–66.
42. Mastenbroek S, Twisk M, van Echten-Arends J, Sikkema-Raddatz B, Korevaar JC, Verhoeve HR, et al. In vitro fertilization with preimplantation genetic screening. N Engl J Med. 2007;357(1):9–17.
43. Rubio C, Bellver J, Rodrigo L, Bosch E, Mercader A, Vidal C, et al. Preimplantation genetic screening using fluorescence in situ hybridization in patients with repetitive implantation failure and advanced maternal age: two randomized trials. Fertil Steril. 2013;99(5):1400–7.
44. Scott RT Jr, Ferry K, Su J, Tao X, Scott K, Treff NR. Comprehensive chromosome screening is highly predictive of the reproductive potential of human embryos: a prospective, blinded, nonselection study. Fertil Steril. 2012;97(4):870–5.
45. Scott RT Jr, Upham KM, Forman EJ, Zhao T, Treff NR. Cleavage-stage biopsy significantly impairs human embryonic implantation potential while blastocyst biopsy does not: a randomized and paired clinical trial. Fertil Steril. 2013;100(3):624–30.

46. Kokkali G, Traeger-Synodinos J, Vrettou C, Stavrou D, Jones GM, Cram DS, et al. Blastocyst biopsy versus cleavage stage biopsy and blastocyst transfer for preimplantation genetic diagnosis of beta-thalassaemia: a pilot study. Hum Reprod. 2007;22(5):1443–9.

47. Handyside AH, Montag M, Magli MC, Repping S, Harper J, Schmutzler A, et al. Multiple meiotic errors caused by predivision of chromatids in women of advanced maternal age undergoing in vitro fertilisation. Eur J Hum Genet. 2012;20(7):742–7.

48. Salvaggio CN, Forman EJ, Garnsey HM, Treff NR, Scott RT Jr. Polar body based aneuploidy screening is poorly predictive of embryo ploidy and reproductive potential. J Assist Reprod Genet. 2014;31:1221.

49. Forman EJ, Treff NR, Stevens JM, Garnsey HM, Katz-Jaffe MG, Scott RT Jr, et al. Embryos whose polar bodies contain isolated reciprocal chromosome aneuploidy are almost always euploid. Hum Reprod. 2013;28(2):502–8.

50. Scott RT Jr, Treff NR, Stevens J, Forman EJ, Hong KH, Katz-Jaffe MG, et al. Delivery of a chromosomally normal child from an oocyte with reciprocal aneuploid polar bodies. J Assist Reprod Genet. 2012;29(6):533–7.

51. Scott KL, Hong KH, Scott RT Jr. Selecting the optimal time to perform biopsy for preimplantation genetic testing. Fertil Steril. 2013;100(3):608–14.

52. Yang Z, Liu J, Collins GS, Salem SA, Liu X, Lyle SS, et al. Selection of single blastocysts for fresh transfer via standard morphology assessment alone and with array CGH for good prognosis IVF patients: results from a randomized pilot study. Mol Cytogenet. 2012;5(1):24.

53. Treff NR, Tao X, Ferry KM, Su J, Taylor D, Scott RT Jr. Development and validation of an accurate quantitative real-time polymerase chain reaction-based assay for human blastocyst comprehensive chromosomal aneuploidy screening. Fertil Steril. 2012;97(4):819–24.e2.

54. Scott RT Jr, Upham KM, Forman EJ, Hong KH, Scott KL, Taylor D, et al. Blastocyst biopsy with comprehensive chromosome screening and fresh embryo transfer significantly increases in vitro fertilization implantation and delivery rates: a randomized controlled trial. Fertil Steril. 2013;100(3):697–703.

55. Forman EJ, Hong KH, Ferry KM, Tao X, Taylor D, Levy B, et al. In vitro fertilization with single euploid blastocyst transfer: a randomized controlled trial. Fertil Steril. 2013;100(1):100–7.e1.

56. Forman EJ, Hong KH, Franasiak JM, Scott RT Jr. Obstetrical and neonatal outcomes from the BEST trial: single embryo transfer with aneuploidy screening improves outcomes after in vitro fertilization without compromising delivery rates. Am J Obstet Gynecol. 2014;210:157.e1.

57. Dahdouh EM, Balayla J, Garcia-Velasco JA. Comprehensive chromosome screening improves embryo selection: a meta-analysis. Fertil Steril. 2015;104(6):1503–12.

58. Dahdouh EM, Balayla J, Garcia-Velasco JA. Impact of blastocyst biopsy and comprehensive chromosome screening technology on preimplantation genetic screening: a systematic review of randomized controlled trials. Reprod Biomed Online. 2015;30(3):281–9.

59. Harton GL, Munne S, Surrey M, Grifo J, Kaplan B, McCulloh DH, et al. Diminished effect of maternal age on implantation after preimplantation genetic diagnosis with array comparative genomic hybridization. Fertil Steril. 2013;100(6):1695–703.

60. Rabinowitz M, Ryan A, Gemelos G, Hill M, Baner J, Cinnioglu C, et al. Origins and rates of aneuploidy in human blastomeres. Fertil Steril. 2012;97(2):395–401.

61. Ledger WL. Measurement of antimullerian hormone: not as straightforward as it seems. Fertil Steril. 2014;101(2):339.

62. Franasiak JM, Forman EJ, Hong KH, Werner MD, Upham KM, Treff NR, et al. Aneuploidy across individual chromosomes at the embryonic level in trophectoderm biopsies: changes with patient age and chromosome structure. J Assist Reprod Genet. 2014;31(11):1501–9.

63. Werner MD, Leondires MP, Schoolcraft WB, Miller BT, Copperman AB, Robins ED, et al. Clinically recognizable error rate after the transfer of comprehensive chromosomal screened euploid embryos is low. Fertil Steril. 2014;102(6):1613–8.

64. Tiegs AW, Hodes-Wertz B, McCulloh DH, Munne S, Grifo JA. Discrepant diagnosis rate of array comparative genomic hybridization in thawed euploid blastocysts. J Assist Reprod Genet. 2016;33(7):893–7.

65. Kung A, Munne S, Bankowski B, Coates A, Wells D. Validation of next-generation sequencing for comprehensive chromosome screening of embryos. Reprod Biomed Online. 2015;31(6):760–9.

66. Maxwell SM, Colls P, Hodes-Wertz B, McCulloh DH, McCaffrey C, Wells D, et al. Why do euploid embryos miscarry? A case-control study comparing the rate of aneuploidy within presumed euploid embryos that resulted in miscarriage or live birth using next-generation sequencing. Fertil Steril. 2016;106:1414.

67. Sher G, Keskintepe L, Keskintepe M, Maassarani G, Tortoriello D, Brody S. Genetic analysis of human embryos by metaphase comparative genomic hybridization (mCGH) improves efficiency of IVF by increasing embryo implantation rate and reducing multiple pregnancies and spontaneous miscarriages. Fertil Steril. 2009;92(6):1886–94.

68. Keltz MD, Vega M, Sirota I, Lederman M, Moshier EL, Gonzales E, et al. Preimplantation genetic screening (PGS) with comparative genomic hybridization (CGH) following day 3 single cell blastomere biopsy markedly improves IVF outcomes while lowering multiple pregnancies and miscarriages. J Assist Reprod Genet. 2013;30(10):1333–9.

Chapter 6
Immune Factors in Recurrent Implantation Failure

Diana Alecsandru and Juan A. Garcia-Velasco

Abbreviations

ART   Assisted reproductive treatments
DET   Double embryo transfer
EVT   Invading extravillous trophoblast
HLA   Human leukocyte antigen
IVF   In vitro fertilization
KIR   Killer immunoglobulin-like receptor
NK cells Natural killer cells
Pb   Peripheral blood
RIF   Recurrent implantation failure
RM   Recurrent miscarriage
SET   Single embryo transfer
uNK cells Uterine natural killer cells

In the last decades, substantial progress has been made to improve the outcome of the assisted reproductive treatments (ART). Our knowledge about folliculogenesis, in vitro embryo culture and their chromosomal composition, as well as endometrial receptivity has undergone a huge improvement during the last few years. Despite this, a high percentage of embryos are still lost right after being transferred (50%) or a bit later, as early miscarriage or clinical miscarriage. A recent study [1] reported a 52% cumulative live birth rate (LBR) after transferring up to five embryos and 79% after 15 embryos had been transferred; but what happens to the rest of the embryos? There might be other factors that contribute to implantation failure or miscarriage, not just embryo aneuploidies—by far, the main contributor to implantation failure, such as endometrial factors, hydrosalpinges, infections or abnormal karyotypes, or even maternal tolerance to pregnancy. At the same time, due to

D. Alecsandru, MD, PhD • J.A. Garcia-Velasco, MD, PhD (✉)
Rey Juan Carlos University, IVI RMA-Madrid, Madrid, Spain
e-mail: juan.garcia.velasco@ivi.es

© Springer International Publishing AG 2018   93
J.M. Franasiak, R.T. Scott Jr. (eds.), *Recurrent Implantation Failure*,
https://doi.org/10.1007/978-3-319-71967-2_6

repeated failed cycles even after gamete donation, we all have witnessed an increasing demand for immune tests and "immune treatments" from our patients. Although this patient's demand may be unjustified, we need to understand if there is a rationale behind to use it, or not, to explain them why not use it. The role of the immune system in recurrent miscarriage (RM) and recurrent implantation failure (RIF) is one of the most controversial issues in assisted reproduction [2]. The controversy, in part, is due to the fact that most of the previous studies about immune system implication in reproduction were focused on finding markers on peripheral blood [3, 4] and quick solutions using different lines of immunomodulation [5, 6]. The main reason that immune treatments have failed so far and immune tests (pbNK or uNK cell testing) have shown very weak or no predictive value is due to poor study design and great patient heterogeneity [2, 7].

Maternal tolerance, as we know, begins at the uterine level, and successful adaptation to the semiallogeneic fetus is more complicated than the initial concept suggested.

Natural Killer Cells

Peripheral blood natural killer (pbNK) cells have become an "immune study core" for women with recurrent miscarriage or RIF, based on the mistaken notion that they are causing reproductive failure by killing or "rejecting" the embryo.

Some reports had a general view [3] as natural killer (NK) cells from the peripheral blood (pbNK) and uterus (uNK) are merged together with the simple marker "NK cells" as the "main immune cells at the maternal–fetal interface." This is, from immunological point of view, an erroneous judgment as pbNK and uNK cells are completely different types of immune cells [8]. pbNK cells are cytotoxic and represent the first line of defense against viruses, tumors, and damaged cells, and they are not trained to "reject" or kill a healthy embryo(s).

In peripheral blood, there are two major types of NK cells [9]; 90% are CD56dim, CD16+, and 10% are CD56bright, CD162 [9, 10]. In contrast, uNK cells are CD56superbright, CD162 and differ radically from pbNK in other phenotype markers and functional assays [8, 11]. uNK killing in vitro assays is very weak compared with pbNK [12]. The uNK cells acquire their functional properties in utero as CD56+ cells do proliferate and differentiate in the specialized progesterone-dominated microenvironment of the secretory endometrium and early deciduas and seem to play an important role in controlling trophoblast invasion and the development of a healthy placenta [10].

Uterine NK (uNK) cells are small and sparse before ovulation, but rapidly proliferate and differentiate into large cells with prominent cytoplasmic granules soon after ovulation. uNK cells are the dominant immune cells in the uterine mucosa and account for 30% of cells in the stroma in the late secretory endometrium in humans [13]. During pregnancy uNK cells are abundant throughout deciduas, and they accumulate particularly at the site of placentation around the infiltrating trophoblast cells in the decidua basalis [14]. They are also particularly prominent around spiral arteries and abundant early in gestation when the placenta is established.

The number of pbNK and uNK cells shows great variability depending on the patient's clinical condition as infections, autoimmunity or tumors, day of the menstrual cycle, treatment condition (ovarian stimulation), stress, time of day, exercise, etc., and previous studies about NK cells and reproductive issues did not take this NK cell physiological variation into consideration.

Using "NK cells" to describe these two contrasting subsets of NK cells, pbNK and uNK, as a unique marker in women with infertility or disorders of pregnancy, contribute only to add more confusion about immune tests in ART.

The fetal cells in direct contact with the mother's immune system in the uterus are trophoblast cells, the layer surrounding the blastocyst [15, 16], and the mother's uterine immune system is dominated by uterine NK (uNK) cells [17], CD56bright CD16dim, which are distinct from peripheral blood NK cells and are the most abundant leukocyte population during the first trimester of human pregnancy [18].

The maternal and fetal circulations do not mix, although transient exchange of cells occurs, particularly during the trauma of delivery [10].

The successful maternal adaptation to the semiallogeneic fetus occurs in the uterus at the site of placentation. The key of the maternofetal tolerance process is the remodeling of the spiral arteries, with destruction of the media by invading extravillous trophoblast (EVT) cells. The EVT cells express major histocompatibility complex molecules: human leukocyte antigen (HLA), class I HLA-C and non-classical HLA-G and HLA-E antigens, whereas the class I antigens HLA-A and HLA-B and class II antigens are absent [19, 20]. Although, HLA-E and HLA-G are oligomorphic, the HLA-C molecules expressed by EVT cells are polymorphic, and ligands for killer immunoglobulin-like receptors (KIRs) are expressed by uNK cells [21]. The EVT invading into the maternal decidua are of fetal not maternal origin, and they express high levels of HLA-C, which is recognized by uterine NK (uNK) cells receptors, also known as KIR. Both polymorphic maternal KIRs and fetal HLA-C molecules are variable and specific to a particular pregnancy [10]. In any pregnancy, the maternal KIR genotype could be AA (non-activating KIRs), AB, BB, or Bx (1–10 activating KIRs) [22]; and the HLA-C ligands for KIRs are divided into two groups: HLA-C1 and HLA-C2. Of the two, C2 is a stronger ligand than C1 [23]. The A haplotypes contain mainly genes for inhibitory KIR, and B haplotypes have additional genes encoding activating KIR. The presence of activating KIR2DS1 (B haplotype) confers protection from pregnancy disorders [24], and its absence (A haplotype) increases the risk of pregnancy complications [14, 25].

Placentation is regulated by interactions (Fig. 6.1) between maternal killer immunoglobulin-like receptors (KIRs) expressed by the uNK and fetal HLA-C molecules expressed by EVT [26, 27]. Hiby et al. showed that invading EVTs are the principal site of HLA-C expression in the decidua basalis and that both maternal and paternal HLA-C allotypes are presented to KIRs [24, 28]. Insufficient invasion of the uterine lining by trophoblasts and vascular conversion in the decidua are thought to be the primary defect in disorders such as recurrent miscarriage (RM), preeclampsia, and fetal growth restriction (FGR) [29], and this process is regulated

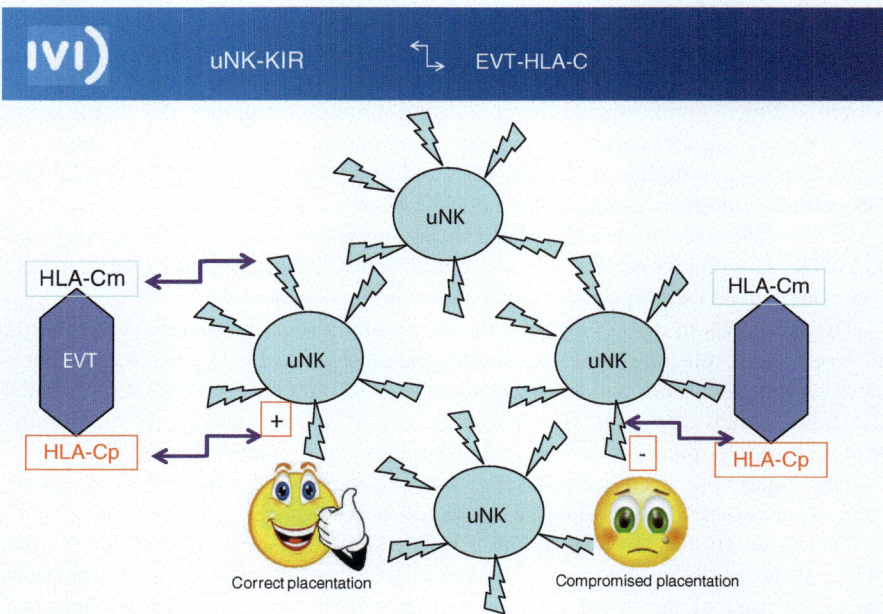

Fig. 6.1 KIR and fetal HLA-C interaction on own oocyte pregnancies. *HLA-Cm* maternal HLA-C; *HLA-Cp* paternal HLA-C. Red color: *nonself* HLA-C (own oocytes), *EVT* invading extravillous trophoblast, *uNK* uterine NK cells

by interaction between maternal KIRs expressed by the uNK and their ligand HLA-C expressed by EVT.

Pregnancies are at increased risk of recurrent miscarriage, preeclampsia, or FGR in mothers who are homozygous for KIR haplotype A (KIR AA) when the fetus has more HLA-C2 genes than the mother and the additional fetal HLA-C2 alleles are of paternal origin [24]. Protection from preeclampsia is likely to be mediated by the activating KIR2DS1 (B haplotype), which also binds HLA-C2.

Thus, depending on the particular KIR-HLA-C interactions, the trophoblast cell invasion will be regulated.

Hiby et al. [27] and Faridi and Agrawal [30] have reported differences in outcomes of medically unassisted pregnancies, increased risk of RM, preeclampsia, and FGR, in mothers with KIR AA carrying a fetus with paternal HLA-C2, and this finding suggests that placentation is deficient when there is a very strong inhibitory signal to uNK cells mediated via the KIR A haplotype gene. Hiby et al. [24, 26, 27, 31, 32] performed larger cohort studies that analyzed both maternal and paternal genotypes, with a large control group, and demonstrated a clear difference between the KIR and HLA-C genotypes in patients with disorders such as RM, preeclampsia, and FGR. Epidemiological studies provide clear evidence that selection for human reproductive success has adapted to the KIR and HLA-C genes and could be responsible for maintaining balanced polymorphisms between the HLA-C1 and HLA-C2 groups and the A and B KIR haplotypes [17, 28, 33, 34].

But What Happens in ART?

Assisted pregnancies differ from medically unassisted pregnancies, in those patients who receive sometimes more than one embryo per transfer, and also donor oocytes, sperm donor or embryo donation, are often used.

After double embryo transfer (DET), the expression of more than one paternal HLA-C per trophoblast cell is induced. In oocyte donor cycles, an increasingly demanded treatment due to advanced maternal age, the oocyte maternal HLA-C, which is genetically different from the mother's receptor, behaves as a paternal HLA-C, and this induces that more nonself HLA antigens are presented to the mother's KIR (per transfer) compared with "normal" pregnancies. After DET in an oocyte donor cycle, the expression of two nonself or "paternal" HLA-C in the EVT (per embryo) is present in the decidua basalis. The trophoblast antigen presentation (HLA-C) to uNK KIRs happens much more frequently than in natural pregnancy, because the embryo transfer is performed even monthly in RIF patients.

In human populations, pregnancy disorders are predicted to reduce the frequency of group A KIR, HLA-C2, or both, and this selection is thought to have originated during human evolution [21, 33, 34]. An inverse correlation between the frequencies of the KIR AA haplotype and HLA-C2 has been observed. Populations with the highest frequency of KIR AA (Japanese and Koreans) have the lowest HLA-C2 frequencies, whereas populations with the lowest frequency of KIR AA (Aboriginal Australians and Asian Indians) have the highest HLA-C2 frequencies. Natural selection seems to have driven an allele-level group A KIR haplotype and HLA-C1 ligand to an unusually high frequency in the Japanese, such that the detrimental KIR AA-HLA-C2 combination does not significantly affect pregnancy outcomes in Japanese and Korean populations [35].

This correlation provides evidence that selection for human reproductive success has adapted to the KIR and HLA-C genes and could be responsible for maintaining balanced polymorphisms between the HLA-C1 and HLA-C2 groups and the A and B KIR haplotypes [21, 28, 33, 34] However, this natural human evolution is not taken into consideration nowadays during ART. Furthermore, donor oocytes are often used in ART, and the literature describes higher maternal morbidity in egg donation pregnancies (pregnancy-induced hypertension, preeclampsia, FGR) [36] and preterm birth compared with pregnancies with own oocyte ART [37–39]. Although part of this increased frequency of complications may be due to the main indication for oocyte donation, which is advanced maternal age, recent age-matched data confirmed this higher frequency of unwanted events, and immunology maladaptation could be the reason [38, 40].

The increased expression of paternal HLA-C after DET could be associated with more pregnancy disorders than single embryo transfer (SET) in mothers with an inhibitory KIR haplotype (AA). A recent study [41] analyzed pregnancy, miscarriage, and LBR/cycle according to KIR haplotype and categorized by DET or SET. A higher rate of early miscarriage after DET when the patient's own oocytes were used occurred in those with the KIR AA (22.8%), followed by those with a KIR AB (16.7%), when compared with mothers with a KIR BB (11.1%) ($p = 0.03$).

A significantly decreased LBR/cycle after DET of donated oocytes was observed in mothers with a KIR AA haplotype (7.5%) compared with those with a KIR AB (26.4%) and KIR BB (21.5%)($p = 0.006$) [41].

The decreased LBR after DET in donor oocyte cycles in mothers KIR AA may be due to increased expression of nonself HLA-C (paternal and oocyte donor HLA-C). In this case, four "paternal" HLA-C would exist per trophoblast cells after DET: one coming from the father and another one coming from the donor, per embryo transferred, as the oocyte donor HLA-C behaves as "paternal" or non-self HLA-C. Expressing four "paternal" HLA-C is more likely to find at least one paternal or oocyte donor HLA-C2 than in own oocytes and SET, and probably implantation or placentation failure occurs in mothers who are KIR AA.

No other report has studied the impact of KIR-HLA-C on donor oocyte cycles. The authors speculate that completing a normal pregnancy was possible only for mothers with the KIR AA haplotype who carry a baby with a least one nonself HLA-C1 (nonself HLA-C1). Recently, they performed a prospective study [42] including 30 women with unknown etiology of RIF and RM and their oocyte donor-assisted reproductive cycles. All women had KIR AA genotype and their partners HLA-C2 genes. They had 54 embryo transfer cycles (82.76% DET; 17.24% SET) with unknown HLA-C oocyte donors and 28 cycles with HLA-C1C1 donors (21.05% DET; 78.95% SET). Pregnancy, miscarriage, and LBR/cycle after embryo transfer (ET) with unknown oocyte donor HLA-C and after transfers with HLA-C1C1 oocyte donor were studied.

Higher pregnancy rate per cycle after HLA-C1C1 oocyte donor transfer (85.71%) compared with unknown HLA-C oocyte donor cycles (31.48%) was observed in the same patients KIR AA with HLA-C2 partners ($p < 0.0001$). Higher miscarriage rate per cycle after unknown HLA-C oocyte donor transfer (94.44%) compared with HLA-C1C1 oocyte donor transfer (8.33%) was observed ($p < 0.0001$).

Significantly increased LBR per cycle was observed after ET with HLA-C1C1 oocyte donor (82.14%) compared with the LBR in the same KIR AA patients and HLA-C2 partners after cycles with unknown HLA-C oocyte donor (0%) ($p < 0.0001$).

This new findings show that the maternal KIR haplotype and fetal HLA-C have an impact on the live birth rate after IVF cycles, especially when donor oocyte and DET are used. Expressing four paternal HLA-C in the EVT cells after DET with donor oocytes is more likely to result in at least one nonself HLA-C2 (even by HLA-C2 allelic frequency on Caucasian population) than with one's own oocyte after SET, and implantation or placentation failure probably occurs in mothers with the KIR AA haplotype. Therefore, selecting HLA-C1, among oocyte and/or sperm donors for patients undergoing egg donation and who express inhibitory KIR haplotypes, could be more efficient and safer. The authors assume that it is a small sample and that is the first report observing differences in LBR by oocyte donor HLA-C in mothers KIR AA with HLA C2 partners. Apart from the statistical significance, the association strength is noticeably high, allowing greater confidence in the findings; however, larger studies are needed and should be replicated by other groups prior to final acceptance of this theory into clinical practice.

The new concept is emerging, and the evidence points to important physiological roles for uNK cells in healthy placentation as well as to abnormal uNK cell function in pregnancy disorders.

The combination of maternal KIR haplotype and parental donor HLA-C could predict which couple can benefit for the selection of SET/DET, or donor selection by HLA-C in ART, in order to increase the LBR/cycle, and it would facilitate the reduction of embryos that are being transferred, facilitating the increase of SET. Therefore, selecting HLA-C1, among oocyte and/or sperm donors for patients undergoing egg donation ART and inhibitory KIR, could be more efficient and safer as identified by epidemiological studies [10, 24, 43]

Other Immune Maternal Cells

The uterine mucosa is the major site where fetal placental cells are directly in contact with maternal tissues, rich in uNK cells, but also contains maternal T cells, effector T cells, and regulatory T cells. The trophoblast cells invading maternal decidua are allogeneic and could be potential targets for T cells. Although the interactions between uNK cells and EVT are clear, how effector T cells might interact with the trophoblast cells is still unclear [44].

Maternal T cells are not immunologically inert, as shown by the presence of fetal-specific T cells and T-cell-dependent humoral responses specific for the rhesus D antigen in rhesus-negative women or for paternally derived allogeneic HLA molecules in multiparous women [27, 45, 46]. Moreover, many studies in mice and humans have described mechanisms that favor T-cell tolerance in the deciduas, among which the expression of receptors that bind the trophoblast HLA-G on decidual antigen-presenting cells, preventing them from being immunogenic [27, 47].

The previous studies have been performed on mice and human spontaneous pregnancies, and questions also remain regarding the mechanisms by which effector T cells cause fetal loss especially in ART in which the fetal antigen presentation happens much more frequently than in natural pregnancy (even monthly), especially in recurrent miscarriage and RIF patients.

Conclusions

A new concept is emerging that the uterine immune system uses NK cell allorecognition to regulate placentation and control the maternofetal interface. In ART, these new insights [41, 42] could have an impact on the selection of SET in patients with recurrent miscarriage or RIF and a KIR AA haplotype. Also, although data are still premature and need to be validated, they may have clinical significance, helping with oocyte and/or sperm donor selection according to HLA-C in patients with recurrent miscarriage or RIF and a KIR AA haplotype as HLA-C1/C1 donors are predicted to be safer and C2/C2 males or oocyte donors may be more "dangerous" as identified by epidemiological studies [24, 43].

This is a new concept and, based on it, it is reasonable to think that the use of different lines of immune therapies (such as prednisolone, intravenous immunoglobulin, intralipid, tumor necrosis factor-a blockers), given in different fertility clinics to decrease the NK cells' activity in infertile women, has to be reconsidered because the scientific principle of the maternofetal tolerance has been misunderstood.

References

1. Garrido N, Bellver J, Remohi J, Simon C, Pellicer A. Cumulative live-birth rates per total number of embryos needed to reach newborn in consecutive in vitro fertilization (IVF) cycles: a new approach to measuring the likelihood of IVF success. Fertil Steril. 2011;96(1):40–6.
2. Alecsandru D, Garcia-Velasco JA. Immune testing and treatment: still an open debate. Hum Reprod. 2015;30(8):1994.
3. Sacks G. Enough! Stop the arguments and get on with the science of natural killer cell testing. Hum Reprod. 2015;30(7):1526–31.
4. Tang AW, Alfirevic Z, Quenby S. Natural killer cells and pregnancy outcomes in women with recurrent miscarriage and infertility: a systematic review. Hum Reprod. 2011;26(8):1971–80.
5. Moffett A, Shreeve N. Reply: First do no harm: continuing the uterine NK cell debate. Hum Reprod. 2015;31(1):218–9.
6. Moffett A, Shreeve N. First do no harm: uterine natural killer (NK) cells in assisted reproduction. Hum Reprod. 2015;30(7):1519–25.
7. Alecsandru D, Garcia-Velasco JA. Immunology and human reproduction. Curr Opin Obstet Gynecol. 2015;27(3):231–4.
8. Koopman LA, Kopcow HD, Rybalov B, Boyson JE, Orange JS, Schatz F, et al. Human decidual natural killer cells are a unique NK cell subset with immunomodulatory potential. J Exp Med. 2003;198(8):1201–12.
9. Caligiuri MA. Human natural killer cells. Blood. 2008;112(3):461–9.
10. Moffett A, Colucci F. Uterine NK cells: active regulators at the maternal-fetal interface. J Clin Invest. 2014;124(5):1872–9.
11. King A, Balendran N, Wooding P, Carter NP, Loke YW. CD3- leukocytes present in the human uterus during early placentation: phenotypic and morphologic characterization of the CD56++ population. Dev Immunol. 1991;1(3):169–90.
12. King A, Birkby C, Loke YW. Early human decidual cells exhibit NK activity against the K562 cell line but not against first trimester trophoblast. Cell Immunol. 1989;118(2):337–44.
13. Bulmer JN, Lash GE. Human uterine natural killer cells: a reappraisal. Mol Immunol. 2005;42(4):511–21.
14. Xiong S, Sharkey AM, Kennedy PR, Gardner L, Farrell LE, Chazara O, et al. Maternal uterine NK cell-activating receptor KIR2DS1 enhances placentation. J Clin Invest. 2013;123(10):4264–72.
15. Moffett A, Loke C. Immunology of placentation in eutherian mammals. Nat Rev Immunol. 2006;6(8):584–94.
16. Moffett A, Loke C. Implantation, embryo-maternal interactions, immunology and modulation of the uterine environment – a workshop report. Placenta. 2006;27(Suppl A):S54–5.
17. Parham P. NK cells and trophoblasts: partners in pregnancy. J Exp Med. 2004;200(8):951–5.
18. Moffett-King A. Natural killer cells and pregnancy. Nat Rev Immunol. 2002;2(9):656–63.

19. King A, Hiby SE, Gardner L, Joseph S, Bowen JM, Verma S, et al. Recognition of tropho-blast HLA class I molecules by decidual NK cell receptors–a review. Placenta. 2000;21(Suppl A):S81–5.
20. Apps R, Murphy SP, Fernando R, Gardner L, Ahad T, Moffett A. Human leucocyte antigen (HLA) expression of primary trophoblast cells and placental cell lines, determined using single antigen beads to characterize allotype specificities of anti-HLA antibodies. Immunology. 2009;127(1):26–39.
21. Parham P, Moffett A. Variable NK cell receptors and their MHC class I ligands in immunity, reproduction and human evolution. Nat Rev Immunol. 2013;13(2):133–44.
22. Uhrberg M, Valiante NM, Shum BP, Shilling HG, Lienert-Weidenbach K, Corliss B, et al. Human diversity in killer cell inhibitory receptor genes. Immunity. 1997;7(6):753–63.
23. Winter CC, Gumperz JE, Parham P, Long EO, Wagtmann N. Direct binding and functional transfer of NK cell inhibitory receptors reveal novel patterns of HLA-C allotype recognition. J Immunol. 1998;161(2):571–7.
24. Hiby SE, Apps R, Sharkey AM, Farrell LE, Gardner L, Mulder A, et al. Maternal activating KIRs protect against human reproductive failure mediated by fetal HLA-C2. J Clin Invest. 2010;120(11):4102–10.
25. Wang S, Li YP, Ding B, Zhao YR, Chen ZJ, Xu CY, et al. Recurrent miscarriage is associated with a decline of decidual natural killer cells expressing killer cell immunoglobulin-like receptors specific for human leukocyte antigen C. J Obstet Gynaecol Res. 2014;40(5):1288–95.
26. Hiby SE, Regan L, Lo W, Farrell L, Carrington M, Moffett A. Association of maternal killer-cell immunoglobulin-like receptors and parental HLA-C genotypes with recurrent miscar-riage. Hum Reprod. 2008;23(4):972–6.
27. Hiby SE, Walker JJ, O'Shaughnessy KM, Redman CW, Carrington M, Trowsdale J, et al. Combinations of maternal KIR and fetal HLA-C genes influence the risk of preeclampsia and reproductive success. J Exp Med. 2004;200(8):957–65.
28. Hiby SE, Ashrafian-Bonab M, Farrell L, Single RM, Balloux F, Carrington M, et al. Distribution of killer cell immunoglobulin-like receptors (KIR) and their HLA-C ligands in two Iranian populations. Immunogenetics. 2010;62(2):65–73.
29. Arck PC, Hecher K. Fetomaternal immune cross-talk and its consequences for maternal and offspring's health. Nat Med. 2013;19(5):548–56.
30. Faridi RM, Agrawal S. Killer immunoglobulin-like receptors (KIRs) and HLA-C allorecogni-tion patterns implicative of dominant activation of natural killer cells contribute to recurrent miscarriages. Hum Reprod. 2011;26(2):491–7.
31. Hiby SE, Apps R, Chazara O, Farrell LE, Magnus P, Trogstad L, et al. Maternal KIR in combi-nation with paternal HLA-C2 regulate human birth weight. J Immunol. 2014;192(11):5069–73.
32. Hiby SE, Ashrafian-Bonab M, Farrell L, Single RM, Balloux F, Carrington M, et al. Distribution of killer cell immunoglobulin-like receptors (KIR) and their HLA-C ligands in two Iranian populations. Immunogenetics. 2009;62(2):65–73.
33. Adams EJ, Parham P. Species-specific evolution of MHC class I genes in the higher primates. Immunol Rev. 2001;183:41–64.
34. Rajalingam R, Parham P, Abi-Rached L. Domain shuffling has been the main mechanism forming new hominoid killer cell Ig-like receptors. J Immunol. 2004;172(1):356–69.
35. Saito S, Takeda Y, Sakai M, Nakabayahi M, Hayakawa S. The incidence of pre-eclampsia among couples consisting of Japanese women and Caucasian men. J Reprod Immunol. 2006;70(1-2):93–8.
36. Savasi VM, Mandia L, Laoreti A, Cetin I. Maternal and fetal outcomes in oocyte donation pregnancies. Hum Reprod Update. 2016;22:620.
37. Pecks U, Maass N, Neulen J. Oocyte donation: a risk factor for pregnancy-induced hyperten-sion: a meta-analysis and case series. Dtsch Arztebl Int. 2011;108(3):23–31.
38. Masoudian P, Nasr A, de Nanassy J, Fung-Kee-Fung K, Bainbridge SA, El Demellawy D. Oocyte donation pregnancies and the risk of preeclampsia or gestational hypertension: a systematic review and metaanalysis. Am J Obstet Gynecol. 2015;214(3):328–39.

39. Blazquez A, Garcia D, Rodriguez A, Vassena R, Figueras F, Vernaeve V. Is oocyte donation a risk factor for preeclampsia? A systematic review and meta-analysis. J Assist Reprod Genet. 2016;33(7):855–63.
40. Jeve YB, Potdar N, Opoku A, Khare M. Three-arm age-matched retrospective cohort study of obstetric outcomes of donor oocyte pregnancies. Int J Gynaecol Obstet. 2016;133(2):156–8.
41. Alecsandru D, Garrido N, Vicario JL, Barrio A, Aparicio P, Requena A, et al. Maternal KIR haplotype influences live birth rate after double embryo transfer in IVF cycles in patients with recurrent miscarriages and implantation failure. Hum Reprod. 2014;29(12):2637–43.
42. Alecsandru D, Barrio A, Aparicio P, Aparicio M, García-Velasco JA, editors. Maternal killer-cell immunoglobulin-like receptor (KIR) and fetal HLA-C compatibility in ART-oocyte donor influences live birth rate. ESHRE. 2016.
43. Skjaerven R, Vatten LJ, Wilcox AJ, Ronning T, Irgens LM, Lie RT. Recurrence of pre-eclampsia across generations: exploring fetal and maternal genetic components in a population based cohort. BMJ. 2005;331(7521):877.
44. Nancy P, Erlebacher A. T cell behavior at the maternal-fetal interface. Int J Dev Biol. 2014;58(2-4):189–98.
45. James E, Chai JG, Dewchand H, Macchiarulo E, Dazzi F, Simpson E. Multiparity induces priming to male-specific minor histocompatibility antigen, HY, in mice and humans. Blood. 2003;102(1):388–93.
46. van Kampen CA, Versteeg-vd Voort Maarschalk MF, Langerak-Langerak J, Roelen DL, Claas FH. Kinetics of the pregnancy-induced humoral and cellular immune response against the paternal HLA class I antigens of the child. Hum Immunol. 2002;63(6):452–8.
47. Apps R, Gardner L, Moffett A. A critical look at HLA-G. Trends Immunol. 2008;29(7):313–21.

Chapter 7
Stress and Implantation Failure

Jeffrey L. Deaton, Bonnie Patel, Erika Johnston-MacAnanny, Jie Yu,
Shannon D. Whirledge, Alexandra Wilson, J. David Wininger, Yimin Shu,
Robert N. Taylor, and Sarah L. Berga

Abbreviations

ACTH	Adrenocorticotropic hormone
ART	Assisted reproductive technology
BMI	Body mass index
CBT	Cognitive behavior therapy
CNS	Central nervous system
CRH	Corticotropin-releasing hormone
DNMT	DNA methyltransferase
FHA	Functional hypothalamic amenorrhea
FSH	Follicle-stimulating hormone
GABA	Gamma-aminobutyric acid
GH	Growth hormone
GnIH	Gonadotropin-inhibitory hormone
hCG	Human chorionic gonadotropin
HPA axis	Hypothalamic-pituitary-adrenal axis
HPO axis	Hypothalamic-pituitary-ovarian axis
IL	Interleukin
IVF	In vitro fertilization
IVF-ET	In vitro fertilization-embryo transfer
KNDy neurons	Kisspeptin-neurokinin B-dynorphin neurons
NMP	Nucleoplasmin
NPY	Neuropeptide Y

J.L. Deaton, MD • B. Patel, MD • E. Johnston-MacAnanny, MD • J. Yu, MD
A. Wilson, MD • J. David Wininger, PhD • Y. Shu, MD
R.N. Taylor, MD, PhD • S.L. Berga, MD (✉)
Department of Obstetrics and Gynecology, Wake Forest School of Medicine, Winston-Salem,
NC, USA
e-mail: sberga@wakehealth.edu

S.D. Whirledge, PhD
Department of Obstetrics, Gynecology and Reproductive Sciences, Yale University School
of Medicine, New Haven, CT, USA

© Springer International Publishing AG 2018
J.M. Franasiak, R.T. Scott Jr. (eds.), *Recurrent Implantation Failure*,
https://doi.org/10.1007/978-3-319-71967-2_7

OS	Oxidative stress
POMC-related peptides	Pro-opiomelanocortin-related peptides
PRL	Prolactin
RCT	Randomized controlled trial
RFRP3	RF-amide-related peptide-3
ROS	Reactive oxygen species
TNF	Tumor necrosis factor
TPO	Thyroid peroxidase antibody
TSH	Thyroid-stimulating hormone
VOC	Volatile organic compound

Stress-Induced Suppression of Folliculogenesis as a Cause of Implantation Failure

Synchronization of the HPO-endometrial axis is crucial for normal human reproduction. Even minimal aberrations compromise fertility. Specifically, factors that alter hypothalamic gonadotropin-releasing hormone (GnRH) drive disrupt HPO functioning, alter the secretion of estradiol and progesterone, and impair endometrial development. Factors that reduce GnRH drive include both insufficient and excessive energy balance and emotional challenges due to acute and chronic psychological stressors. The term functional hypothalamic amenorrhea (FHA), often defined as the absence of menses for 6 or more months without evidence of organic disease, encompasses a myriad of disorders resulting from nonorganic and potentially reversible reductions in GnRH drive. Impaired folliculogenesis is directly attributable to reduced GnRH drive, but FHA is more than insufficient central GnRH drive; FHA is also accompanied by a constellation of other neuroendocrine aberrations that include increased cortisol, reduced thyroxine, and amplified nocturnal melatonin [1, 2]. The behaviors associated with FHA include severe caloric imbalance, excessive exercise, and psychological challenges [3]. Often FHA results from a combination of stressors [4].

GnRH, a decapeptide secreted into the portal vasculature, is absolutely necessary for reproductive function. Approximately 4000 neurons located in the arcuate nucleus of the hypothalamus comprise the GnRH "pulse generator." Both GnRH pulse frequency and amplitude are critical for appropriate HPO function. GnRH pulses occur once every 60–90 min in the follicular phase and about 120–360 min in the luteal phase of the menstrual cycle [5]. GnRH pulsatility is modulated by a multitude of neurotransmitters and neuromodulators emanating from the cerebral cortex, suprahypothalamic centers, other hypothalamic nuclei, and hypothalamic vasculature as well as by metabolic signals that are actively transported by neurovascular cells across the blood-brain barrier [6, 7]. GnRH neurons are endogenously pulsatile, and neurotransmitters and metabolic factors either synchronize or desynchronize the GnRH neuronal cohort [8]. Neurons that release gamma-aminobutyric acid (GABA) primarily inhibit GnRH activity via the kisspeptin-neurokinin B-dynorphin (KNDy) neurons [9]. Kisspeptin, the product of the KiSS-1 gene and its G-protein-coupled receptor GPR54, are the proximate regulators of GnRH release and play a key role in the modulation of the GnRH pulse generator [10]. Administration of exogenous kisspeptin causes transient increase of serum LH and FSH in healthy women [11] and women with FHA [12].

Animal studies have demonstrated that other neurotransmitter systems including dopamine, norepinephrine, and serotonin regulate GnRH secretion. Activation of the noradrenergic system is associated with increased GnRH drive, whereas dopaminergic or serotonergic activation can either inhibit or stimulate GnRH release [13, 14]. These observations may explain the CNS-associated disruption of normal menstrual cycles in patients who take stimulants, antidepressants, and sedatives on a chronic basis. Excitatory amino acids, including aspartate and glutamate, have been found in large concentrations in presynaptic boutons of the arcuate nucleus and appear to activate GnRH secretion [15]. Alternatively, endogenous opiate peptides such as endorphins, enkephalins, and dynorphins appear to inhibit GnRH and LH secretion. KNDy neurons in the arcuate nucleus influence both the GnRH cell body and the neurosecretory terminals [16]. Since KNDy neurons express both neurokinin B receptors and kappa opioid receptors, it has been postulated that the reciprocating interplay of stimulatory neurokinin B and inhibitory dynorphin causes pulsatile release of kisspeptin, which then triggers GnRH pulsatile release [17] (Fig. 7.1).

FHA implies both anovulation and amenorrhea. However, lesser degrees of inhibition of GnRH may result in luteal insufficiency or anovulatory cycling [13]. Persistently low concentrations of gonadotropins in the presence of low estradiol concentrations (<60 pg/mL) suggest hypothalamic hypogonadism.

Given the metabolic demands of reproduction, it is not surprising that nutritional intake regulates reproduction. Identification of neuropeptides that alter feeding behaviors has provided a physiological mechanism to explain alterations in the HPO-endometrial axis of individuals who experience significant changes in nutritional status. Three key peptides, neuropeptide Y (NPY), leptin, and ghrelin, regulate feeding behavior and mediate the link between nutrition and reproduction.

Leptin, the product of the *ob* gene, is a 167 amino acid polypeptide that is primarily synthesized by adipocytes but also by the skeletal muscle, heart, stomach, and the placental-fetal unit. A member of the cytokine family, leptin, is classified as an anorexigenic peptide. In contrast, orexigenic peptides such as neuropeptide Y and the agouti-related peptide antagonize the actions of leptin. Patients suffering from hypothalamic amenorrhea display lower serum leptin concentrations compared with age-, weight-, and body fat-matched eumenorrheic controls. Recovery from FHA is associated with an increase in leptin independent of an increase in body weight [19]. Leptin likely plays a significant role in communicating nutritional status to the cascade that regulates HPO activity. Studies have demonstrated that ultradian fluctuations in leptin levels show pattern synchrony with those of both LH and estradiol [20].

Ghrelin is a polypeptide that stimulates appetite but conversely reduces fat utilization [21]. Additionally, ghrelin inhibits the HPO axis and is the primary peptide

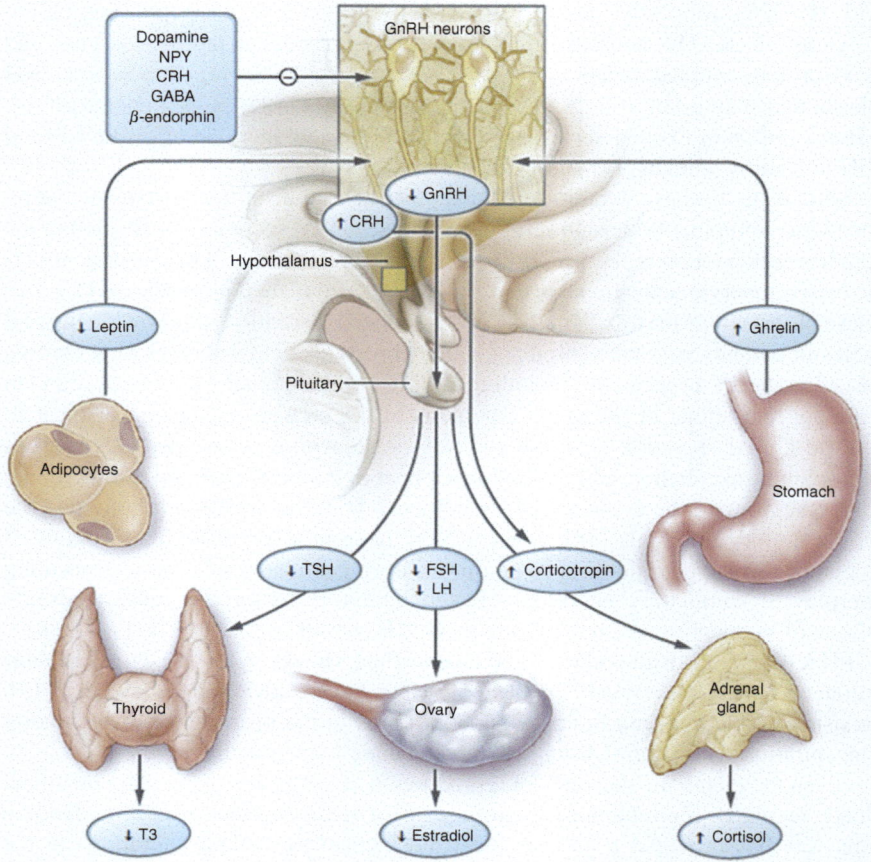

Fig. 7.1 Hormonal changes seen in women with functional hypothalamic amenorrhea (FHA). Three major classes of FHA exist, namely, stress, exercise, or weight loss induced. In addition to a loss of GnRH pulsatility, other changes include an overactive hypothalamic-pituitary-adrenal axis and a thyroid pattern similar to the one seen in chronic illness or starvation [2, 18]

responsible for the prolongation of amenorrhea in subjects who have regained normal weight [22]. Women with FHA are characterized by elevated ghrelin levels compared with eumenorrheic women [23]. Furthermore, heavily exercising or underweight amenorrheic patients have a tendency to exhibit a significantly greater serum ghrelin elevation than those who remain at a stable and healthy weight [24]. Miljic et al. demonstrated that women with anorexia nervosa are resistant to the orexigenic properties of ghrelin [25]. NPY affects the appetite center in the hypothalamus and can stimulate feeding behavior [26] and also directly stimulates GnRH secretion when estradiol levels are high. Conversely, NPY can inhibit GnRH secretion in hypoestrogenic states [27]. Meczekalski et al. observed lower basal serum NPY levels in amenorrheic hypoestrogenic women compared to their eumenorrheic counterparts [28]. Neuropeptides reflect ongoing nutritional status, body habitus, and physical stress and through direct and indirect mechanisms modulate reproductive function including GnRH drive. Further, neuropeptides that regulate the hypothalamus may also directly impact endometrium. Identifying direct endometrial effects will require in vitro models.

Stress and FHA

Physical and emotional stressors result in multiple neuroendocrine adaptations including activation of the hypothalamic-pituitary-adrenal axis (HPA), which manifests as increased circulating and cerebrospinal fluid levels of glucocorticoids [2, 29]. While appropriate levels of cortisol are critical for health, including establishment and maintenance of fertility, stress-induced excess can be detrimental [30]. During stress, the increase in cortisol occurs primarily at night during sleep [2, 19], making it difficult to detect elevated cortisol with a single blood, urine, or salivary sample [29, 31].

Stress alters central GABAergic function [32]; GABA modulates the neuroendocrine cascade that regulates GnRH pulsatility [9, 33]. Figure 7.2 illustrates the anatomy of the regulation of GnRH neurons [9]. Glucocorticoids also have direct effects on hypothalamic function. For instance, Kiss1 neurons in the anteroventral periventricular nucleus and periventricular nucleus continuum of the preoptic area of the hypothalamus express glucocorticoid receptors at relatively robust concentrations in rats, suggesting that glucocorticoids can act directly on these neurons [34]. In

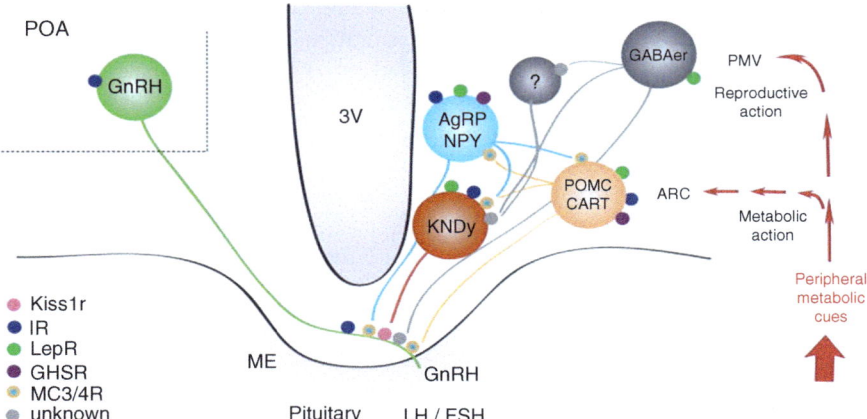

Fig. 7.2 Schematic representation of the neural interactions between metabolic and reproductive functions depicting the likely sites of action of leptin, insulin, and ghrelin to control gonadotropin-releasing hormone (GnRH) release. *3V* third ventricle, *ARC* arcuate nucleus, *ME* median eminence, *PMV* ventral pre-mammillary nucleus, *POA* preoptic area [9]

mice, in situ hybridization analyses revealed that corticosterone treatment diminishes both the absolute number of Kiss1 neurons as well as the levels of *Kiss1* mRNA per cell [35]. Furthermore, corticosterone treatment blunts pituitary expression of the genes encoding the GnRH receptor and LHβ, indicating a direct inhibition of gonadotropes. This represents a novel mechanism by which stress-induced increases in glucocorticoids may alter GnRH pulsatility. A newly discovered mammalian neuropeptide, RF-amide-related peptide-3 (RFRP3), may inhibit GnRH secretion and gonadotrope responsiveness through direct effects on GnRH and Kiss1 neurons [36]. Neuronal pathways secreting this hormone, also known as gonadotropin-inhibitory hormone (GnIH), may directly affect GnRH and Kiss1 neurons. Recent data demonstrate that acute and chronic stressors in sheep increase the function of GnIH neurons [37]. In mice, immobilization stress-induced upregulation of GnIH and inhibited LH releases from the pituitary. Adrenalectomy blocked the expression of GnIH [38].

Stress does more than inhibit GnRH drive. The "stress response complex" includes CRH, ACTH, GH, PRL, oxytocin, vasopressin, norepinephrine, and epinephrine [39]. Physical or mental stress causes acute release of CRH secretion centrally, leading to pituitary secretion of ACTH and other pro-opiomelanocortin (POMC)-related peptides such as beta-endorphin [40]. Both animal models and human studies demonstrate a direct antagonistic effect of CRH on GnRH pulsatility [41]. In one study, prolonged and intermittent infusion of CRH into the third cerebral ventricle of follicular phase ewes resulted in a significant decrease in GnRH mRNA levels in the hypothalamus. Conversely, institution of a CRH signaling blockade through administration of CRH receptor antagonists results in an increase in GnRH transcriptional activity. Michopoulos et al. showed that administration of a CRH antagonist to monkeys reversed the GABAergic activation caused by the stress of subordination [32]. Modification of the stress response may restore physiologic HPO activity and is associated with restoration of other neuroendocrine and metabolic aberrations. A randomized controlled trial of 16 women treated with cognitive behavior therapy (CBT) versus observation showed that CBT not only restored normal ovulatory function but also simultaneously reduced nocturnal cortisol secretion [32, 42]; this RCT provides additional validation of the notion that FHA is caused by stress. Additionally, other neuroendocrine and metabolic components such as TSH and leptin levels were increased in CBT-treated women compared to controls. This study not only underscores the effect of stress on reproductive function, it also highlights the therapeutic importance of active stress management for stress-induced infertility.

Endometrial Exposure to Glucocorticoids as a Model to Explore Causes of Implantation Failure

The detrimental effects of psychological and physical stress on endometrial function are increasingly recognized and can occur via direct or indirect pathways. Partial or complete suppression of the HPO axis results in lower estradiol and progesterone secretion which, in turn, alters endometrial development. Subtle alterations may diminish endometrial receptivity. For instance, restraint stress for as little as 2 h causes significant decreases in estradiol and progesterone levels in murine models [43]. As a consequence, the psychogenic stress caused by restraint results in decreased endometrial receptivity, and thereby pregnancy rates, in mice. However, the story is likely much more complex than exposure of the endometrium to lower estradiol and progesterone levels.

Direct, local, uterine mediators include reactive oxygen species [44], endoplasmic reticulum stress [45], catecholamines, and glucocorticoid hormones [46]. Cytotoxic cytokines, such as IL-1β and TNF-α, predominantly derived from infiltrating uterine macrophages, also can interfere with the epithelioid differentiation of decidualized endometrium as a result of inflammatory stress [47]. Alternatively, stress can indirectly impact the uterus via the HPO axis, inhibiting gonadotropins and perturbing physiological patterns of estradiol and progesterone secretion required for endometrial receptivity [48].

In the early days of assisted reproductive technologies, a number of practitioners postulated that local endometrial inflammation in the peri-implantation environment might compromise uterine receptivity and early pregnancy establishment. Immunosuppressive doses of glucocorticoids (e.g., 60 mg/day of methylprednisolone for 4 days) became a standard of care and were advocated, initially, based on a nonrandomized study of women undergoing IVF-ET [49]. However, subsequent randomized, prospective, double-blinded clinical trials [50, 51] failed to show either a benefit or risk of a short course of peri-implantation glucocorticoids. Despite these findings, the habit of routine corticosteroid administration during the peri-implantation persists in some practices. A recent report from a single, large center compared a historical cohort of 442 subjects from 2014, when methylprednisolone and doxycycline were routinely given for 4 days, to a cohort of 434 women treated the following year without the supplemental medications. Their findings showed a nonsignificant trend ($P = 0.10$) for higher clinical pregnancy rates (56.1 vs. 61.5%) in the unmedicated cohort, but blastocyst stage embryos, frozen transfers, and lower age at transfer were all more prevalent in the latter group [52].

As biochemical mediators of chronic stress have long been suspected to reduce embryonic implantation success in women, and glucocorticoids are known to antagonize estrogen-regulated genes in endometrial cell lines [53], we undertook a study in our translational model of decidualized human endometrial stromal cells (ESC). Human ESC cultures were treated for 7 days with 10 nM estradiol, 100 nM progesterone, and 0.5 mM dibutyryl cAMP (E/P/c) to induce decidualization [54]. Some cultures were co-incubated with cortisol (1 μM) or methylprednisolone (267 nM) for up to 7 days. Cortisol alone increased the secretion of IL-11 and the combination of E/P/c and glucocorticoids resulted in a small (~50%) increase in prolactin secretion. As IL-11 and prolactin are markers of decidual differentiation, these results suggest that supplementation of glucocorticoids in the in vitro paradigm might accelerate ESC decidualization.

Given that the extant molecular and in vitro data are divergent and the clinical data show no benefit of methylprednisolone treatment, we believe that the prudent practice currently is to avoid the use of glucocorticoid exposure to the peri-implantation endometrium. One limitation of the cellular studies is that they do not necessarily mimic stress per se. Thus, one can conclude that understanding the effects of chronic stress and its myriad mediators will require more sophisticated in vitro and in vivo models of endometrial function.

Obesity as a Reproductive Stressor and Contributor to Implantation Failure

Obesity may result from psychogenic stress and simultaneously can cause metabolic stress. Obesity is common among women of reproductive age and has many reproductive consequences including anovulation, infertility, menorrhagia, and adverse pregnancy outcomes. Significant debate exists as to which components of the reproductive process are affected most by obesity. While some investigators have focused on the adverse effects of obesity on oocyte quality, others have delineated the impact upon endometrium [55]. However, obesity is not uniformly adverse and may represent adaption to low fuel environments that thereby allows pregnancy to occur in more extreme environments.

Obesity is typically assessed by body mass index (BMI), but the type of obesity plays a role in determining its health effects. In general, abdominal adiposity is associated with greater risks of diabetes and cardiovascular disease than is gynecoid obesity. In most modern societies, consumption of refined sugars drives obesity. Evaluation of the effect of consumption of refined sugars on oocyte and embryo quality was studied in rhesus monkeys. Monkeys fed a low-dose sucrose diet were compared to those fed a standard high protein biscuit diet for 6 months followed by controlled ovarian stimulation. The ability of oocytes to resume meiosis was significantly impaired in the high-sucrose group [56], although the differentiation of the somatic component of the ovarian follicle into progesterone-producing cells was not altered. While a small subset of oocytes in the high-sucrose group were fertilized in vitro and developed into preimplantation blastocysts, there were >1100 changes in blastocyst gene expression. Because sucrose treatment ended before fertilization, the effects of sugar intake by healthy primates were attributed to epigenetic modifications in the immature oocyte that are manifest in the preimplantation embryo [56].

Obesity may be an easily recognized marker of stress. For instance, subordinated monkeys ate more food than the dominant monkeys if they had access to high-fat, high-sugar chow [57]. Michopoulos and Wilson found that subordinated monkeys not only ate more high-fat, high-sugar chow but also displayed higher cortisol reactions to stressors; this coupling has been termed "emotional feeding." Antagonism of stress with the CRH receptor antagonist antalarmin attenuated the caloric intake of subordinated rhesus monkeys [58]. Further, higher cortisol levels after dexamethasone suppression predicted increased consumption of a high-fat, high-sugar diet over the low-fat, high-fiber diet. Surprisingly, a choice of diets amplified the cortisol response to the stress of social separation [59]. When stressed monkeys have ready access to energy dense foods, overeating and weight gain result. Taken together, the above observations suggest that stress causes overeating of high-calorie foods and that obesity may be an easily recognized marker of stress in fuel-replete environments.

The effect of elevated BMI on oocyte quality was investigated in women undergoing in vitro fertilization (IVF). A higher percentage of oocytes with granular cytoplasm, which is typically a marker of poor quality, was found in women with BMI ≥ 25 ($p = 0.04$). However, percentages of mature, immature oocytes and germinal vesicles were similar in overweight and normal weight patients. No differences were found in fertilization and cleavage rates and percentages of embryo quality. The implantation rate ($p < 0.001$) was significantly lower in the overweight group than in the normal weight group. The amount of gonadotropins used was significantly higher in the overweight group ($p = 0.003$). These findings suggest that the poor reproductive outcome of obese women is influenced by the release of ova with reduced fertilization potential [60].

Impact of Stress on Oocyte Epigenetics and Impaired Implantation

Normal Oocyte Development and Epigenetics

Epigenetics was first introduced by Conrad Waddington [61] as "the branch of biology which studies the causal interactions between genes and their products which bring phenotypes into being." Epigenetic regulation of the oocyte has implications for both its health and the success of the future pregnancy. In essence, oocyte gene products (e.g., mRNAs, proteins) can linger for indefinite amounts of time, only to be activated at a precise moment, often at fertilization, to sustain embryonic health. These entities are called effector genes and are critical for the success of the oocyte, embryo, and pregnancy.

Successful folliculogenesis and oocyte growth, necessary components of normal fertilization and early embryo development, have fascinated biologists for centuries. The interplay between the ovarian somatic components and the oocyte is carefully mediated by hormones and growth factors in the HPO axis [62]. There appears to be a complex bidirectional communication, under control of the oocyte [63], Via local factors exchanged between the oocyte and its surrounding somatic cells that is essential for the future health of a pregnancy (Fig. 7.3).

The process of oocyte growth, taking up to 150 days, begins as primordial follicles emerge from quiescence. Early morphologic changes in the follicle are marked by proliferation of the granulosa cells, growth of the oocyte, and initial formation of the zona pellucida. Secondary oocytes (e.g., pre-antral follicles) form with the emergence of theca cells as well as the development of FSH and steroid receptors

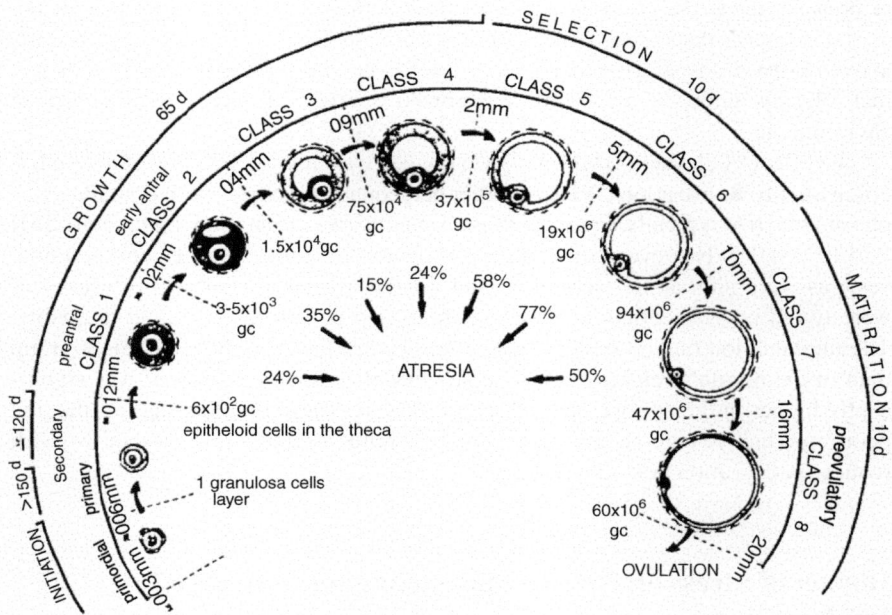

Fig. 7.3 Stages of follicular growth in the adult human ovary. Folliculogenesis is divided into two major periods, pre-antral (FSH independent) and antral (FSH dependent). Primordial follicles are defined by a single layer of granulosa cells and the development of the zona pellucida. Secondary or pre-antral follicles are defined by the presence of theca cells as well as FSH and steroid receptors on the granulosa cells [64]

on the granulosa cells. The growth of these early primordial and pre-antral follicles is FSH independent but represents the pool from which FSH recruitment and ultimate oocyte dominance occur [64]. In hypophysectomized animals, early oocyte growth and development occurs without FSH, but perhaps at a slower rate [65].

While there is often a focus on improper meiotic segregation which can lead to aneuploidy, especially in the older woman [66], the early pre-antral oocyte is a metabolically active and dynamic cell, forming most of the cytoplasm, nuclear components, and organelles that will be relayed to the embryo at fertilization. The epigenetic modifications essential for fetal development, such as the cytoplasmic skeleton and the intracellular distribution of organelles, begin to be established during the pre-antral stage [67].

For many of these epigenetic regulators, the oocyte gene products as proteins are often selectively localized in the cytoplasm and protected from degradation, thereby leading to their function at the precise time in early embryo development. This appears to be an important principle in epigenetics; namely, oocyte protein products are better regulators than mRNA due to the ability of the oocyte and embryo to selectively localize and protect proteins until their use as well as the depletion of maternal mRNA at embryo gene activation.

Ratnam et al. demonstrated the importance of protein localization during embryo development [68]. An important methylation enzyme, DMNT1, is translated during oogenesis but is localized in the oocyte cortex where it remains inactive. At specifically the 8-cell embryo stage, Dmnt1 moves into the nucleus to cause its effect on the dimethyl-transferase gene. Knocking out the Dnmt1 gene leads to embryo arrest at the morula stage. This protein is produced during oocyte maturation but remains inactive until the eight-cell stage of the embryo, when it moves into the nucleus to effect remethylation of the genome. This is a prime example of how ovarian health, more than just having the correct chromosome complement, is vital to the success of the pregnancy.

The transition from secondary follicle to an antral follicle and resultant FSH dependence is an important and vital step in the maturation of the oocyte and subsequent successful development of the embryo. Promoted by FSH, the process involves influx of fluid and development of the antrum which appears to be an important factor in growth and maturation of the oocyte-cumulus complex and its subsequent release at ovulation [69]. A few days prior to ovulation, granulosa cells proliferate in combination with a rapid accumulation of antral fluid, turning the complex into a preovulatory Graafian follicle.

Final oocyte maturation is a complex process involving both the cumulus cells and the actual oocyte. Both the nuclear changes and the cytoplasmic changes are critical in the development of an egg that can be fertilized and develop to a healthy blastocyst. While the focus of this section involves epigenetic changes, a brief overview of nuclear developments is in order. First, the preovulatory oocyte is arrested in prophase of meiosis I. Following development of LH receptors on the granulosa cells of the dominant follicle, an LH surge (in response to a critical level and duration of estrogen from the follicle) leads to three important events. First, there is the resumption of meiosis I with subsequent arrest in metaphase of meiosis II. Second, there is luteinization of the granulosa cells with subsequent production of progesterone. Third, there is the proteolytic release of the egg from the ovary in response to the LH surge.

Furthermore, the LH surge leads to an important cytoplasmic maturation that occurs in concert with the genetic changes noted above. Specific genes, oocyte mRNAs, and subsequent proteins reorder the cytoskeleton to promote successful early embryo development and implantation. The endoplasmic reticulum and mitochondria move toward the oocyte cortex [70], while the egg loses its ability to synthesize new proteins. By moving between active and quiescent, maternal mRNAs provide important proteins at key times in the life of the individual.

The journey from a primordial follicle to an embryo involves a precise interplay of cytoplasmic and genetic events, involving both critical timing and critical proteins. While the overall time frame from primordial follicle to egg maturity is important, there are also key moments in the life of the egg that are vital for successful fertilization. For example, knockout mice lacking oocyte zona pellucida protein 3 show defective follicle development and cumulus-oocyte complex formation [71]. Essential trophic factors appear to be important in preventing atresia [72], and several cytoplasmic proteins have been implicated in the process of atresia, including sphingomyelinase, Fas, and Caspase-12 [73–75]. Fertilization is also under epigenetic control, as evidenced by knockout of the cMOS gene which leads to parthenogenetic activation of the egg [76].

While epigenetics are critical for successful ovulation and fertilization, this is not the end of the story. There are also multiple maternal effector genes that are activated at critical moments in the life of the early embryo. In addition to DMNT1 noted above, the absence of nucleoplasmin 2 (NMP2) leads to arrest at the one cell stage [77], and E-cadherin and gamma tubulin have been shown to be important in the compaction of the embryo at the morula stage [78]. It certainly appears to be a continuum from primordial follicle to healthy individual, with the actual number of chromosomes representing only a small part of the story. As shown above, the precise timing of key oocyte effector genes is critical in the life and health of the individual.

Environment, Stress, and Epigenetics

Since Waddington first introduced the concept of epigenetics, there are increasing data suggesting that the egg and embryo environment are important factors in the later health of the individual. Barker et al. laid the groundwork for a fetal basis of adult disease in 1992 [79]. Perera and Herbstman provided evidence that prenatal exposure to environmental chemicals can lead to both developmental disorders and disease that present in childhood or later in adulthood [80]. Several retrospective studies have linked periods of caloric restriction during early pregnancy to disease states in the adult, providing some of the earliest evidence for epigenetic effects during the postfertilization period [81, 82]. These studies demonstrate the ability of the fetus to adjust its metabolic pathways based on its environment within its mother, thereby preparing itself for its future survival.

Evidence continues to mount revealing the importance of the maternal diet to the health of the oocyte and the embryo. During the peri-implantation window, even a modest reduction in maternal protein consumption can lead to hypertension in the adult [83]. Furthermore, enzymes important in methylation of the genome are known to be regulated by maternal folate intake [84]. As discussed earlier, Chaffin et al. showed that increased dietary sugar inhibits oocyte maturation and early embryo development even though the oocytes were removed and fertilized under euglycemic conditions [56]. In addition, higher BMI is associated with lower IVF success rates, but this effect is reversed with the use of donor oocytes, suggesting an important impact of obesity on the developing egg [85]. Since obesity may be a marker of stress, it is unclear whether the detrimental effect on oocytes is due primarily to stress or some other underlying metabolic conditions.

There is also increasing evidence linking the important role of thyroid function in the success of both natural conceptions and those conceived via IVF. With regard to thyroid antibodies, Weghofer et al. correlated rising TSH levels and possibly TPO antibodies to impaired embryo quality [86], while Scoccia et al. showed that despite levothyroxine treatment, women with hypothyroidism have a decreased chance of achieving pregnancy following IVF [87]. Furthermore, a recent meta-analysis correlated thyroid supplementation to improved clinical outcome in women with subclinical hypothyroidism [88]. While further studies are needed to elucidate the mechanism, many authors support lowering TSH levels to below 2.5 to optimize pregnancy rates in IVF as well as term delivery rates and birthweight [89, 90]. While the mechanism may remain unclear, it appears that the thyroid has an important epigenetic role in the health of the embryo and future pregnancy.

The impact of stress on the oocyte and early embryo is becoming increasingly important due in part to the emerging role of IVF in our society. In 2015, there were 72,913 live born infants in the USA alone from IVF, accounting for roughly 1.8% of all babies born [91]. This number continues to increase year by year. Babies born from IVF have been shown to have an increased incidence of preterm birth and low birth weight for gestational age. In 2015, roughly 21.9% of the births from IVF were preterm, compared to only 9.6% in the general population [92]. While unproven, preterm births and low birth weight remain as possible predictors of the onset of adult metabolic diseases. While studies are conflicting, there is also the suggestion of an increased incidence of birth defects in babies born from IVF, namely, imprinting disorders such as Beckwith-Wiedemann and Prader-Willi syndromes [93]. Epigenetic dysregulation of the methylation silencing of the genome is theorized as a possible cause of these imprinting disorders.

In vitro produced embryos show clear effects of the culture medium on gene expression [94]. Also, methylation of the embryo genome is impacted by the culture media ingredients, revealing a susceptibility of the early embryo to epigenetic programming [95]. Embryo growth factors can also be used in culture media to aid embryonic survival and health [96]. Embryo culture conditions have also been shown to alter blastomere allocation between the inner cell mass and trophectoderm [97] as well as placental morphology and function [98], leading to adverse fetal development and the onset of adult diseases [99]. Whether these alterations which lead to low birth weight and future disease states are purely the result of embryo culture versus abnormal oocyte epigenetics remains to be seen. But in either regard, gene expression in the preimplantation embryo is vital to the future health of the pregnancy and offspring. Which critical epigenetic factors in oocytes and embryos are important remain to be identified.

In 2002, Leese postulated that an embryo with a "calm" metabolic state is more viable than the embryo with an overactive metabolism [100]. Mitochondrial DNA levels have been proposed as a marker of a stressed embryo, such that conditions which deviate from normal (i.e., aneuploidy, chemical stress, maternal age) tend to show higher mitochondrial DNA levels and lower frequency of a live birth [101]. Since distressed embryos may be prone to a higher energy level as a compensatory mechanism, mitochondrial DNA has been proposed as a biomarker for embryo viability [102]. However, a recent report questioned the current technology of determining mitochondrial DNA content and found an equal amount of mitochondrial DNA between blastocysts stratified by age and implantation potential [103]. In addition to possible use in determining embryo viability, there are also data suggesting that stressed oocytes show a marked alteration in mitochondrial function and distribution, once again revealing the epigenetic importance of a healthy oocyte to the viability of the pregnancy [104]. More studies are needed to determine the usefulness of mitochondrial DNA as a marker of embryo viability.

There is further evidence that stress plays an epigenetic role in the process from early oocyte to healthy embryo. Information can be transmitted from parent to offspring through epigenetic marks in germ cells, including microRNA. Rodgers et al. demonstrated that sperm microRNAs, identified in a stress model, functionally reduce maternal mRNA stores in early embryos, thereby altering gene expression in the offspring [105]. Furthermore, stress in the form of heat shock has been shown to disrupt nuclear maturation through cytoskeletal defects, leading to either failed fertilization or abnormal embryo development [106]. Other authors have proposed that stress-related epigenetic modifications work through disruption of heterochromatin structure [107].

Other epigenetic effects are expressed through corticosteroids. Their action in target organs is regulated by relative activities of enzymes responsible for conversion of cortisone to cortisol or inactivation of cortisol. A recent study showed that the bovine cumulus ovarian complex can modulate the level of cortisol through relative activities of these enzymes, thereby creating an environment conducive to fertilization and subsequent embryo development [108]. Furthermore, the enzyme responsible for cortisol degradation appears to increase activity during oocyte maturation, leading to lower levels of functional corticosteroids in the early embryo [109]. In chickens, corticosteroids have been shown to reduce the length of erythrocyte telomeres [110].

Finally, Nesan and Vijayan showed that in the zebrafish model, cortisol plays an important role in corticosteroid receptors that in turn are transcription factors able to modulate downstream gene expression in a host of developmental events [111]. For example, increased cortisol in the newly fertilized embryo causes a disruption in cardiogenesis. They further postulate that this epigenetic modification in early embryos is due to maternal cortisol, since the embryo begins synthesizing cortisol only at the hatching stage. If glucocorticoids are developmental regulators, then maternal stress during folliculogenesis could disrupt the normal development of the early embryo through impaired organogenesis and growth. They also argue that proper regulation of embryo cortisol levels is important for a normal stress response in the adult. An appropriate level of cortisol, the key stress hormone in women, appears crucial for both normal fertilization and subsequent normal development in the early embryo. In other words, an abnormal stress pattern in women can lead to ovulation disorders as well as faulty early embryo development.

In summary, oocyte epigenetics play a key role in the future health of the preimplantation embryo, and environmental conditions surrounding the early embryo influence the health of the future offspring. The oocyte and the preimplantation embryo need to sequester maternal effector genes and, at the right moment, express proteins for successful health and development. This is accomplished through timely cytoskeletal remodeling and gene activation. Stress likely impacts many if not all of the processes delineated above.

Reproductive aging is an increasing problem in the field of infertility, and stress has been shown to accelerate the aging process. Most research in the field of reproductive aging centers on the oocyte DNA during oogenesis and the impact of chromosome segregation both before and after fertilization. Many steps in oogenesis are at risk for epigenetic alterations that can have long-lasting impact on the offspring. In addition to aneuploidy, we need to also consider the effects of hormonal imbalance, lifestyle modifications, and culture conditions on the developmental competence of the oocyte and preimplantation embryo. The health of the offspring is not only dependent on the right number of chromosomes but also on the appropriate expression of genes at critical moments of oocyte and embryo maturation. These critical moments in the life of the oocyte and embryo can be greatly affected by epigenetic imprinting which in turn reflects the sum of exposures including environmental toxins and behavioral stressors of all types.

Impact of Lab Stress upon Embryo Health and Implantation

Healthy embryos have a higher probability of implantation, and many of the advances in IVF relate to minimizing the stress of embryo culture. The IVF process, including embryo culture, not only distorts the innate physiological processes that promote embryo health, but it also introduces many additional stressors. Oocytes and embryos are always exposed to oxidative stress (OS), but antioxidants present in the reproductive tissues protect embryos in vivo. Oxidative stress has been implicated as one of the factors responsible for unsatisfactory outcomes in ART. During in vitro culture, there are several sources of oxidative stress including:

- High oxygen tension
- Composition and pH of the culture media
- Exposure to light
- Air quality

Oxygen Concentration

In ART laboratories, embryos are either cultured in an atmospheric oxygen concentration of 20% or reduced oxygen concentration of 5–6%. Oxygen plays an essential role in cell growth and differentiation, but the presence of high concentrations of oxygen during incubation activates various cellular oxidase enzymes. Multiple reports have demonstrated that compared to embryos cultured under atmospheric oxygen conditions, those cultured at 5% oxygen yielded better embryo quality during IVF cycles. Production of reactive oxygen species (ROS) during embryo culture has been attributed to atmospheric oxygen conditions and also has been implicated as a main contributor to poor embryo development. However, cause and effect have not been demonstrated. While an increase in antioxidant gene expression under 20% oxygen has not been observed, reducing oxygen tension promotes better embryo development in vitro than treatment with detoxifying enzymes [112].

Culture Media

The high energy demands of the mammalian preimplantation embryo are critical to creating vulnerability to preimplantation metabolic stressors. In vitro, the accumulation of metabolic derivatives, including carbohydrate substrates or toxic byproducts, may contaminate culture media and affect energy usage by embryos. In vitro culture is a closed system compared with the metabolic waste dissipation capacities provided by the oviduct (which to an embryo are essentially infinite [113]. Variations in nutrient availability alter developmental competence [114], implying that culture in vitro is a source of great stress. The pH of culture media is also a source of in vitro stress. The pH of culture conditions is often unstable, and pH is a powerful modulator of metabolic activity. Changes to pH (or lack thereof) could perturb metabolic homeostasis, stimulate or prevent induction of specific molecular pathways, and facilitate potentially irreversible metabolic changes.

Exposure to Light

There are several ways that light might affect a cell. There may be a direct effect where light "stresses" the cell, activates stress genes, or even damages DNA directly via ionization. Light has been linked to increased production of ROS and to DNA damage. Light has also been implicated in the oxidation of oil used in the culture of human embryos [115]. Embryology laboratories should not be located in areas where direct sunlight might damage them. Care should be taken with hood lights, ambient lights, headlamps, and microscope lamps [116]. It is important to continue to evaluate the role light might play in the production and growth of human embryos.

Air Quality

Volatile organic compounds (VOCs) are a major stressor to the development of embryos in vitro. Their removal should be an integral element of air cleanliness in IVF. Removal of VOCs is achieved by potassium permanganate-impregnated, activated carbon filters. In vitro fertilization laboratories aiming to control air pollution should integrate both air particle and VOC filtration. Better air quality conditions are associated with higher embryo development, implantation, and live birth rates [117].

Summary

Stress is the product of a complex integration of physiological reactions that seek to promote survival of the individual. The panoply of biological consequences initiated by stress, only some of which are delineated above, may compromise not only acute reproductive function but also future reproductive potential. Identification and management of stressors have the potential to improve reproductive outcomes.

References

1. Berga SL, Mortola JF, Yen S. Amplification of nocturnal melatonin secretion in women with functional hypothalamic amenorrhea. J Clin Endocrinol Metab. 1988;66(1):242–4.
2. Berga SL, Mortola JF, Girton L, Suh B, Laughlin G, Pham P, Yen SS. Neuroendocrine aberrations in women with functional hypothalamic amenorrhea. J Clin Endocrinol Metab. 1989;68(2):301–8.
3. Liu JH. Hypothalamic amenorrhea: clinical perspectives, pathophysiology, and management. Am J Obstet Gynecol. 1990;163:1732–6.
4. Berga SL. Stress and reproduction: a tale of false dichotomy? Endocrinology. 2008;149(3):867–8. https://doi.org/10.1210/en.2008-0004.
5. Clarke IJ. Control of GnRH secretion. J Reprod Fertil Suppl. 1987;34:1–8.
6. Prevot V. GnRH neurons directly listen to the periphery. Endocrinology. 2011;152(10):3589–91. https://doi.org/10.1210/en.2011-1544.
7. Prevot V. Glial-neuronal-endothelial interactions are involved in the control of GnRH secretion. J Neuroendocrinol. 2002;14(3):247–55.
8. Zsarnovszky A, Horvath TL, Garcia-Segura LM, Horvath B, Naftolin F. Oestrogen-induced changes in the synaptology of the monkey (Cercopithecus aethiops) arcuate nucleus during gonadotropin feedback. J Neuroendocrinol. 2001;13:22–8.
9. Navarro VM, Kaiser UB. Metabolic influences on neuroendocrine regulation of reproduction. Curr Opin Endocrinol Diabetes Obes. 2013;20(4):335–41. https://doi.org/10.1097/MED.0b013e32836318ce.
10. Funes S, Hedrick JA, Vassileva G, Markowitz L, Abbondanzo S, Golovko A, Yang S, Monsma FJ, Gustafson EL. The KiSS-1 receptor GPR54 is essential for the development of the murine reproductive system. Biochem Biophys Res Commun. 2003;312(4):1357–63.
11. Roa J, Tena-Sempere M. KiSS-1 system and reproduction: comparative aspects and roles in the control of female gonadotropic axis in mammals. Gen Comp Endocrinol. 2007;153(1-3):132–40.
12. Sills ES, Walsh AP. The GPR54-Kisspeptin complex in reproductive biology: neuroendocrine significance and implications for ovulation induction and contraception. Neuro Endocrinol Lett. 2008;29(6):846–51.
13. Berga S, Naftolin F. Neuroendocrine control of ovulation. Gynecol Endocrinol. 2012;28(Suppl 1):9–13.
14. Filicori M, Santoro N, Merriam GR, Crowley WF. Characterization of the physiological pattern of episodic gonadotropin secretion throughout the human menstrual cycle. J Clin Endocrinol Metab. 1986;62:1136–44.
15. Brann DW, Mahesh VB. Excitatory amino acids: function and significance in reproduction and neuroendocrine regulation. Front Neuroendocrinol. 1994;15:3.
16. Goodman RL, Lehman MN, Smith JT, Coolen LM, de Oliveira CV, Jafarzadehshirazi MR, Pereira A, Iqbal J, Caraty A, Ciofi P, et al. Kisspeptin neurons in the arcuate nucleus of the ewe express both dynorphin A and neurokinin B. Endocrinology. 2007;148(12):5752–60.

17. Rance NE, Krajewski SJ, Smith MA, Cholanian M, Dacks PA. Neurokinin B and the hypothalamic regulation of reproduction. Brain Res. 2010;1364(116–28.
18. Gordon CM. Clinical practice. Functional hypothalamic amenorrhea. N Engl J Med. 2010;363(4):365–71.
19. Michopoulos V, Mancini F, Loucks TL, Berga SL. Neuroendocrine recovery initiated by cognitive behavioral therapy in women with functional hypothalamic amenorrhea: a randomized, controlled trial. Fertil Steril. 2013;99(7):2084–91.e1.
20. Licinio J, Negrão AB, Mantzoros C, Kaklamani V, Wong ML, Bongiorno PB, Mulla A, Cearnal L, Veldhuis JD, Flier JS, McCann SM, Gold PW. Synchronicity of frequently sampled, 24-h concentrations of circulating leptin, luteinizing hormone, and estradiol in healthy women. Proc Natl Acad Sci U S A. 1998;95(5):2541–6.
21. Barreiro ML, Tena-Sempere M. Ghrelin and reproduction: a novel signal linking energy status and fertility? Mol Cell Endocrinol. 2004;226(1-2):1–9.
22. Schneider LF, Warren MP. Functional hypothalamic amenorrhea is associated with elevated ghrelin and disordered eating. Fertil Steril. 2006;86(6):1744–9.
23. Tolle V, Kadem M, Bluet-Pajot MT, Frere D, Foulon C, Bossu C, Dardennes R, Mounier C, Zizzari P, Lang F, Epelbaum J, Estour B. Balance in ghrelin and leptin plasma levels in anorexia nervosa patients and constitutionally thin women. J Clin Endocrinol Metab. 2003;88(1):109–16.
24. De Souza MJ, Leidy HJ, O'Donnell E, Lasley B, Williams NI. Fasting ghrelin levels in physically active women: relationship with menstrual disturbances and metabolic hormones. J Clin Endocrinol Metab. 2004;89(7):3536–42.
25. Miljic D, Pekic S, Djurovic M, Doknic M, Milic N, Casanueva FF, Ghatei M, Popovic V. Ghrelin has partial or no effect on appetite, growth hormone, prolactin, and cortisol release in patients with anorexia nervosa. J Clin Endocrinol Metab. 2006;91(4):1491–5.
26. Pedrazzini T, Pralong F, Grouzmann E. Neuropeptide Y: the universal soldier. Cell Mol Life Sci. 2003;60(2):350–77.
27. Kalra SP, Crowley WR. Neuropeptide Y: a novel neuroendocrine peptide in the control of pituitary hormone secretion, and its relation to luteinizing hormone. Front Neuroendocrinol. 1992;13(1):1–46.
28. Meczekalski B, Genazzani AR, Genazzani AD, Warenik-Szymankiewicz A, Luisi M. Clinical evaluation of patients with weight loss-related amenorrhea: neuropeptide Y and luteinizing hormone pulsatility. Gynecol Endocrinol. 2006;22(5):239–43.
29. Brundu B, Loucks TL, Adler LJ, Cameron JL, Berga SL. Increased cortisol in the cerebrospinal fluid of women with functional hypothalamic amenorrhea. J Clin Endocrinol Metab. 2006;91:1561–5.
30. Erichsen MM, Husebye ES, Michelsen TM, Dahl AA, Løvås K. Sexuality and fertility in women with Addison's disease. J Clin Endocrinol Metab. 2010;95(9):4354–60.
31. Berga SL, Daniels TL, Giles DE. Women with functional hypothalamic amenorrhea but not other forms of anovulation display amplified cortisol concentrations. Fertil Steril. 1997;67(6):1024–30.
32. Michopoulos V, Embree M, Reding K, Sanchez MM, Toufexis D, Votaw JR, Voll RJ, Goodman MM, Rivier J, Wilson ME, Berga SL. CRH receptor antagonism reverses the effect of social subordination upon central GABAA receptor binding in estradiol-treated ovariectomized female rhesus monkeys. Neuroscience. 2013;250:300–8.
33. Martin C, Navarro VM, Simavli S, Vong L, Carroll RS, Lowell BB, Kaiser UB. Leptin-responsive GABAergic neurons regulate fertility through pathways that result in reduced kisspeptinergic tone. J Neurosci. 2014;34(17):6047–56. https://doi.org/10.1523/JNEUROSCI.3003-13.2014.
34. Takumi K, Iijima N, Higo S, Ozawa H. Immunohistochemical analysis of the colocalization of corticotropin-releasing hormone receptor and glucocorticoid receptor in kisspeptin neurons in the hypothalamus of female rats. Neurosci Lett. 2012;531(1):40–5.

35. Luo E, Stephens SB, Chaing S, Munaganuru N, Kauffman AS, Breen KM. Corticosterone blocks ovarian cyclicity and the LH surge via decreased kisspeptin neuron activation in female mice. Endocrinology. 2016;157(3):1187–99.
36. Ubuka T, Morgan K, Pawson AJ, Osugi T, Chowdhury VS, Minakata H, Tsutsui K, Millar RP, Bentley GE. Identification of human GnIH homologs, RFRP-1 and RFRP-3, and the cognate receptor, GPR147 in the human hypothalamic pituitary axis. PLoS One. 2009;4(12):e8400.
37. Clarke IJ, Bartolini D, Conductier G, Henry BA. Stress increases gonadotropin inhibitory hormone cell activity and input to GnRH cells in ewes. Endocrinology. 2016;157(11):4339–50.
38. Kirby ED, Geraghty AC, Ubuka T, Bentley GE, Kaufer D. Stress increases putative gonadotropin inhibitory hormone and decreases luteinizing hormone in male rats. Proc Natl Acad Sci U S A. 2009;106(27):11324–9.
39. Liu JH, Patel B, Collins G. Central causes of amenorrhea. In: De Groot LJ, Chrousos G, Dungan K, Feingold KR, Grossman A, Hershman JM, Koch C, Korbonits M, McLachlan R, New M, Purnell J, Rebar R, Singer F, Vinik A, editors. Endotext [internet]. South Dartmouth: MDText.com, Inc.; 2000–2016.
40. Rivier C, Brownstein M, Spiess J, Rivier J, Vale W. In vivo corticotropin-releasing factor-induced secretion of adrenocorticotropin, beta-endorphin, and corticosterone. Endocrinology. 1982;110(1):272–8.
41. Ciechanowska M, Łapot M, Malewski T, Mateusiak K, Misztal T, Przekop F. Effects of corticotropin-releasing hormone and its antagonist on the gene expression of gonadotrophin-releasing hormone (GnRH) and GnRH receptor in the hypothalamus and anterior pituitary gland of follicular phase ewes. Reprod Fertil Dev. 2011;23(6):780–7.
42. Berga SL, Marcus MD, Loucks TL, Hlastala S, Ringham R, Krohn MA. Recovery of ovarian activity in women with functional hypothalamic amenorrhea (FHA) treated with cognitive behavior therapy (CBT). Fertil Steril. 2003;80:976–81.
43. Zhao LH, Cui XZ, Yuan HJ, Liang B, Zheng LL, Liu YX, Luo MJ, Tan JH. Restraint stress inhibits mouse implantation: temporal window and the involvement of HB-EGF, estrogen and progesterone. PLoS One. 2013;8(11):e80472.
44. Sugino N. The role of oxygen radical-mediated signaling pathways in endometrial function. Placenta. 2007;28(Suppl A):S133–6.
45. Taylor RN, Yu J, Torres PB, Schickedanz AC, Park JK, Mueller MD, Sidell N. Mechanistic and therapeutic implications of angiogenesis in endometriosis. Reprod Sci. 2009;16(2):140–6.
46. Whirledge S, Cidlowski JA. Glucocorticoids and reproduction: traffic control on the road to reproduction. Trends Endocrinol Metab. 2017;28(6):399–415.
47. Weiss G, Goldsmith LT, Taylor RN, Bellet D, Taylor HS. Inflammation in reproductive disorders. Reprod Sci. 2009;16(2):216–29.
48. Breen KM, Mellon PL. Influence of stress-induced intermediates on gonadotropin gene expression in gonadotrope cells. Mol Cell Endocrinol. 2014;385(1–2):71–7.
49. Polak de Fried E, Blanco L, Lancuba S, Asch RH. Improvement of clinical pregnancy rate and implantation rate of in-vitro fertilization-embryo transfer patients by using methylprednisone. Hum Reprod. 1993;8(3):393–5.
50. Moffitt D, Queenan JT Jr, Veeck LL, Schoolcraft W, Miller CE, Muasher SJ. Low-dose glucocorticoids after in vitro fertilization and embryo transfer have no significant effect on pregnancy rate. Fertil Steril. 1995;63(3):571–7.
51. Mottla GL, Smotrich DB, Gindoff PR, Stillman RJ. Increasing clinical pregnancy rates after IVF/ET. Can immunosuppression help? J Reprod Med. 1996;41(12):889–91.
52. Kaye L, Bartels C, Bartolucci A, Engmann L, Nulsen J, Benadiva C. Old habits die hard: retrospective analysis of outcomes with use of corticosteroids and antibiotics before embryo transfer. Fertil Steril. 2017;107(6):1336–40.
53. Whirledge S, Xu X, Cidlowski JA. Global gene expression analysis in human uterine epithelial cells defines new targets of glucocorticoid and estradiol antagonism. Biol Reprod. 2013;89(3):66.

54. Yu J, Berga SL, Johnston-MacAnanny EB, Sidell N, Bagchi IC, Bagchi MK, Taylor RN. Endometrial stromal decidualization responds reversibly to hormone stimulation and withdrawal. Endocrinology. 2016;157(6):2432–46.
55. Jungheim ES, Moley KH. Current knowledge of obesity's effects in the pre- and periconceptional periods and avenues for future research. Am J Obstet Gynecol. 2010;203(6):525–30.
56. Chaffin CL, Latham KE, Mtango NR, Midic U, VandeVoort CA. Dietary sugar in healthy female primates perturbs oocyte maturation and in vitro preimplantation embryo development. Endocrinology. 2014;155(7):2688–95.
57. Arce M, Michopoulos V, Shepard KN, Ha QC, Wilson ME. Diet choice, cortisol reactivity, and emotional feeding in socially housed rhesus monkeys. Physiol Behav. 2010;101(4):446–55.
58. Moore CJ, Johnson ZP, Higgins M, Toufexis D, Wilson ME. Antagonism of corticotrophin-releasing factor type 1 receptors attenuates caloric intake of free feeding subordinate female rhesus monkeys in a rich dietary environment. J Neuroendocrinol. 2015;27(1):33–43.
59. Michopoulos V, Toufexis D, Wilson ME. Social stress interacts with diet history to promote emotional feeding in females. Psychoneuroendocrinology. 2012;37(9):1479–90.
60. Depalo R, Garruti G, Totaro I, Panzarino M, Vacca MP, Giorgino F, Selvaggi LE. Oocyte morphological abnormalities in overweight women undergoing in vitro fertilization cycles. Gynecol Endocrinol. 2011;27(11):880–4.
61. Waddington CH. The epigenotype. Endeavor. 1942;1:18–20.
62. Combelles CM, Carabatsos MJ, Kumar TR, et al. Hormonal control of somatic cell oocyte interactions during ovarian follicle development. Mol Reprod Dev. 2004;69:347–55.
63. Matzuk MM, Burns KH, Viveiros MM, Eppig JJ. Intercellular communication in the mammalian ovary: oocytes carry the conversation. Science. 2002;296:2178–80.
64. Gougeon A. Dynamics of follicular growth in the human: a model from preliminary results. Hum Reprod. 1986;1:81–7.
65. Oktay K, Newton H, Mullen J, Gosden RG. Development of human primordial follicles to antral stages in SCID/hpg mice stimulated with follicle stimulating hormone. Hum Reprod. 1998;13:1133–8.
66. Volarcik K, Sheean L, Goldfarb J, et al. The meiotic competence of in-vitro matured human oocytes is influenced by donor age: evidence that folliculogenesis is compromised in the reproductively aged ovary. Hum Reprod. 1998;13:154–60.
67. Pozo J, Corral E, Pereda J. Subcellular structure of prenatal human ovary: mitochondrial distribution during meiotic prophase. J Submicrosc Cytol Pathol. 1990;22:601–7.
68. Ratnam S, Mertineit C, Ding F, et al. Dynamics of Dnmt1 methyltransferase expression and intracellular localization during oogenesis and preimplantation development. Dev Biol. 2002;245:304–14.
69. Irving-Rogers RJ, van Wezel IL, Krupa M, Lavranos TC. Dynamics of the membrane granulosa during expansion of the ovarian follicular antrum. Mol Cell Endocrinol. 2001;171:41–8.
70. Stastna J, Dvorak M, Pilka L. Electron microscopic and cytochemical study of the cortical cytoplasm in the preovulatory human oocyte. Z Mikrosk Anat Forsch. 1983;97:675–87.
71. Rankin T, Familari M, Lee E, et al. Mice homozygous for an insertional mutation in the ZP-3 gene lack a zona pellucida and are infertile. Development. 1996;122:2903–10.
72. Hsueh AJ, Billig H, Tsafriri A. Ovarian follicle atresia: a hormonally controlled apoptotic process. Endocr Rev. 1994;15:707–24.
73. Himelstein-Braw R, Byskov AG, Peters H, Faber M. Follicular atresia in the infant human ovary. J Reprod Fertil. 1976;46:55–9.
74. Pru JK, Tilly JL. Programmed cell death in the ovary: Insights and future prospects using genetic technologies. Mol Endocrinol. 2001;15:845–53.
75. Kondo H, Maruo T, Peng X, Mochizuki M. Immunological evidence for the expression of the Fas antigen in the infant and adult human ovary during follicular regression and atresia. J Clin Endocrinol Metab. 1996;81:2702–10.
76. Colledge W, Carlton MB, Udy GB, Evans MJ. Disruption of c-mos causes parthenogenetic development of unfertilized mouse eggs. Nature. 1994;370:65–8.

77. Burns KH, Viveiros MM, Ren Y, et al. Roles of NMP2 in chromatin and nucleolar organization in oocytes and embryos. Science. 2003;300:633–6.
78. Yuba-Kubo A, Kubo A, Hata M, Tsukita S. Gene knockout analysis of two gamma-tubulin isoforms in mice. Dev Biol. 2005;282:361–73.
79. Law CM, Barker DJ, Osmond C, et al. Early growth and abdominal fatness in adult life. J Epidemiol Community Health. 1992;46:184–6.
80. Perera F, Herbstman J. Prenatal environmental exposures, epigenetics, and disease. Reprod Toxicol. 2011;31:363–73.
81. Elias SG, van Noord PA, Peeters PH, et al. The 1944-1945 Dutch famine and subsequent overall cancer incidence. Cancer Epidemiol Biomark Prev. 2005;14:1981–5.
82. Roseboom TJ, van der Meulen JH, Ravelli AC, et al. Effects of prenatal exposure to the Dutch famine on adult disease in later life: an overview. Mol Cell Endocrinol. 2001;185:93–8.
83. Kwong WY, Wild AE, Roberts P, et al. Maternal under nutrition during the preimplantation period of rat development causes blastocyst abnormalities and programming of postnatal hypertension. Development. 2000;127:4195–202.
84. van Engeland M, Weijenberg MP, et al. Effects of dietary folate and alcohol intake on promoter methylation in sporadic colorectal cancer: the Netherlands cohort study on diet and cancer. Cancer Res. 2003;63:3133–7.
85. Jungheim ES, Schon SB, Schulte MB, et al. IVF outcomes in obese donor oocyte recipients: a systemic review and meta-analysis. Hum Reprod. 2013;28:2720–7.
86. Weghofer A, Himaya E, Kushnir VA, et al. The impact of thyroid function and thyroid autoimmunity on embryo quality in women with low functional ovarian reserve: a case-control study. Reprod Biol Endocrinol. 2015;13:43.
87. Scoccia B, Demir H, Kang Y, et al. In vitro fertilization pregnancy rates in levothyroxine-treated women with hypothyroidism compared to women without thyroid dysfunction disorders. Thyroid. 2012;22:631–6.
88. Velkeniers B, Van Meerhaeghe A, Poppe K, et al. Levothyroxine treatment and pregnancy outcome in women with subclinical hypothyroidism undergoing assisted reproduction technologies: systematic review and meta-analysis of RCTs. Hum Reprod Update. 2013;19:251–8.
89. Fumarola A, Grani G, Romanzi D, et al. Thyroid function in infertile patients undergoing assisted reproduction. Am J Reprod Immunol. 2013;70:336–41.
90. Baker VL, Rone HM, Pasta DJ, et al. Correlation of thyroid stimulating hormone (TSH) level with pregnancy outcome in women undergoing in vitro fertilization. Am J Obstet Gynecol. 2006;194:1668–74.
91. Assisted Reproductive National Data, Centers for Disease Control and Prevention, 2015.
92. National Vital Statistics Reports, Volume 66, Number 1, January 5, 2017.
93. Lazaraviciute G, Kauser M, Bhattacharya S, et al. A systematic review and meta-analysis of DNA methylation levels and imprinting disorders in children conceived by IVF/ICSI compared with children conceived spontaneously. Hum Reprod Update. 2014;20:840–52.
94. Niemann H, Wrenzycki C. Alterations of expression of developmentally important genes in preimplantation bovine embryos by in vitro culture conditions: implications for subsequent development. Theriogenology. 2000;53:21–34.
95. Khosla S, Dean W, Brown D, et al. Culture of preimplantation mouse embryos affects fetal development and the expression of imprinted genes. Biol Reprod. 2001;64:918–26.
96. Rinaudo PF, Schultz RM. Effects of embryo culture on global pattern of gene expression in preimplantation mouse embryos. Reproduction. 2004;128:301–11.
97. Lee ES, Fukui Y, Lee BC, et al. Promoting effect of amino acids added to a chemically defined medium on blastocyst formation and blastomere proliferation of bovine embryos cultured in vitro. Anim Reprod Sci. 2004;84:257–67.
98. Sjoblom C, Roberts CT, Wikland M, Robertson SA. Granulocyte-macrophage colony stimulating factor alleviates adverse consequences of embryo culture on fetal growth trajectory and placental morphogenesis. Endocrinology. 2005;146:2142–53.

99. Anderson CM, Lopez F, Zimmer A, Benoit JN. Placental insufficiency leads to developmental hypertension and mesenteric artery dysfunction in two generations of Sprague-Dawley rat offspring. Biol Reprod. 2006;74:538–44.
100. Leese HJ. Quiet please, do not disturb: a hypothesis of embryo metabolism and viability. BioEssays. 2002;24:845–9.
101. Fragouli E, Spath K, Alfarawati S, et al. Altered levels of mitochondrial DNA are associated with female age, aneuploidy, and provide an independent measure of embryonic implantation potential. PLoS Genet. 2015;11:e1005241.
102. Diez-Juan A, Rubio C, Marin C, et al. Mitochondrial DNA content as a viability score in human euploid embryos: less is better. Fertil Steril. 2015;104:534–41.
103. Victor AR, Brake AJ, Tyndall BA, et al. Accurate quantitation of mitochondrial DNA reveals uniform levels in human blastocysts irrespective of ploidy, age, or implantation potential. Fertil Steril. 2016;107:34–42.
104. Tatone C, Heizenrieder T, Emidio GD, et al. Evidence that carbonyl stress by methylglyoxal exposure induces DNA damage and spindle aberrations, affects mitochondrial integrity in mammalian oocytes and contributes to oocyte aging. Hum Reprod. 2011;26:1843–59.
105. Rodgers AB, Morgan CP, Leu NA, Bale TL. Transgenerational epigenetic programming via sperm microRNA recapitulates effects of paternal stress. Proc Natl Acad Sci. 2015;112:44–9.
106. Roth Z, Hansen PJ. Disruption of nuclear maturation and rearrangement of cytoskeletal elements in bovine oocytes exposed to heat shock during maturation. Reproduction. 2005;129:235–44.
107. Seong KH, Li D, Shimizu H, et al. Inheritance of stress-induced, ATF-2-dependent epigenetic change. Cell Press. 2011;145:1049–61.
108. Tetsuka M, Takagi R, Ambo N, et al. Glucocorticoid metabolism in the bovine cumulus oocyte complex matured in vitro. Reproduction. 2016;151:73–82.
109. Webb RJ, Sunak N, Wren L, Michael AE. Inactivation of glucocorticoids by 11-beta-hydroxysteroid dehydrogenase enzymes increases during the meiotic maturation of porcine oocytes. Reproduction. 2008;136:725–32.
110. Hausmann MF, Longenecker AS, Marchetto NM, Juliano SA, Bowden RM. Embryonic exposure to corticosterone modifies the juvenile stress response, oxidative stress, and telomere length. Proc Biol Sci. 2012;279:1447–56.
111. Nesan D, Vijayan MM. Role of glucocorticoid in developmental programming: evidence from zebrafish. Gen Comp Endocrinol. 2013;181:35–44.
112. Bontekoe S, Mantikou E, van Wely M, Seshadri S, Repping S, Mastenbroek S. Low oxygen concentrations for embryo culture in assisted reproductive technologies. Cochrane Database Syst Rev. 2012;7:CD008950.
113. Gardner DK, Lane M. Culture of viable human blastocysts in defined sequential serum-free media. Hum Reprod. 1998;13(Supp 3):148–59. discussion 160
114. Edwards LJ, Williams DA, Gardner DK. Intracellular pH of the mouse preimplantation embryo: amino acids act as buffers of intracellular pH. Hum Reprod. 1998;13:3441–8.
115. Otsuki J, Nagai Y, Chiba K. Damage of embryo development caused by peroxidized mineral oil and its association with albumin in culture. Fertil Steril. 2009;91:1745–9.
116. Pomeroy K, Reed M. The effect of light on embryos and embryo culture. J Reprod Stem Cell Biotechnol. 2013;3(2):46–54.
117. Heitmann RJ, Hill MJ, James AN, Schimmel T, Segars JH, et al. Live births achieved via IVF are increased by improvements in air quality and laboratory environment. Reprod Biomed Online. 2015;31:364–71.

Chapter 8
Hematologic Disease in Implantation Failure

Shelby A. Neal, Jason M. Franasiak, and Richard T. Scott

Introduction

As treatment strategies in assisted reproduction have evolved over time, success rates have progressively increased. Nevertheless, a substantial number of embryos, even those determined to be chromosomally normal, fail to implant. The process of embryo implantation is complex and involves a number of events that occur at the microvascular level. Hematologic pathology, specifically inherited and acquired thrombophilias, has been proposed as a potential etiology for implantation failure. This idea has largely evolved from the robust body of literature surrounding thrombophilias and obstetric outcomes. The underlying pathophysiology behind this association relates to the concept that thrombophilic conditions create a predisposition to thrombosis beyond that which already exists during pregnancy. Microthromboses can result in reduced uteroplacental blood flow, leading to a myriad of obstetric complications.

The most prominent connection between hematologic pathology and decreased reproductive success is antiphospholipid antibody syndrome, an acquired thrombophilia. The presence of these antibodies has been associated with an increased risk of recurrent pregnancy loss (RPL) [1–4]. Women with RPL are three times more likely to test positive for antiphospholipid antibodies than the general obstetric population [5]. The proposed mechanism involves the binding of antiphospholipid antibodies to trophoblast cells, resulting in abnormal endovascular trophoblastic invasion in early pregnancy. In addition, antiphospholipid antibodies have been noted to reduce production of vascular endothelial growth factor (VEGF), thereby

S.A. Neal, MD • J.M. Franasiak, MD, HCLD (✉) • R.T. Scott, MD, HCLD
Sidney Kimmel Medical College, Thomas Jefferson University Philadelphia,
Philadelphia, PA, USA

IVI-RMA of New Jersey, Basking Ridge, NJ, USA
e-mail: jfranasiak@rmanjs.com

© Springer International Publishing AG 2018
J.M. Franasiak, R.T. Scott Jr. (eds.), *Recurrent Implantation Failure*,
https://doi.org/10.1007/978-3-319-71967-2_8

limiting the formation of blood vessels [6]. In addition to recurrent pregnancy loss, several obstetric complications including preeclampsia and intrauterine growth restriction (IUGR) have an established association with antiphospholipid antibodies [7, 8]. Women with antiphospholipid antibodies have a fivefold increased risk of developing preeclampsia [9] and 1.5–3-fold risk of developing IUGR [7, 8]. Thrombosis in the placental circulation is the most plausible mechanism in these cases.

Once antiphospholipid antibodies were established as a cause of RPL, inherited thrombophilias were explored as an etiology with a similar underlying mechanism in mind. While some studies have reported an association between inherited thrombophilias and RPL with an approximately threefold increased risk of loss [10–12], multiple other studies have failed to establish a link [13, 14]. Additionally, there is conflicting evidence regarding their impact on adverse obstetric outcomes such as preeclampsia, intrauterine growth restriction, and placental abruption. Some studies report an association [15–17], while others do not [14, 18]. These conflicting data make this topic a challenging one for both patients and providers. We will discuss what evidence exists for and against their contribution to reproductive failure and what, if anything, can or should be done if a hematologic abnormality is present.

Despite the prevalence of literature surrounding thrombophilias and recurrent pregnancy loss, their impact on implantation failure is less clear. The proposed mechanism is similar to that underlying RPL, namely, that microthrombosis causes disturbed blood flow to the endometrium and, in the case of recurrent implantation failure, impairs the initial vascularization process that is necessary for successful implantation to occur [19]. Some data in the literature support this association; however, they are mostly in the form of case-control studies, and a number of cohort studies have found conflicting results. Large randomized controlled trials are needed despite the fact they are challenging to implement in this setting. In this chapter, the available literature regarding the potential role of thrombophilias in implantation failure and the evidence for possible therapeutic options will be reviewed.

Physiology and Pathophysiology of Hemostasis

Hemostasis is the physiologic mechanism that curtails bleeding following vascular injury. Normal hemostasis depends upon the presence of tissue factor and activation of the coagulation cascade, which involves a number of critical clotting factors and cofactors. Inappropriate activation of this system is prevented by the anticoagulant system. Thrombophilic states can occur when there is an alteration in one of these processes.

Inherited Thrombophilias

Thrombophilias can be classified as either inherited or acquired. Inherited thrombophilias are due to genetic mutations in various components of the coagulation cascade, the majority of which are inherited in an autosomal dominant fashion. Each one has its own unique effect on the coagulation cascade (Fig. 8.1).

Factor V Leiden is the most common known mutation, resulting from a substitution of guanine by adenine at nucleotide 1691. As a result of this mutation, factor V is rendered resistant to cleavage by activated protein C. Although a case-control study did identify factor V Leiden as a risk factor for pregnancy loss [10], a larger prospective study found no association [14].

Other frequently studied mutations include mutations in the prothrombin gene (substitution of guanine by adenine at nucleotide 20210) and methylenetetrahydrofolate reductase (MTHFR) (cytosine to thymine substitution at nucleotide 677). In the setting of a prothrombin gene mutation, there is increased translation resulting in increased circulating levels of prothrombin. The same case-control study that identified factor V Leiden as a risk factor for pregnancy loss also implicated prothrombin gene mutation G20210A as a risk factor [10]; however, a larger prospective study found no association [13].

Mutant forms of MTHFR are the most common cause of hyperhomocysteinemia. There are conflicting data on the association of hyperhomocysteinemia and pregnancy loss. A meta-analysis suggested the possibility of an increased risk with

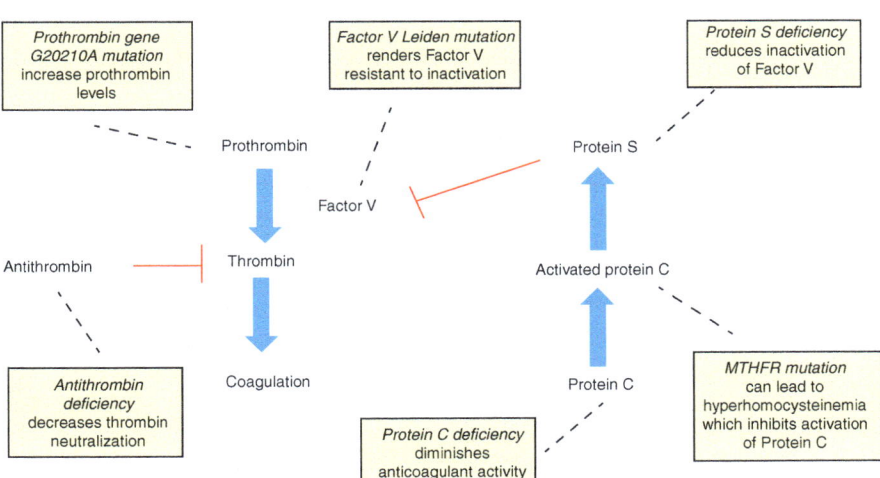

Fig. 8.1 Overview of the inherited thrombophilias and their effects on the coagulation cascade

OR 1.4 (95% CI 1.0–2.0) [20]. However, subsequent meta-analyses have concluded that MTHFR mutations are not associated with pregnancy loss [12, 21].

Deficiencies in natural anticoagulants, such as antithrombin III, protein C, and protein S, also result in a thrombophilic state. Data regarding the association with anticoagulant deficiencies and recurrent pregnancy loss is lacking, but a meta-analysis of the few studies available only revealed an increased risk of recurrent pregnancy loss in the setting of protein S deficiency (OR 14.72) [12].

Acquired Thrombophilias

In contrast, antiphospholipid antibody syndrome (APAS) is considered an acquired thrombophilia. Diagnosis requires at least one clinical criterion (either obstetric or thrombotic) and one laboratory criterion. Acceptable laboratory criteria include the presence of certain antiphospholipid antibodies (APAs), namely, anticardiolipin antibody, anti-β2 glycoprotein I antibody, or lupus anticoagulant. At least one of these antibodies must be preset on two separate occasions, at least 12 weeks apart [22]. A number of mechanisms by which antiphospholipid antibodies activate coagulation have been proposed including resistance to natural anticoagulants, impairment of fibrinolysis, and activation of endothelial cells, platelets, and the coagulation cascade [23]. Many studies support an association between antiphospholipid antibodies and recurrent pregnancy loss [1–4]. In patients with APAs, 50% of pregnancy losses occur after the tenth week [24].

Embryo Implantation and Vascular Invasion

Understanding the process of embryo implantation, specifically as it relates to invasion of the microvasculature, is fundamental to understanding the possible mechanisms by which hematologic abnormalities may influence implantation. Normal implantation occurs approximately 7 days after fertilization and is comprised of three distinct stages [25]. The first stage involves the initial apposition of the embryo to the uterine wall via interdigitation of microvilli on the syncytiotrophoblasts and uterine epithelium. In the second stage, the embryo becomes more stably adhered to the uterine epithelium. The final stage is characterized by invasion of the syncytiotrophoblasts into the uterine wall and vasculature. Alterations in this process may result in a wide spectrum of pathology, from failed implantation or placental insufficiency (secondary to inadequate trophoblastic invasion) to morbidly adherent placenta (due to excessive trophoblastic invasion).

Recurrent Implantation Failure

Although there is a robust body of knowledge regarding the association of thrombophilias with recurrent pregnancy loss and obstetric outcomes, less is known with respect to recurrent implantation failure. Furthermore, most of the available data comes from case-control studies, and the results have been conflicting.

Inherited Thrombophilias

Several investigators have proposed an association between inherited thrombophilic conditions and recurrent implantation failure. In a case-control study, examining the prevalence of prothrombotic mutations among 18 women who underwent at least three IVF cycles with subsequent fetal loss or implantation failure compared to 24 randomly selected women undergoing their first or second IVF cycle at the same center, the first group had more mutation carriers (27.7 versus 0%, $p = 0.010$) [26]. Another case-control study had similar results when comparing 45 women with $\geq$4 failed IVF cycles to 44 age-matched controls, with thrombophilic mutations identified in 26.7% of the study group versus 9.1% of the controls ($p = 0.003$) [27]. Yet another case-control study revealed that women with $\geq$3 failed IVF cycles were more likely to have at least one inherited or acquired thrombophilia when compared to women with successful pregnancy after their first IVF cycle and women who conceived spontaneously (68.9 versus 25% and 25.6%, $p < 0.01$) [28]. A more recent systematic review and meta-analysis examined eight case-control studies and two cohort studies and concluded that factor V Leiden is more prevalent among women with ART failure (OR 3.08, 95% CI 1.77–5.36) [29].

Equally compelling is the evidence from studies that have found no difference in the prevalence of inherited thrombophilia in women who experience recurrent implantation failure when compared to control groups [30–33]. The previously mentioned meta-analysis did not find a significant association between ART failure and prothrombin gene mutation, MTHFR mutation, or deficiencies in protein C, protein S, or antithrombin [29].

Acquired Thrombophilias

Given the association of antiphospholipid antibodies with recurrent pregnancy loss and obstetric complications, it is not unexpected that there are data to support an association with implantation failure as well. Multiple case-control studies have noted a higher prevalence of antiphospholipid antibodies in women with implantation failure when compared to controls [2, 28, 33–36]. In addition, a prospective cohort study found that patients with antiphospholipid antibodies had a lower pregnancy rates than those without, although this difference was not statistically significant (5.4 versus 26.1%, $p = 0.07$) [37]. Lastly, a systematic review and meta-analysis of the literature involving 29 studies concluded that antiphospholipid antibodies are more prevalent among women with ART failure (OR 3.33, 95% CI 1.77–6.26) [29]. However, the majority of the studies were case-control designs, and the authors concluded that the overall methodologic quality was poor secondary to inappropriate control group selection.

There are also ample data to suggest that antiphospholipid antibodies do not have an association with implantation failure. These include a number of case-control studies [30, 38], retrospective cohort studies [39, 40], and prospective cohort studies [41, 42]. In 2006, the Practice Committee of the American Society for Reproductive Medicine published a committee opinion entitled "Anti-phospholipid antibodies do not affect IVF success," in which they reviewed seven studies with over 2000 patients in total, all of which concluded that there is no statistically significant impact of the presence of APAs on IVF outcomes [43]. The authors conclude that assessment of antiphospholipid antibodies is not indicated in couples undergoing IVF and therapy is not justified on the basis of the existing data. However, many of these studies did not specifically examine patients with recurrent IVF failure but rather failure in one cycle. Perhaps the studies examining those with recurrent failure enrich the population and make the effect more readily apparent.

Therapeutic Options

Despite the conflicting data available regarding the association of inherited and acquired thrombophilias with implantation failure, testing for these conditions remains an important consideration when evaluating these patients as potential therapeutic options exist. When identified, therapeutic interventions for these conditions are aimed at altering the coagulation cascade in hopes of correcting the perturbation.

Both aspirin and heparin have been explored as treatment for antiphospholipid antibodies in the setting of recurrent implantation failure, based largely on the data that support their use for patients with RPL [44–48]. Aspirin inhibits platelet aggregation via antithromboxane effects and may counteract antiphospholipid antibody-mediated hypercoagulability in the choriodecidual space (Fig. 8.2) [49]. Heparin is theorized to exert its protective effects by inhibiting the binding of phospholipid antibodies, thereby protecting the trophoblast from injury [50].

Mixed evidence exists to suggest that treatment may be beneficial for patients with both recurrent implantation failure and diagnosed thrombophilia. One randomized controlled trial found that implantation rates were doubled in patients treated

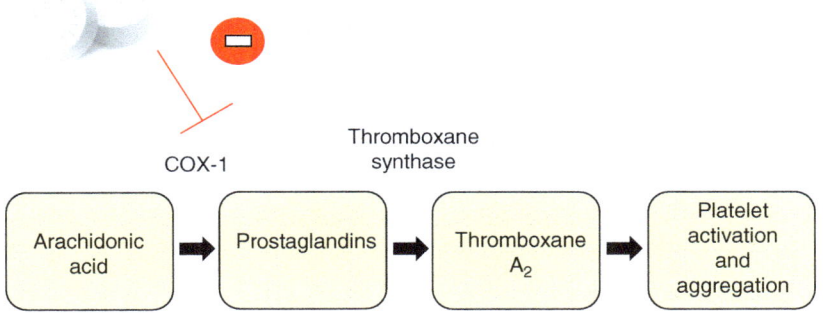

Fig. 8.2 Mechanism of action of aspirin

with low molecular weight heparin (LMWH) in comparison with placebo [51]. In this particular study, recurrent implantation failure was defined as ≥3 failed IVF cycles, and patients had at least one inherited or acquired thrombophilia. However, another randomized controlled trial found no difference in pregnancy, implantation, or live birth rates following treatment with aspirin and heparin [52]. This study only examined patients with antiphospholipid antibodies, and the authors defined recurrent implantation failure as ≥10 embryos transferred without pregnancy.

Although treatment with heparin and aspirin may be associated with increased implantation rates in patients with known thrombophilia, there is currently no evidence to suggest empiric treatment for patients without diagnosed thrombophilia. Multiple prospective randomized controlled trials have found that treatment with LMWH in patients with ≥2 failed IVF cycles did not improve live birth rates [53, 54]. It is possible that patients with ≥3 failed IVF cycles may benefit from empiric LMWH; however, the improvement in pregnancy rates did not reach statistical significance in the study that evaluated this subgroup [54].

Summary

The relationship between thrombophilia and implantation failure remains largely inconclusive. The idea that there is an association is largely based on the literature for recurrent pregnancy loss. This association has been supported by a number of small case-control and cohort studies but refuted by many others. Until larger prospective studies are undertaken, it is difficult to make a strong recommendation for routine screening of IVF patients or empiric treatment in the setting of thrombophilia. However, there is some evidence to suggest that treatment of individuals with a known thrombophilic condition *and* recurrent implantation failure may benefit from treatment. It is therefore reasonable to test for thrombophilia in patients with recurrent implantation failure and consider treatment if a thrombophilic disorder is identified.

References

1. Parazzini F, Acaia B, Faden D, Lovotti M, Marelli G, Cortelazzo S. Antiphospholipid antibodies and recurrent abortion. Obstet Gynecol. 1991;77(6):854–8.
2. Balasch J, Creus M, Fábregues F, Reverter JC, Carmona F, Tàssies D, et al. Antiphospholipid antibodies and human reproductive failure. Hum Reprod. 1996;11(10):2310–5.
3. Rai RS, Regan L, Clifford K, Pickering W, Dave M, Mackie I, et al. Antiphospholipid antibodies and beta 2-glycoprotein-I in 500 women with recurrent miscarriage: results of a comprehensive screening approach. Hum Reprod. 1995;10(8):2001–5.
4. MacLean MA, Cumming GP, McCall F, Walker ID, Walker JJ. The prevalence of lupus anticoagulant and anticardiolipin antibodies in women with a history of first trimester miscarriages. Br J Obstet Gynaecol. 1994;101(2):103–6.
5. Branch DW, Gibson M, Silver RM. Clinical practice. Recurrent miscarriage. N Engl J Med. 2010;363(18):1740–7.
6. Di Simone N, D'Ippolito S, Marana R, Di Nicuolo F, Castellani R, Pierangeli SS, et al. Antiphospholipid antibodies affect human endometrial angiogenesis: protective effect of a synthetic peptide (TIFI) mimicking the phospholipid binding site of β2glycoprotein I. Am J Reprod Immunol. 2013;70(4):299–308.
7. Lima F, Khamashta MA, Buchanan NM, Kerslake S, Hunt BJ, Hughes GR. A study of sixty pregnancies in patients with the antiphospholipid syndrome. Clin Exp Rheumatol. 1996;14(2):131–6.
8. Branch DW, Silver RM, Blackwell JL, Reading JC, Scott JR. Outcome of treated pregnancies in women with antiphospholipid syndrome: an update of the Utah experience. Obstet Gynecol. 1992;80(4):614–20.
9. Yamada H, Atsumi T, Kobashi G, Ota C, Kato EH, Tsuruga N, et al. Antiphospholipid antibodies increase the risk of pregnancy-induced hypertension and adverse pregnancy outcomes. J Reprod Immunol. 2009;79(2):188–95.
10. Lissalde-Lavigne G, Fabbro-Peray P, Cochery-Nouvellon E, Mercier E, Ripart-Neveu S, Balducchi J-P, et al. Factor V Leiden and prothrombin G20210A polymorphisms as risk factors for miscarriage during a first intended pregnancy: the matched case-control "NOHA first" study. J Thromb Haemost. 2005;3(10):2178–84.
11. Dudding TE, Attia J. The association between adverse pregnancy outcomes and maternal factor V Leiden genotype: a meta-analysis. Thromb Haemost. 2004;91(4):700–11.
12. Rey E, Kahn SR, David M, Shrier I. Thrombophilic disorders and fetal loss: a meta-analysis. Lancet Lond Engl. 2003;361(9361):901–8.
13. Silver RM, Zhao Y, Spong CY, Sibai B, Wendel G, Wenstrom K, et al. Prothrombin gene G20210A mutation and obstetric complications. Obstet Gynecol. 2010;115(1):14–20.
14. Dizon-Townson D, Miller C, Sibai B, Spong CY, Thom E, Wendel G, et al. The relationship of the factor V Leiden mutation and pregnancy outcomes for mother and fetus. Obstet Gynecol. 2005;106(3):517–24.
15. Alfirevic Z, Roberts D, Martlew V. How strong is the association between maternal thrombophilia and adverse pregnancy outcome? A systematic review. Eur J Obstet Gynecol Reprod Biol. 2002;101(1):6–14.
16. Kupferminc MJ, Eldor A, Steinman N, Many A, Bar-Am A, Jaffa A, et al. Increased frequency of genetic thrombophilia in women with complications of pregnancy. N Engl J Med. 1999;340(1):9–13.
17. Nurk E, Tell GS, Refsum H, Ueland PM, Vollset SE. Factor V Leiden, pregnancy complications and adverse outcomes: the Hordaland homocysteine study. QJM Mon J Assoc Physicians. 2006;99(5):289–98.
18. D'Elia AV, Driul L, Giacomello R, Colaone R, Fabbro D, Di Leonardo C, et al. Frequency of factor V, prothrombin and methylenetetrahydrofolate reductase gene variants in preeclampsia. Gynecol Obstet Investig. 2002;53(2):84–7.

19. Simon A, Laufer N. Assessment and treatment of repeated implantation failure (RIF). J Assist Reprod Genet. 2012;29(11):1227–39.
20. Nelen WL, Blom HJ, Steegers EA, den Heijer M, Eskes TK. Hyperhomocysteinemia and recurrent early pregnancy loss: a meta-analysis. Fertil Steril. 2000;74(6):1196–9.
21. Paidas MJ, D-HW K, Langhoff-Roos J, Arkel YS. Inherited thrombophilias and adverse pregnancy outcome: screening and management. Semin Perinatol. 2005;29(3):150–63.
22. Miyakis S, Lockshin MD, Atsumi T, Branch DW, Brey RL, Cervera R, et al. International consensus statement on an update of the classification criteria for definite antiphospholipid syndrome (APS). J Thromb Haemost. 2006;4(2):295–306.
23. Vlachoyiannopoulos PG, Routsias JG. A novel mechanism of thrombosis in antiphospholipid antibody syndrome. J Autoimmun. 2010;35:248–55.
24. Oshiro BT, Silver RM, Scott JR, Yu H, Branch DW. Antiphospholipid antibodies and fetal death. Obstet Gynecol. 1996;87(4):489–93.
25. Norwitz ER, Schust DJ, Fisher SJ. Implantation and the survival of early pregnancy. N Engl J Med. 2001;345(19):1400–8.
26. Grandone E, Colaizzo D, Lo Bue A, Checola MG, Cittadini E, Margaglione M. Inherited thrombophilia and in vitro fertilization implantation failure. Fertil Steril. 2001;76(1):201–2.
27. Azem F, Many A, Ben Ami I, Yovel I, Amit A, Lessing JB, et al. Increased rates of thrombophilia in women with repeated IVF failures. Hum Reprod. 2004;19(2):368–70.
28. Qublan HS, Eid SS, Ababneh HA, Amarin ZO, Smadi AZ, Al-Khafaji FF, et al. Acquired and inherited thrombophilia: implication in recurrent IVF and embryo transfer failure. Hum Reprod. 2006;21(10):2694–8.
29. Di Nisio M, Rutjes AWS, Ferrante N, Tiboni GM, Cuccurullo F, Porreca E. Thrombophilia and outcomes of assisted reproduction technologies: a systematic review and meta-analysis. Blood. 2011;118(10):2670–8.
30. Martinelli I, Taioli E, Ragni G, Levi-Setti P, Passamonti SM, Battaglioli T, et al. Embryo implantation after assisted reproductive procedures and maternal thrombophilia. Haematologica. 2003;88(7):789–93.
31. Rudick B, Su HI, Sammel MD, Kovalevsky G, Shaunik A, Barnhart K. Is factor V Leiden mutation a cause of in vitro fertilization failure? Fertil Steril. 2009;92(4):1256–9.
32. Simur A, Ozdemir S, Acar H, Colakoğlu MC, Görkemli H, Balci O, et al. Repeated in vitro fertilization failure and its relation with thrombophilia. Gynecol Obstet Investig. 2009;67(2):109–12.
33. Vaquero E, Lazzarin N, Caserta D, Valensise H, Baldi M, Moscarini M, et al. Diagnostic evaluation of women experiencing repeated in vitro fertilization failure. Eur J Obstet Gynecol Reprod Biol. 2006;125(1):79–84.
34. Coulam CB, Kaider BD, Kaider AS, Janowicz P, Roussev RG. Antiphospholipid antibodies associated with implantation failure after IVF/ET. J Assist Reprod Genet. 1997;14(10): 603–8.
35. Kaider BD, Price DE, Roussev RG, Coulam CB. Antiphospholipid antibody prevalence in patients with IVF failure. Am J Reprod Immunol. 1996;35(4):388–93.
36. Geva E, Yaron Y, Lessing JB, Yovel I, Vardinon N, Burke M, et al. Circulating autoimmune antibodies may be responsible for implantation failure in in vitro fertilization. Fertil Steril. 1994;62(4):802–6.
37. el-Roeiy A, Gleicher N, Friberg J, Confino E, Dudkiewicz A. Correlation between peripheral blood and follicular fluid autoantibodies and impact on in vitro fertilization. Obstet Gynecol. 1987;70(2):163–70.
38. Martinuzzo M, Iglesias Varela ML, Adamczuk Y, Broze GJ, Forastiero R. Antiphospholipid antibodies and antibodies to tissue factor pathway inhibitor in women with implantation failures or early and late pregnancy losses. J Thromb Haemost. 2005;3(11):2587–9.
39. Buckingham KL, Stone PR, Smith JF, Chamley LW. Antiphospholipid antibodies in serum and follicular fluid—is there a correlation with IVF implantation failure? Hum Reprod. 2006;21(3):728–34.

40. Birdsall MA, Lockwood GM, Ledger WL, Johnson PM, Chamley LW. Antiphospholipid antibodies in women having in-vitro fertilization. Hum Reprod. 1996;11(6):1185–9.
41. Denis AL, Guido M, Adler RD, Bergh PA, Brenner C, Scott RT. Antiphospholipid antibodies and pregnancy rates and outcome in in vitro fertilization patients. Fertil Steril. 1997;67(6):1084–90.
42. Chilcott IT, Margara R, Cohen H, Rai R, Skull J, Pickering W, et al. Pregnancy outcome is not affected by antiphospholipid antibody status in women referred for in vitro fertilization. Fertil Steril. 2000;73(3):526–30.
43. Practice Committee of the American Society for Reproductive Medicine. Anti-phospholipid antibodies do not affect IVF success. Fertil Steril. 2006;86(5 Suppl 1):S224–5.
44. Kutteh WH. Antiphospholipid antibody-associated recurrent pregnancy loss: treatment with heparin and low-dose aspirin is superior to low-dose aspirin alone. Am J Obstet Gynecol. 1996;174(5):1584–9.
45. Ziakas PD, Pavlou M, Voulgarelis M. Heparin treatment in antiphospholipid syndrome with recurrent pregnancy loss: a systematic review and meta-analysis. Obstet Gynecol. 2010;115(6):1256–62.
46. Backos M, Rai R, Baxter N, Chilcott IT, Cohen H, Regan L. Pregnancy complications in women with recurrent miscarriage associated with antiphospholipid antibodies treated with low dose aspirin and heparin. Br J Obstet Gynaecol. 1999;106(2):102–7.
47. Empson M, Lassere M, Craig J, Scott J. Prevention of recurrent miscarriage for women with antiphospholipid antibody or lupus anticoagulant. Cochrane Database Syst Rev. 2005;2:CD002859.
48. Rai R, Cohen H, Dave M, Regan L. Randomised controlled trial of aspirin and aspirin plus heparin in pregnant women with recurrent miscarriage associated with phospholipid antibodies (or antiphospholipid antibodies). BMJ. 1997;314(7076):253–7.
49. Harris EN, Gharavi AE, Hughes GR. Anti-phospholipid antibodies. Clin Rheum Dis. 1985;11(3):591–609.
50. Ermel LD, Marshburn PB, Kutteh WH. Interaction of heparin with antiphospholipid antibodies (APA) from the sera of women with recurrent pregnancy loss (RPL). Am J Reprod Immunol. 1995;33(1):14–20.
51. Qublan H, Amarin Z, Dabbas M, Farraj A-E, Beni-Merei Z, Al-Akash H, et al. Low-molecular-weight heparin in the treatment of recurrent IVF-ET failure and thrombophilia: a prospective randomized placebo-controlled trial. Hum Fertil (Camb). 2008;11(4):246–53.
52. Stern C, Chamley L, Norris H, Hale L, Baker HWG. A randomized, double-blind, placebo-controlled trial of heparin and aspirin for women with in vitro fertilization implantation failure and antiphospholipid or antinuclear antibodies. Fertil Steril. 2003;80(2):376–83.
53. Urman B, Ata B, Yakin K, Alatas C, Aksoy S, Mercan R, et al. Luteal phase empirical low molecular weight heparin administration in patients with failed ICSI embryo transfer cycles: a randomized open-labeled pilot trial. Hum Reprod. 2009;24(7):1640–7.
54. Berker B, Taşkin S, Kahraman K, Taşkin EA, Atabekoğlu C, Sönmezer M. The role of low-molecular-weight heparin in recurrent implantation failure: a prospective, quasi-randomized, controlled study. Fertil Steril. 2011;95(8):2499–502.

Chapter 9
Endocrine Causes of Implantation Failure

Scott Morin, Baris Ata, and Emre Seli

Introduction

Successful implantation is dependent upon a highly coordinated sequence of hormonal stimuli to prepare the endometrium for pregnancy. In the natural setting, this complex but logical process is beautifully designed to mirror the progress of the preimplantation embryo as it traverses the oviduct and uterotubal junction and approaches the endometrium. However, given the reliance of this delicate system on endocrine signaling, inadequate support or disturbed timing of hormonal stimuli may cause the endometrium to become inhospitable to the preimplantation embryo. Furthermore, alterations in these signals as a result of exogenous gonadotropin administration in modern infertility treatment can have major implications on the receptivity of the endometrium. Additionally, other endocrine processes separate from the hypothalamo-pituitary-ovarian (HPO) axis are involved in optimizing this process, and pathology in these systems can also negatively impact implantation.

While considerable progress has been made in elucidating the mechanisms underlying this complex system, many questions still remain. This chapter seeks to (1) describe the normal coordination of endocrine stimuli required to achieve

S. Morin, MD
Sidney Kimmel Medical College, Thomas Jefferson University Philadelphia, Philadelphia, PA, USA

IVI-RMA of New Jersey, Basking Ridge, NJ, USA
e-mail: scottjmorin@gmail.com

B. Ata, MD
Department of Obstetrics and Gynecology, Koc University School of Medicine, Istanbul, Turkey
e-mail: barisata@ku.edu.tr

E. Seli, MD (✉)
Department of Obstetrics Gynecology and Reproductive Sciences, Yale School of Medicine, New Haven, CT, USA
e-mail: emre.seli@yale.edu; emreseli65@gmail.com

© Springer International Publishing AG 2018
J.M. Franasiak, R.T. Scott Jr. (eds.), *Recurrent Implantation Failure*,
https://doi.org/10.1007/978-3-319-71967-2_9

implantation, (2) review our current understanding of how this system is affected by modern infertility treatment, (3) discuss how pathological endocrine processes disrupt implantation, and (4) discuss treatment options for optimizing the chance for successful implantation.

Endocrine Regulation of Endometrial Growth and Regeneration

For the vast majority of women, the menstrual cycle demonstrates little variability from cycle to cycle, with a normal range of 25–35 days [1]. In the absence of pregnancy, this cycle is repeated approximately 400 times during the adult life of a normally menstruating female. This consistency reflects a predictable cascade of events originating in the hypothalamus and resulting in ovarian sex steroid production. A foundational understanding of the processes coordinating each step is required when attempting to optimize each patient's chance for successful pregnancy.

Neuroendocrine Control of Menstrual Cycle

Any discussion of the menstrual cycle must begin with an understanding of the neuroendocrine mechanisms underlying its function. This system begins with pulsatile secretion of GnRH from the arcuate nucleus of the hypothalamus under the regulation of kisspeptin. Both pulse frequency and amplitude vary significantly over the course of the menstrual cycle. Early in follicular phase, GnRH pulses slow to every 90–100 min. This period is marked by pituitary FSH production and secretion, which supports follicular recruitment. In the midfollicular phase, GnRH pulse frequency increases to every 60 min. While amplitude is initially low, it increases in parallel with increased estradiol secretion from the follicular unit. The rising estradiol level also induces an increase in pituitary gonadotrope responsiveness to GnRH in the midfollicular phase. At midcycle, this increased responsiveness ultimately facilitates the LH surge, followed by ovulation approximately 36 h later. Following ovulation, progesterone secretion from the corpus luteum slows GnRH pulse frequency to every 4–8 h. Pulse amplitude increases, however, resulting in the persistence of adequate LH levels to support corpus luteum function.

Two-Cell Theory of Ovarian Sex Steroid Production

There is compelling evidence for a cooperative relationship between theca and granulosa cells that is based on specialization of androgen substrate production in the theca for eventual aromatization in the granulosa cells. This process begins in the preceding luteal phase, as FSH levels begin to rise. A slight increase in FSH rescues a cohort of preantral follicles from atresia and initiates growth. As levels continue to rise during the early follicular phase, FSH stimulates granulosa cell proliferation and increases gap junction formation producing a syncytium of granulosa cells in the developing follicle. This mitogenic activity of FSH on granulosa cells works in combination with an FSH-induced increase in aromatase activity to facilitate an increased capacity for estrogen production. Simultaneously, as follicular growth proceeds, theca cells begin to produce an increasing number of LH receptors. In the theca cells, LH binding facilitates cholesterol uptake and conversion into androgens. Preovulatory granulosa cells are unable to complete conversion of the 21-carbon substrates into androgens, and as a result ovarian steroidogenesis is largely dependent on this LH activity in the theca cells. Thus, as follicular development progresses, increasing amounts of androgen substrate are produced as a result of increasing LH activity. These substrates diffuse into adjacent granulosa cells where they are aromatized to estradiol. As the follicular phase advances, increasing LH levels result in additional androgen substrate and ultimately increasing estradiol secretion from the follicular unit. Throughout this process, FSH also increases the number of LH receptors present on the granulosa cells preparing the follicular unit for ovulation.

Ovulation

Ovulation is ultimately facilitated by the increased estradiol produced by the dominant follicle. This increased estradiol causes increased pituitary responsiveness to GnRH and induces the LH surge. The LH surge not only triggers resumption of meiosis in the oocyte and induces ovulation but also induces a significant shift in the activity of the follicular unit. Prior to ovulation, granulosa cell activity is dominated by estradiol production. While progesterone production is initiated in the hours leading up to ovulation, its secretion is significantly increased following ovulation— reaching a peak at approximately 8 h after the LH surge. Progesterone levels remain elevated as long as the corpus luteum is supported by LH stimulus. Meanwhile, estradiol levels decrease to a steady but reduced level following ovulation.

Luteinization and Postovulation Steroid Secretion

The process of luteinization is facilitated by a wide array of mechanisms. The previously avascular follicular unit is transformed into a highly vascular tissue which allows increased exposure to cholesterol substrate for progesterone production. This process is further facilitated by an increased expression of steroidogenic acute regulatory protein (StAR) and side-chain cleavage enzyme which regulate cholesterol transfer into the inner mitochondrial membrane and eventual conversion to pregnenolone. Increased progesterone production is the result of increased 3-beta-hydroxysteroid dehydrogenase activity in the granulosa cells. All of these processes require continued tonic secretion of LH from the anterior pituitary. Thus, the efficiency of the corpus luteum is determined by the extent to which LH receptor accumulation occurred prior to ovulation. An inefficient follicular unit prior to ovulation forebodes a poorly functioning corpus luteum following ovulation. Whether this can be overcome by exogenous support of corpus luteum function or progesterone supplementation is discussed in detail later in this chapter.

Because progesterone secretion is dependent upon the pulsatile release of LH, levels vary throughout the luteal phase. Thus, attempts at correlating progesterone levels with luteal function are limited by the frequent changes in progesterone levels relative to its episodic production from the corpus luteum. This reality has limited the applicability of progesterone measurements in predicting the chance of ongoing gestation. Instead, it appears as though as long as progesterone levels reach a threshold for inducing secretory change in the endometrium, increasing levels due not improve chances at implantation. The more clinically relevant measure of progesterone's impact on the chance of successful implantation involves determining when progesterone crosses this threshold in relation to when the embryo approaches the endometrium. This concept of endometrial-embryo synchrony is discussed in great detail in Chap. 2 and will also be considered briefly below.

Endometrial Response to Sex Hormone Secretion in the Normal Menstrual Cycle

In the clinical setting, the dynamic changes of ovarian sex steroid production receive the majority of focus when considering the physiology of the menstrual cycle. Providers are prone to focusing on the HPO axis because measuring hormones provides data with which to base treatment decisions during treatment cycles. In contrast, the endometrium provides relatively less information in a given cycle. However, when considering the effect of the endocrine system on implantation, the endometrium must be considered the final recipient of the cascade of messages produced during the menstrual cycle. Without a coordinated endometrial response to the cyclic changes in sex steroid production by the follicular unit, pregnancy will not ensue.

The endometrial cycle is the result of three stages of development in response to ovarian estrogen and progesterone exposure—proliferation, differentiation, and tissue breakdown. At the molecular level, these sex steroids act via cognate receptors to initiate expression of specific cascades of genes and to induce shifts in autocrine, paracrine, and intracrine communication in the endometrium. Estrogen is responsible for the proliferative changes during the follicular phase of the ovarian cycle. Progesterone is required for the establishment and maintenance of pregnancy consequent upon the transformation of the estrogen-primed endometrium into the secretory phase. Menstruation results from withdrawal of both hormones upon demise of the corpus luteum.

Endometrial Structure

A full appreciation of endometrial preparations for implantation requires an under-standing of the structure and function of the endometrium. The endometrium is comprised of two major layers: the functionalis and the basalis. The functionalis is a transient and proliferative layer that comprises the upper two-thirds of the endo-metrium. The basalis is the bottom one-third of the endometrium directly adjacent to the myometrium and is responsible for regenerating the functionalis after men-strual shedding. The basalis contains the basal arteries, which are branches of the radial arteries and are unresponsive to the hormonal changes of follicular unit. The spiral arteries are separate branches of the radial arteries which extend into the func-tionalis layer and are responsive to cyclic hormonal changes. The other major struc-tural feature of the endometrium is its rich and dynamic endowment of glands. These glands originate in the basalis and extend to the luminal surface of the endo-metrium. Their presence indicates an important functional component of the endo-metrium, in that their secretory products serve to communicate with the preimplantation embryo to promote the events leading up to implantation.

A significant body of literature exists for describing the histologic changes that accompany shifts in hormonal stimuli in the endometrium. These morphological changes have been reviewed in detail in classical experiments [2]. The proliferative phase is characterized by a transition from cuboidal, ragged surface epithelium fol-lowing menstruation to a columnar, pseudostratified luminal epithelium. Gland morphology also develops in the proliferative endometrium from short and narrow in shape to more undulant surfaces with increasing tortuosity. The stromal compo-nent demonstrates active mitoses, and its density begins to increase throughout this phase of the cycle.

Due to the fact that most investigations of endometrial histology were primarily carried out in infertile patients in an effort to describe alterations in the timing of endometrial structural changes, more attention has been paid to the subtle, daily changes in the secretory endometrium. In a classic paper, Noyes et al. [3] argued that an increased rate of structural change in the secretory endometrium allowed assignment of specific endometrial dating based on histologic assessment. The first, easily identifiable morphologic change due to progesterone exposure occurs on day 3 following ovulation. Prominent subnuclear vacuoles appear and increase in size resulting in loss of pseudostratification and generation of an orderly row of nuclei in the luminal epithelium. On day 4 following ovulation, these vacuoles slip past the nuclei and localize near the luminal surface of the endometrial glands. By day 5 postovulation, few vacuoles are evident indicating intraluminal secretion of their contents. By this time, nuclei are impressively aligned at the basal portion of the glandular epithelium. During this process, gland diameter and tortuosity increases.

The primary morphologic feature at the time of implantation is an appreciable increase in stromal edema, which begins on day 6 postovulation. This feature is responsible for the familiar uniformly echogenic appearance of the endometrium on ultrasound in the secretory phase. Stromal edema reaches its height on days 7 and 8 after ovulation and is accompanied by increased coiling of spiral arterioles. Soon after, polymorphonuclear leukocytes—primarily uterine natural killer cells and macrophages—infiltrate the stroma. A process of pseudodecidualization under the influence of progesterone is also established around the time of implantation. So-called predecidual cells characterized by cytonuclear enlargement, increased mitotic activity, and development of a basement membrane can initially be identified surrounding blood vessels. These cells act in concert with decidual leukocytes to control trophoblastic invasion. At this time, the secretory endometrium is organized into three distinct layers—the unchanged basalis, the lace-like stratum spongiosum (composed of edematous stroma, tightly coiled spiral vessels, and dilated glands), and the superficial stratum compactum (resulting from predecidual transformation).

In the absence of pregnancy and the sustaining actions of human chorionic gonadotropin, the corpus luteum ultimately reaches the end of its predetermined life span. The resulting withdrawal of progesterone and estrogen results in a series of events leading up to menstruation. The primary mechanism responsible for this phenomenon is vasospasm of the spiral arterioles resulting in endometrial ischemia. Furthermore, lytic enzymes including matrix metalloproteinases previously confined to lysosomes under the control of progesterone are released upon progesterone withdrawal. This leads to enzymatic autodigestion of the cellular components, extracellular matrix, and basement membrane of the functionalis. Menstrual sloughing results.

Limitations in Endometrial Dating as a Clinical Tool

Despite significant progress in describing the histologic changes that accompany the sequential hormonal shifts in the menstrual cycle, the utility of endometrial dating as a tool to optimize timing in fertility treatments has been questioned on multiple grounds. First, significant inter- and intra-observer variability on the dating of a given endometrial biopsy sample has been described in multiple papers [4–6]. Much of these discrepancies result from difficulties assigning accurate endometrial dating in the case of glandular-stromal dyssynchrony [7]. Furthermore, the utility of endometrial dating as part of the infertility work up was significantly challenged when Coutifaris et al. [8] demonstrated in a large, multicentered prospective trial that out-of-phase biopsy results failed to discriminate between fertile and infertile couples. Thus, while description of endometrial dating has proven a useful framework for studying the effect of modern treatments on endometrial progression, it provides very little clinical value as a screening tool for infertility. As a result, these efforts are not recommended as part of the modern infertility work up.

The Impact of the Supraphysiologic Hormonal Milieu on Endometrial Development in Controlled Ovarian Hyperstimulation

Multifollicular development is the goal of exogenous gonadotropin treatment in an IVF cycle. However, multifollicular development results in supraphysiologic concentrations of estradiol and progesterone. Thus, the endocrine stimuli responsible for the chronologic changes in endometrial histology over the course of the physiologic menstrual cycle are inherently different following administration of exogenous gonadotropins. Not surprisingly, endometrial histology is often also altered. This phenomenon has been extensively described, and the changes in endometrial structure in stimulated cycles are generally divided into two categories: (1) accelerated transition to the secretory changes of the endometrium associated with premature progesterone rise and (2) lack of synchrony of development between the different cellular and structural compartments of the endometrium [9] (Fig. 9.1).

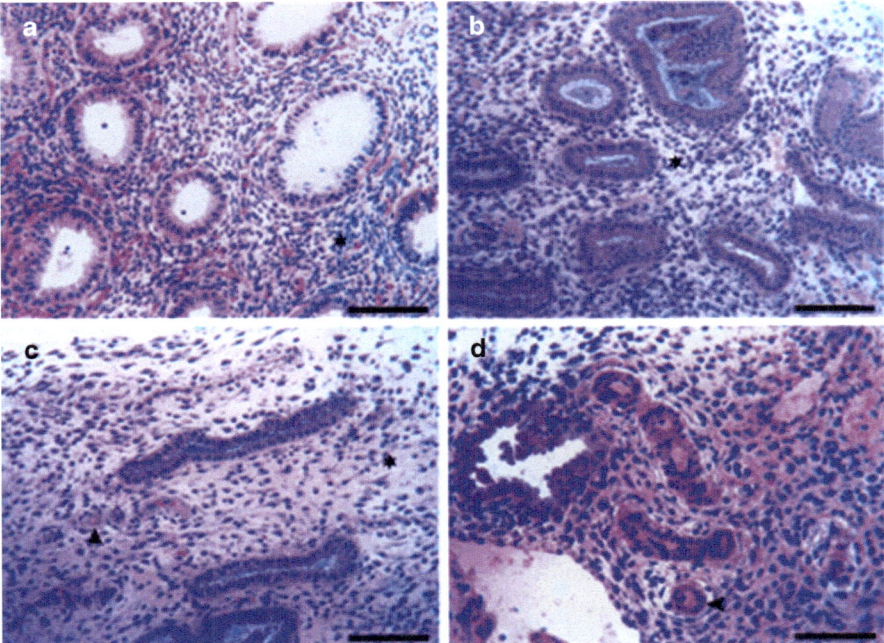

Fig. 9.1 Morphology of the endometrium showing variable stages of glandular and stromal development in the natural cycles and ovarian stimulation cycles of moderate responders and high responders. (**a**) Natural cycle endometrial biopsy showing in-phase glandular development and lowest amounts of stromal edema (asterisk). (**b**) Moderate responder: in-phase endometrium showing coordinated development of glands and stroma (asterisk) after ovarian stimulated. (**c, d**) High responders demonstrating glands stromal dyssynchrony: delayed glandular development and edematous stromal features (asterisk). This arrows show spiral arterial maturation appropriate to the late secretory phase. Bar = 100 μm

The effect of COH on endometrial development has also been demonstrated by identifying aberrations in the endometrial transcriptome following stimulation [10, 11]. Of the identified altered genes, those with known roles in implantation such as leukemia inhibition factor (LIF) and glycodelin have been demonstrated to be downregulated following stimulation. Additional alterations, including microRNA dysregulation have also been described [12]. Most studies attribute these issues to premature progesterone exposure following COH. Indeed, advancement in endometrial histology of >2 days has been reported in 45–100% of cycles with premature progesterone elevations [13, 14]. This advancement in endometrial structure and function has a significant impact on the likelihood of achieving implantation. This conclusion is supported by clinical data that demonstrate a restoration of normal pregnancy rates when embryos created in cycles with prematurely elevated progesterone levels are vitrified and transferred in a subsequent cycle [15, 16]. This issue is explored in much greater detail in Chap. 2.

The question of whether or not supraphysiologic estradiol levels alone following exogenous gonadotropin administration affect endometrial receptivity has also been debated. Marchini et al. [17] performed biopsies prior to oocyte retrieval and described accentuated proliferative characteristics and early secretory changes even prior to premature progesterone rise. Furthermore, some have suggested that although estradiol levels at different concentrations can support implantation, the window of uterine receptivity can be narrowed by supraphysiologic estradiol levels. Using a mouse model, Ma et al. [18] demonstrated that LIF, PTGS2, and HEGFL were downregulated sooner when the endometrium was exposed to a higher level of circulating estradiol levels. These authors suggested that this aberrant expression of key genes associated with implantation in the presence of supraphysiologic estradiol levels indicate an accelerated endometrial refractoriness to implantation [18].

This logic has been applied to the clinical setting as well. Paulson et al. initially postulated that higher implantation rates noted in oocyte donation cycles were in part a product of a more physiologic hormonal milieu present in cycles involving recipients of donated oocytes. Supraphysiologic estradiol levels in fresh non-donor IVF cycles were suggested as a potential culprit. This argument was corroborated to some degree by recent data that demonstrated superior live birth rates for frozen transfer compared to fresh embryo transfer in patients with polycystic ovarian syndrome (PCOS) [19]. Patients in the fresh embryo transfer arm in this study had an average maximum estradiol level of 4288 pg/mL [20]. However, it is unclear in this study whether the decrement in pregnancy rates following fresh embryo transfer is solely due to elevated estradiol levels or partially due to the chronic inflammation or aberrant hormonal milieu in PCOS patients. Other studies have failed to demonstrate an association between peak estradiol levels and pregnancy outcomes in fresh IVF cycles. One compelling study comparing implantation rates between patients utilizing autologous oocytes produced in cycles with peak estradiol levels >3000 pg/mL against recipients of donated oocytes produced in cycles with similar peak estradiol levels demonstrated no improvement in implantation rates for recipients of donated oocytes, despite their more physiologic estradiol levels [21]. Multiple additional studies subsequently produced similar findings [19, 20, 22].

Thus, while there exists some evidence of alterations in endometrial histology in the presence of supraphysiologic estradiol levels alone, it is still unclear that this is the primary cause of implantation failure in the most patients. Instead, the primary mechanism by which controlled ovarian hyperstimulation impacts implantation rates in IVF cycles appears to be premature elevation in progesterone and a shift in the window of endometrial receptivity prior to embryo transfer. However, no well-designed studies have been performed by controlling for premature progesterone elevations to isolate the impact of supraphysiologic estradiol levels alone on the incidence of recurrent implantation failure. Thus, more data is needed to definitively answer this question.

Estrogen Administration in Frozen Embryo Transfer Cycles

If supraphysiologic estradiol levels and an increased risk of premature progesterone rise do impact the chance of implantation in fresh cycle following exogenous gonadotropin administration, this can be avoided by proceeding with a frozen embryo transfer. However, a similar debate regarding the optimal endometrial preparation for embryo transfer exists. If the goal is to avoid supraphysiologic estradiol levels, then replacement in a natural cycle would be the ideal choice. Indeed, estradiol levels do tend to be higher in so-called artificial FET cycles than unmedicated cycles [23, 24].

Multiple studies have compared clinical outcomes between natural FET cycles, modified natural FET cycles (with hCG trigger and/or progesterone supplementation), and artificial FET cycles. These studies have been combined into a systematic review [25], and a meta-analysis [26]—neither of which revealed a significant advantage of one specific approach over another. It is important to note that the vast majority of data on this subject comes from retrospective studies, and thus there is still a significant need for more high-quality data. Only two prospective randomized trials on artificial versus natural cycle FET have been performed, and no difference in pregnancy rates was observed in either [27, 28]. One additional prospective trial compared modified natural cycle with an artificial cycle with GnRH agonist downregulation. Similarly, no difference in pregnancy rates was found between the groups [29].

Thus, the available evidence suggests that the typically higher levels of estradiol seen in artificial FET cycles do not result in detrimental outcomes. Furthermore, there is no evidence to support the notion that changing the strategy for endometrial preparation should be expected to improve implantation efficiency. It is also important to note that none of the above studies have focused specifically on patients with recurrent implantation failure. It is possible that RIF represents a unique population of patients that require more specific optimization of the endometrium to achieve pregnancy. This is not clear at the current time, however.

Luteal Phase Deficiency

Given the importance of progesterone production in preparing the endometrium for implantation, it seems logical that suboptimal corpus luteum function may be responsible for some instances of implantation failure. This conclusion is supported by observations that cycles that lead to normal early pregnancy development tend to have higher midluteal progesterone levels than those that result in failed implantation or loss [30]. These lines of thinking have helped generate the concept of luteal phase deficiency (LPD) as cause of infertility in some patients. However, despite being first described in 1949 [31], there is still a lack of high-quality data to support LPD as a plausible and common cause of implantation failure. This section will review the available evidence for LPD and discuss the utility of progesterone supplementation as a therapeutic strategy.

Pathophysiology of LPD

Given that ovarian progesterone secretion follows a cascade of signaling originating in the central nervous system, many authors have proposed that some instances of inadequate luteal progesterone secretion originates with disorders in the neuroendocrine support of the corpus luteum. These mechanisms include disorders associated with altered GnRH pulsatility (including hypothalamic amenorrhea, thyroid disease, and hyperprolactinemia) and dysregulated LH secretion (obesity). Others have suggested that ovarian aging alone may result in suboptimal luteal function. However, while the mechanistic changes associated with these pathologies have biologic plausibility, the pulsatile secretion of progesterone and associated challenges of obtaining accurate measurements makes direct evidence of luteal deficiency as the primary mechanism of poor outcomes in these patients difficult to establish.

Furthermore, there is not a widely accepted profile of ideal progesterone secretion required for implantation. While it is well established that progesterone levels peak 6–8 days after ovulation, these levels demonstrate rapid and significant variability according to LH pulsatility in the luteal phase [32]. Levels as low as 2.3 and as high as 40.1 ng/mL have been observed in the same patient in a 90-min interval [33]. This presents challenges for determining peak progesterone concentrations in the luteal phase in any given cycle. In addition, low progesterone levels early in pregnancy may be more reflective of poor hCG secretion from an abnormal early pregnancy than poor corpus luteum function.

The other logical strategy for evaluating luteal phase function is an assessment of luteal dating via endometrial biopsy. However, the same shortcomings for endometrial histology described above apply for diagnosing LPD. These include (1) high intercycle variability in dating for individual patients [34], (2) high interobserver diagnostic variability among pathologists [4], and (3) no difference in the incidence of delayed endometrial maturation between infertile patients and fertile controls [8]. Furthermore, once progesterone levels cross a given threshold for inducing secretory changes, it is unclear whether low normal and high normal levels have different impact on endometrial histology [35].

Therapeutic Strategies for Optimizing the Luteal Phase

In the absence of evidence for the above noted pathologies' association with poor central support of corpus luteal function, all strategies for enhancing luteal function are empiric in nature. Multiple different therapeutic approaches have been examined in many different clinical contexts. One approach is to increase progesterone and/or estrogen exposure of the endometrium by directly supplying these hormones exogenously during the luteal phase. One study demonstrated that increasing serum progesterone levels in the luteal phase after controlled ovarian hyperstimulation were associated with an increased clinical pregnancy rate. In this study [36], higher serum levels were achieved with vaginal progesterone. While the overall pregnancy rates between the routes of administration were no different, higher levels were associated with an increase in pregnancy rates. Another strategy is to artificially augment corpus luteum function by administering hCG. Some practitioners argue that tailoring the route of administration of progesterone or enhancing endogenous progesterone may be a consideration in patients with recurrent implantation failure to achieve high levels of progesterone due to the limited downside. However, there is limited data to suggest improvement in outcomes.

Direct progesterone supplementation is often utilized in COH cycles. While supplementation can be administered in multiple ways, vaginal progesterone is the most commonly utilized strategy. However, while there is little downside to administering supplemental progesterone, there is also no evidence to suggest that luteal phase progesterone supplementation is beneficial in increasing COH cycle implantation rates, though this is common practice due to the presumption that increased sex steroid production associated with multifollicular growth may suppress LH support of luteal function [37]. The only clinical scenario with high-quality evidence for progesterone supplementation is for use in ART cycles utilizing GnRH agonists [38] and antagonists [39] due to their strong association with premature luteolysis. Use in these cycles significantly improves clinical pregnancy rates.

Administration of hCG to support endogenous production of progesterone from the corpus luteum is another strategy for improving luteal function. Many programs measure progesterone levels following ovulation in COH cycles and administer an additional dose of hCG if progesterone remains below a predefined threshold. This is physiologically sound but again has not been demonstrated outside of ART to improve the chances of pregnancy. Like exogenous progesterone supplementation, hCG administration has been demonstrated to improve success rates in IVF cycles utilizing GnRH analogues. However, the increased risk of OHSS makes this a less desirable strategy than direct progesterone supplementation in ART cycles [40].

Thyroid

Physiology of Thyroid Signaling and Implantation

There is substantial experimental and clinical evidence that implicate thyroid hormones (TH) in the implantation process. While it is unclear whether these actions are mediated through classical endocrine regulation of the hypothalamic-pituitary-thyroid axis, or through paracrine and intracrine signaling at the implantation site, there is little doubt that thyroid hormones help regulate the cascade of events culminating in implantation. Interestingly, there is convincing evidence that TH influences both embryonic and endometrial activity. The following will review the physiology of thyroid hormone actions at the implantation site and discuss recommendations for clinical thyroid management in the infertile patient.

The best evidence for thyroid regulation of implantation is the variation in endometrial expression of nuclear thyroid hormone receptors (TR) and G protein-coupled thyroid stimulating hormone receptors (TSHR) across the menstrual cycle [41]. TRα1, TRβ1, and TSHR are present in the glandular and luminal epithelium of the endometrium, and all demonstrate an increase in expression during the secretory phase followed by a subsequent decrease. Each receptor reaches peak expression at the same time that endometrial pinopodes appear and receptivity is established. Whether these receptors respond primarily to hormones secreted by the thyroid gland or to locally produced TH is still up for debate as evidence exists for TH production in the endometrium. Transcripts encoding deiodinases, thyroglobulin, and thyroid peroxidase are all expressed in the endometrium [42]. Additionally, there is strong evidence suggesting that the endometrium serves as a target tissue of pituitary TSH. During the window of implantation, TSH increases leukemia inhibitory factor (LIF) and LIF receptor expression—both of which are essential components in the implantation cascade. TSH also regulates glucose transport by increasing expression of glucose transporter-1 (GLUT-1) [43]. This biosynthetic activity in the endometrium appears to be partially regulated by the presence of progesterone, as mifepristone administration reduces expression of TR and thyroglobulin. This theory may also explain, in part, menstrual irregularity experienced by patients with thyroid dysfunction [44].

Experimental evidence also suggests that the embryo responds to thyroid hormone both prior to and during implantation. Oocytes, cleavage-stage embryos, and blastocysts all possess TRα mRNA. The preimplantation blastocyst expresses deiodinases and thyroid hormone transporters, such as monocarboxylate transporter 8 (MCT8). Multiple studies have suggested that TH exposure augments early embryo development. Experiments in bovine embryo culture have reported improved embryo cleavage, blastulation rates, and hatching rates when culture media is supplemented with TH [45, 46] Others have theorized that thyroid hormone utilization may result in blastocyst secretion of human chorionic gonadotropin (hCG), thus facilitating embryo-endometrial communication during the time of implantation [43] (Fig. 9.2). After implantation, TH promotes normal placental growth and

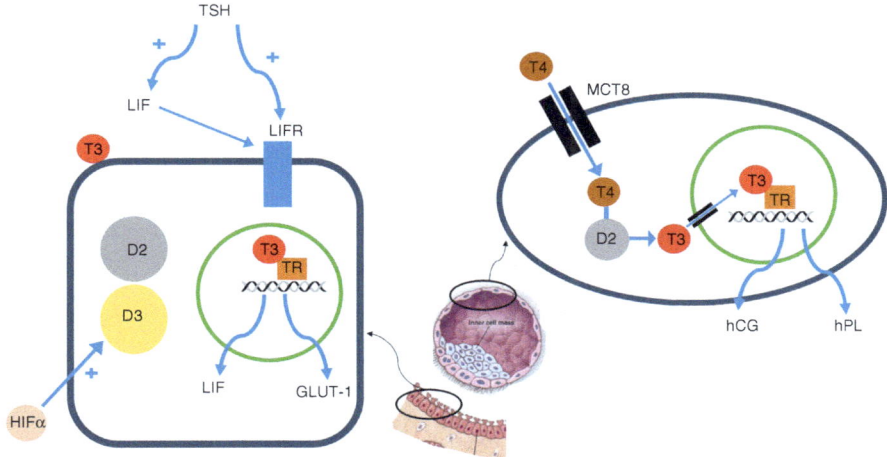

Fig. 9.2 During the window of implantation, TSH increases LIF and LIFR expression and regulates glucose transport by increasing GLUT-1 expression. Low oxygen tension at the implantation site increases HIFα expression which increases deiodinases. The trophectoderm cells express TRs, thyroid hormone transporters, such as MCT8 and deiodinases. T3 helps regulate the production of hCG and later, hPL

invasion by inhibiting expression of pro-apoptotic factors Fas, Fas ligand, and Bcl-2 and preventing cleavage of caspase-3 in the trophoblast [47].

Clinical Management of Thyroid Dysfunction

A substantial body of literature has developed to address the optimal clinical management of thyroid dysfunction in the context of reproduction. This literature has been challenging to interpret due to disagreements in definitions of thyroid pathologies and discrepancies in recommendations for clinical management among national and international professional organizations. However, there is little doubt that gross abnormalities in thyroid function negatively impacts implantation and that treatment improves outcomes. The controversy lies in the more subtle interruptions in thyroid homeostasis.

Overt hypothyroidism is associated with a number of reproductive pathologies. Abnormal thyroid homeostasis can interfere with normal LH pulsatility and can cause hyperprolactinemia [48]. Furthermore, hypothyroidism is associated with an increased risk of miscarriage, preterm birth, gestational hypertension, placental abruption, fetal growth restriction, and impaired neuropsychological development of the offspring [49]. Thus, there is no debate regarding the utility of levothyroxine replacement in patients with overt hypothyroidism.

There is less clarity, however, regarding the proper management subclinical hypothyroidism (SCH) in the context of reproduction. Much of the confusion has stemmed from a disagreement regarding the proper definition of subclinical hypothyroidism. The upper limit of the reference range for TSH levels was established by the National Health and Nutritional Examination Survey (NHANES III) to be 4.5–5 mIU/L [50]. Thus, the classical definition of subclinical hypothyroidism is a TSH level >4.5 mIU/L, with normal free thyroxine (T4) levels. However, the National Academy of Clinical Biochemistry suggested in 2002 that the normal reference range for TSH be reduced to 2.5 mIU/L after reporting that 95% of rigorously screened euthyroid individuals had serum TSH values between 0.4 and 2.5 mIU/L [51]. In addition, the Endocrine Society and the American Society for Reproductive Medicine recommend that 2.5 mIU/L be used as the upper limit of normal for the first trimester of pregnancy [52, 53]. As a result, most IVF programs treat patients with levothyroxine if they demonstrate a TSH value above this range prior to initiating treatment.

The best data in support improved implantation rates in levothyroxine treated SCH patients comes from two randomized controlled trials. Using a cutoff of >4.5 mIU/L, Kim et al. [54] randomized patients with SCH to either levothyroxine (50 micrograms daily) versus no treatment. The implantation rate was significantly higher in the treatment arm than in the control group (26.9 vs. 14.9%, $p = 0.044$). A similar study by Abdel Rahman et al. [55] used a TSH cutoff of 4.2 mIU/L to diagnose SCH and randomized 70 patients to levothyroxine or placebo. In this study, the clinical pregnancy rate was also significantly higher in the treatment group (35 vs. 10%, $p = 0.02$). Thus, there is high-quality data demonstrating that untreated SCH negatively impacts implantation rate after IVF. However, no studies have evaluated whether this effect persists at TSH levels >2.5 mIU/L but <4.2 mIU/L. Furthermore, tighter control of TSH levels below 2.5 do not appear to impact implantation or live birth rates.

One study did evaluate IVF outcomes according to TSH levels in the first 11 weeks of pregnancy. In this study, levels between 2.5 and 5 mIU/L were associated with a significant increase in pregnancy loss (6.1 vs. 3.6%, $p = 0.006$) [56]. However, this study did not control for the chromosomal status of the embryo. Thus, it is possible that the lower hCG levels associated with aneuploid gestations may have contributed to the failure of TSH to fall below 2.5 mIU/L in this cohort. Thus, the ideal TSH level within the normal range for optimizing implantation success is unclear, but levels about 2.5 mIU/L during early pregnancy may increase miscarriage risk.

Multiple studies have addressed whether the evidence of thyroid autoimmunity (anti-thyroperoxidase or antithyroglobulin antibodies) impacts IVF success. A meta-analysis of seven studies including 330 thyroid antibody-positive patients and 1430 controls demonstrated no difference in implantation rate after IVF (odds ratio 0.67, 95% confidence interval 0.36–1.4, $p = 0.67$) [57]. One prospective, randomized controlled trial evaluated empiric treatment with levothyroxine in euthyroid patients with evidence of thyroid autoimmunity. In that study, there was a trend to improvement in clinical pregnancy rates between the treated and untreated patients (56 vs. 49%); however, transfer order was not reported in each group, limiting the conclusion [58]. Furthermore, this data has not been replicated in other trials, and thus further evaluation is merited. However, both the meta-analysis and prospective trials listed above suggested that thyroid autoimmunity increased the risk of miscarriage and preterm delivery, which could be prevented by replacement therapy. Thus, if a decision is made to not treat women with TSH levels between 2.5 and 5.0 mIU/L, it may be prudent to measure thyroid peroxidase antibodies and treat if positive [59].

Summary

A proper endocrine stimulus is required to allow the endometrium to accept and support pregnancy. A significant body of literature has contributed to our understanding of how this complex system coordinates endometrial development and prepares the uterus for implantation. However, many of the current tools for improving the efficiency of a given cycle, such as exogenous gonadotropins, may negatively impact endometrial receptivity. Thus, special attention is required in patients with recurrent implantation failure to ensure that modern therapies are not inadvertently decreasing their chances of achieving sustained implantation. More data is needed in this regard.

Furthermore, our tools for assessing the health of the endocrine system in relation to implantation remain limited. Many new and exciting diagnostic methods are currently in development that may help elucidate the effect of endocrine stimuli on the endometrial receptivity. As with many aspects of modern infertility care, it is likely that a strong understanding of the physiologic basis of normal implantation, combined with state of the art molecular technologies, will help develop treatments strategies that mimic the natural setting while harnessing the power of modern assisted reproductive techniques. These advanced diagnostics are needed as we push to optimize outcomes.

References

1. Treloar AE, Boynton RE, Begn BG, Brown BW. Variation of the human menstrual cycle through reproductive life. Int J Fertil. 1967;12:77–126.
2. Rock J, Bartlett MK. Biopsy studies of human endometrium. JAMA. 1937;108(24):2022–8.
3. Noyes RW, Hertig AT, Rock J. Dating the endometrial biopsy. Fertil Steril. 1950;1:3–25.
4. Murray MJ, Meyer WR, Zaino RJ, Lessey BA, Novotny DB, Ireland K, Zeng D, Fritz MA. A critical analysis of the accuracy, reproducibility, and clinical utility of histologic endometrial dating in fertile women. Fertil Steril. 2004;81:1333–43.
5. Scott RT, Snyder RR, Strickland DM, Tyburski CC, Bagnall JA, Reed KR, Adair CA, Hensley SB. The effect of interobserver variation in dating endometrial histology of the diagnosis of luteal phase defects. Fertil Steril. 1988;50:888–92.
6. Smith S, Hosid S, Scott L. Endometrial biopsy dating. Interobserver variation and its impact on clinical practice. J Reprod Med. 1995;76:782–91.
7. Deglidisch L. Hormonal pathology of the endometrium. Mod Pathol. 2000;13:285–94.

8. Coutifaris C, Myers ER, Guzick DS, Diamond MP, Carson SA, Legro RS, McGovern PG, Schlaff WD, Carr BR, Steinkampf MP, Silva S, Vogel DL, Leppert PC. Histological dating of timed endometrial biopsy tissue is not related to fertility status. Fertil Steril. 2004;82:1264–72.

9. Evans J, Hannan NJ, Edgell TA, Vollenhoven BJ, Lutjen PJ, Osianlis T, Salamonsen LA, Rombauts LJF, Hincks C, Rombauts LJ, Salamonsen LA. Fresh versus frozen embryo transfer: backing clinical decisions with scientific and clinical evidence. Hum Reprod Update. 2014;0:1–14.

10. Horcajadas JA, Riesewijk A, Polman J, van Os R, Pellicer A, Mosselman S, Simon C. Effect of controlled ovarian hyperstimulation in IVF on endometrial gene expression profiles. Mol Hum Reprod. 2005;11:195–205.

11. Van Vaerenbergh I, Van Lommel L, Ghislain V, In't Veld P, Schuit F, Fatemi HM, Devroey P, Bourgain C. In GnRH antagonist/rec-FSH stimulated cycles, advanced endometrial maturation on the day of oocyte retrieval correlates with altered gene expression. Hum Reprod. 2009;24:1085–91.

12. Li R, Qiao J, Wang L, Li L, Zhen X, Liu P, Zheng X. MicroRNA array and microarray evaluation of endometrial receptivity in patients with high serum progesterone levels on the day of hCG administration. Reprod Biol Endocrinol. 2011;9:29.

13. Kolibianakis EM, Bourgain C, Papanikolaou EG, Camus M, Tournaye H, Van Steirteghem AC, Devroey P. Prolongation of follicular phase by delaying hCG administration results in higher incidence of endometrial advancement on the day of oocyte retrieval in GnRH antagonist cycles. Hum Reprod. 2005;20:2453–6.

14. Ubaldi F, Bourgain C, Tournaye H, Smitz J, Van Steirteghem A, Devroey P. Endometrial evaluation by aspiration biopsy on the day of oocyte retrieval in the embryo transfer cycles in patients with serum progesterone rise during the follicular phase. Fertil Steril. 1997;67:521–6.

15. Shapiro BS, Daneshmand ST, Garner FC, Aguirre M, Hudson C, Thomas S. Evidence of impaired endometrial receptivity after ovarian stimulation for in vitro fertilization: a prospective randomized trial comparing fresh and frozen-thawed embryo transfer in normal responders. Fertil Steril. 2011;96(2):344–8.

16. Yang S, Pang T, Li R, Yang R, Zhen X, Chen X, Wang H, Ma C, Liu P, Qiao J. The individualized choice of embryo transfer timing for patients with elevated serum progesterone level on the HCG day in IVF/ICSI cycles: a prospective randomized clinical study. Gynecol Endocrinol. 2015;31(5):355–8.

17. Marchini M, Fedele L, Bianchi S, Losa GA, Ghisletta M, Gandiani GB. Secretory changes in preovulatory during controlled ovarian hyperstimulation with buserelin acetate and human gonadotropins. Fertil Steril. 1991;55:717–21.

18. Ma WG, Song H, Das SK, Paria BC, Dey SK. Estrogen is a critical determinant that specifies the duration of the window of uterine receptivity for implantation. Proc Natl Acad Sci U S A. 2003;100:2963–8.

19. Chen ZJ, Shi Y, Sun Y, Zhang B, Liang X, Cao Y, Yang J, Liu J, Wei D, Weng N, Tian L, Hao C, Yang D, Zhou F, Shi J, Xu Y, Li J, Yan J, Qin Y, Zhao H, Zhang H, Legro R. Fresh versus frozen embryos for infertility in the polycystic ovary syndrome. N Engl J Med. 2016;375:523–33.

20. Chen HC, Zhang X, Barnes R, Confino E, Milad M, Puscheck E, Kazer R. Relationship between peak serum estradiol levels and treatment outcome in in vitro fertilization cycles after embryo transfer on day 3 or day 5. Fertil Steril. 2003;80:75–9.

21. Levi AJ, Drews MR, Bergh PA, Miller BT, Scott RT Jr. Controlled ovarian hyperstimulation does not adversely affect endometrial receptivity in in vitro fertilization cycles. Fertil Steril. 2001;76(4):670.

22. Papageorgiou T, Guibert J, Goffinet F, Patrat C, Fulla Y, Janssens Y, Zorn AR. Percentile curves of serum estradiol levels during controlled ovarian stimulation in 905 cycles stimulated with recombinant FSH show that high estradiol is not detrimental to IVF outcome. Hum Reprod. 2001;17:2846–50.

23. Hancke K, More S, Kreienberg R, Weiss JM. Patients undergoing frozen-thawed embryo transfer have similar live birth rates in spontaneous and artificial cycles. J Assist Reprod Genet. 2012;29:403–7.

24. Tomax C, Alsbjerg B, Martikainen H, Humaidan P. Pregnancy loss after frozen-embryo transfer – a comparison of three protocols. Fertil Steril. 2012;98:1165–9.
25. Ghobara T, Vandekerckhove P. Cycle regimens for frozen-thawed embryo transfer. Cochrane Database Syst Rev. 2008;7:CD003414.
26. Groenewoud ER, Cantineau AEP, Kollen BJ, Mackon NS, Cohlen BJ. What is the optimal means of preparing the endometrium in frozen-thawed embryo transfer cycles? A systematic review and meta-analysis. Hum Reprod Update. 2013;19:458–70.
27. Cattoli M. A randomized prospective study on cryopreserved-thawed embryo transfer: natural versus hormone replacement cycles. Abstracts of the 10th Annual Meeting of the ESHRE Brussels 1994;356:139.
28. Mounce G, McVeigh E, Turner K, Child TJ. Randomized, controlled pilot trial of natural versus hormone replacement therapy cycles in frozen embryo replacement in vitro fertilization. Fertil Steril. 2015;104:915–20.
29. Greco E, Litwicka K, Arrivi C, Varrichio MT, Caragia A, Greco A, Minasi MG, Fiorentino G. The endometrial preparation for frozen thawed euploid blastocyst transfer: a prospective randomized trial comparing clinical results from natural modified cycle with exogenous hormone stimulation with GnRH agonist. J Assist Reprod Genet. 2016;33:873–84.
30. Baird DD, Weinberg CR, Wilcox AJ, McConnaughey DR, Musey PL, Collins DC. Hormonal profiles of natural conception cycles in ending in early, unrecognized pregnancy loss. New Engl J Med. 1999;340:1796–9. Nonsupplemented luteal phase characteristics after the administration of recombinant human chorionic gonadotropin, recombinant luteinizing hormone, or gonadotropin-releasing hormone (GnRH) agonist to induce final oocyte maturation in in vitro fertilization patients after ovarian stimulation with recombinant follicle-stimulating hormone and GnRH antagonist cotreatment. J Clin Endocrinol Metab. 2003;88(9):4186–92
31. Jones GES. Some newer aspects of management of infertility. JAMA. 1949;141:1123–9.
32. Speroff L, Fritz MA. Clinical gynecologic endocrinology and infertility. 8th ed. Philadelphia: Lippincott Williams & Wilkins; 2014.
33. Filicori M, Butler JP, Crowley WF Jr. Neuroendocrine regulation of the corpus luteum in the human. Evidence for pulsatile progesterone secretion. J Clin Invest. 1984;73:1638–47.
34. Davis OK, Berkeley AS, Naus GJ, Cholst IN, Freedman KS. The incidence of luteal phase defect in normal, fertile women, determine by serial endometrial biopsies. Fertil Steril. 1989;51:582–56.
35. Usadi RS, Groll JM, Lessey BA, Lininger RA, Zaino RJ, Fritz MA. Endometrial development and function in experimentally induced luteal phase deficiency. J Clin Endocrinol Metab. 2008;93:4058–64.
36. Mitwally MF, Diamond MP, Abuzeid M. Vaginal micronized progesterone versus intramuscular progesterone for luteal support in women undergoing in vitro fertilization-embryo transfer. Fertil Steril. 2010;93(20):554–69.
37. American Society for Reproductive Medicine Practice Committee. Current clinical irrelevance of luteal phase deficiency: a committee opinion. Fertil Steril. 2015;103:327–e32.
38. Pritts EA, Atwood AK. Luteal phase support in infertility treatment: a meta-analysis of the randomized trials. Hum Reprod. 2002;17:2287–99.
39. Beckers NG, Latteau P, Eijkemans MJ, Macklon NS, de Jong FH, Devroey P, Fauser BC. The early luteal phase administration of estrogen and progesterone does not induce premature luteolysis in normo-ovulatory women. Eur J Endocrinol. 2006;1559(2):355–63.
40. Daya S, Gunby J. Luteal phase support in assisted reproduction cycles. Cochrane Database Syst Rev. 2004;10:CD004830.
41. Aghajanova L, Stavreus-Evers A, Lindeberg M, Landgren BM, Skjoldebrand Sparre L, Hovatta O. Thyroid-stimulating hormone receptor and thyroid hormone-receptors are involved in human endometrial physiology. Fertil Steril. 2011;95:230–7.
42. Catalano RD, Critchley HO, Heikinheimo O, Baird DT, Hapangama D, Sherwin JRA, Charnock-Jones DS, Smith SK, Sharkey AM. Mifepristone induced progesterone withdrawal reveals novel regulatory pathways in the human endometrium. Mol Hum Reprod. 2007;13:641–54.

43. Colicchia M, Campagnolo L, Baldini E, Ulisse S, Valensise H, Moretti C. Molecular basis of thyrotropin and thyroid hormone action during implantation and early development. Hum Reprod Update. 2014;20(6):884–904.
44. Scoccia B, Demir H, Kang Y, Fierro MA, Winston NJ. In vitro fertilization pregnancy rates in levothyroxine-treated women with hypothyroidism compared to women without thyroid dysfunction disorders. Thyroid. 2012;22:631–6.
45. Ashkar FA, Semple E, Schmidt CH, St John E, Bartlewski PM, King WA. Thyroid hormone supplementation improves bovine embryo development in vitro. Hum Reprod. 2010;25:334–44.
46. Costa NN, Cordeiro MS, Silva TV, Sastre D, Santana PP, Sa AL, Sampaio RV, Santos SS, Adona PR, Miranda MS. Effect of triiodothyronine on developmental competence of bovine oocytes. Theriogenology. 2013;80:295–301.
47. Laoag-Fernandez JB, Matsuo H, Murakoshi H, Hamada AL, Tsang BK, Maruo T. 3,5,3′-Triiodothyronine down-regulates Fas and Fas ligand expression and suppresses caspase-3 and poly (adenosine 5′-diphosphate-ribose) polymerase cleavage and apoptosis in early placental extravillous trophoblasts in vitro. J Clin Endocrinol Metab. 2004;89:4069–77.
48. Krassas GE, Poppe K, Glinoer D. Thyroid function and human reproductive health. Endocr Rev. 2010;31:702–55.
49. Vissenberg R, van den Boogaard E, van Wely M, van der Post JA, Filers E, Bisschop PH, Goddijn M. Treatment of thyroid disorders before conception and in early pregnancy: a systematic review. Hum Reprod Update. 2012;18:360–73.
50. Hollowell JG, Staehling NW, Flanders WD, Hannon WH, Gunter EW, Spencer CA, et al. Serum TSH, T(4), and thyroid antibodies in the United States population (1988 to 1994): National Health and Nutrition Examination Survey (NHANES III). J Clin Endocrinol Metab. 2002;87:489–99.
51. National Academy of Clinical Biochemistry. Laboratory medicine practice guidelines. Laboratory support for the diagnosis of thyroid disease, vol. 13. Washington, DC: The National Academy of Clinical Biochemistry; 2002.
52. American Society for Reproductive Medicine Practice Committee. Subclinical hypothyroidism in the infertile female population: a guideline. Fertil Steril. 2015;104:545–53.
53. De Groot L, Abalovich M, Alexander EK, Amino N, Barbour L, Cobin RH, Eastman CJ, Lazarus JH, Luton D, Mandel SJ, Mestman J, Rovet J, Sullivan S. Management of thyroid dysfunction during pregnancy and postpartum: an Endocrine Society clinical practice guideline. J Clin Endocrinol Metab. 2012;97:2543–65.
54. Kim CH, Ahn JW, Kang SP, Kim SH, Chae HD, Kang BM. Effect of levothyroxine treatment on in vitro fertilization and pregnancy outcome in infertile women with subclinical hypothyroidism undergoing in vitro fertilization/intracytoplasmic sperm injection. Fertil Steril. 2011;95(5):1650–4.
55. Abdel Rahman AH, Aly Abbassy H, Abbassy AA. Improved in vitro fertilization outcomes after treatment of subclinical hypothyroidism in infertile women. Endocr Pract. 2010;16:792–7.
56. Negro R, Mangieri T, Coppola L, Presicce G, Casavola EC, Gismondi R, Locorotondo G, Caroli P, Pezzarossa A, Dazzi D, Hassan H. Levothyroxine treatment in thyroid peroxidase antibody-positive women undergoing assisted reproduction technologies: a prospective study. Hum Reprod. 2005;20:1529–33.
57. van den Boogaard E, Vissenberg R, Land JA, van Wely M, van der Post JA, Goddijn M, Bisschop PH. Significance of (sub)clinical thyroid dysfunction and thyroid autoimmunity before conception and in early pregnancy: a systematic review. Hum Reprod Update. 2011;17:605–19.
58. Negro R, Schwartz A, Gismondi R, Tinelli A, Mangieri T, Stagnaro-Green A. Increased pregnancy loss rate in thyroid antibody negative women with TSH levels between 2.5 and 5.0 in the first trimester of pregnancy. J Clin Endocrinol Metab. 2010;95:E44–8.
59. Fox C, Morin S, Jeong JW, Scott RT Jr, Lessey BA. Local and systemic factors and implantation: what is the evidence? Fertil Steril. 2016;105:873–84.

Chapter 10
Anatomic Abnormalities and Recurrent Implantation Failure

Jeffrey M. Goldberg, Julian Gingold, and Natalia Llarena

Fibroids

Uterine myomas are the most common uterine abnormality with a lifetime incidence of up to 70% among white women and 80% in black women and an annual incidence that increases with age up to menopause [1]. They have been classified by International Federation of Gynecology and Obstetrics (FIGO) stage as submucosal, intramural, subserosal, and cervical [2–4] (Fig. 10.1).

Fibroids arise as benign monoclonal tumors of the smooth muscle cells of the myometrium, frequently due to a single event involving multiple chromosomal breaks with random reassembly [5]. Myoma origin has also been traced to point mutations in the mediator complex subunit MED12 [6]. In addition to causing anatomical distortions of the uterine cavity, leiomyomas are known to express higher levels of TGF-β mRNA [7]. Stro-1/CD44 has been proposed as a putative human fibroid (as well as myometrial) stem cell marker based on formation of fibroid-like lesions in xenotransplantation mouse models [8].

Infertility Associated with Fibroids

It is clear based on multiple prospective trials and systematic reviews that submucosal myomas adversely impact fertility, decreasing successful IVF outcomes by approximately 70%, whereas subserosal myomas appear to have minimal impact on fertility [9–11]. Although some early data on intramural myomas showed no adverse effect on fertility [9, 12, 13], several systematic reviews have since revealed a

J.M. Goldberg, MD (✉) • J. Gingold, MD • N. Llarena, MD
Department of Gynecology and Obstetrics, Cleveland Clinic, Cleveland, OH, USA
e-mail: goldbej@ccf.org

© Springer International Publishing AG 2018
J.M. Franasiak, R.T. Scott Jr. (eds.), *Recurrent Implantation Failure*,
https://doi.org/10.1007/978-3-319-71967-2_10

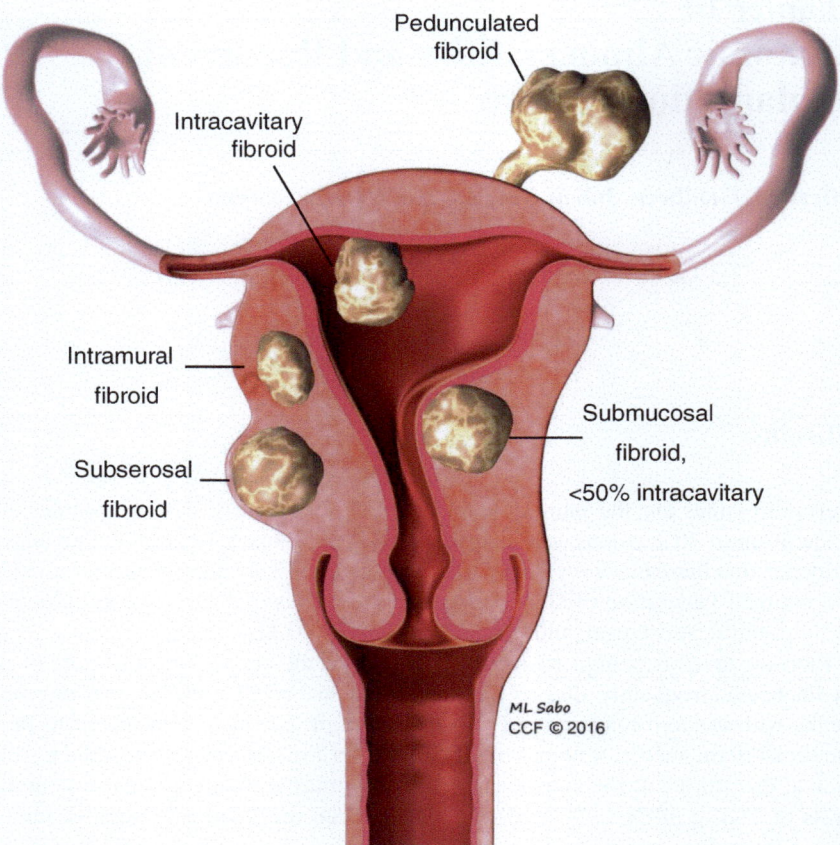

Fig. 10.1 Uterine fibroids. Fibroids may be present as submucosal, intramural, or subserosal lesions and may be located anywhere in the uterus, including the cervix. Myomectomy for fibroids distorting the endometrial cavity is recommended to improve fertility and reduce recurrent pregnancy loss. ©ML Sabo CCF 2016

reduction in IVF success rates of 20–30% associated with intramural fibroids [10, 11, 14]. A 2009 meta-analysis of 23 studies evaluated IVF outcomes among patients with and without uterine fibroids. Significantly decreased clinical pregnancy (RR, 0.363; 95% CI, 0.179–0.737) and live birth rates (RR, 0.283; 95% CI, 0.123–0.649) as well as an increased miscarriage rate (RR, 1.678; 95% CI, 1.373–2.051) were observed in patients with submucosal fibroids compared to controls [10]. There was no significant difference in clinical pregnancy, live birth, or miscarriage rates among patients with subserosal fibroids [10]. In patients with intramural myomas, the review reported decreased pregnancy (RR, 0.810; 95% CI, 0.696–0.941) and live birth (RR, 0.684; 95% CI, 0.587–0.796) rates, as well as an increased miscarriage rate (RR, 1.747; 95% CI, 1.226–2.489) [10]. Other systematic reviews reported similar findings [11, 14].

Pathophysiology

Infertility associated with fibroids has been attributed to a number of mechanisms, but the most significant effects of fibroids on fertility are thought to result from impaired implantation. Mechanical distortion of the uterine cavity may adversely affect implantation by obstructing fallopian tubes, increasing the presence of blood and clots in the uterine cavity, and disturbing normal uterine contractility [15–17]. Increased uterine contractility may prevent sperm migration, embryo transport, and ovum capture [18–21]. MRI studies show altered uterine contractility during the mid-luteal phase among infertile patients with intramural fibroids [17]. In a follow-up study, this increased contractility improved after myomectomy and was associated with improved pregnancy rates [22]. In addition to causing mechanical endometrial distortion, there is also evidence that fibroids may impair implantation at the histologic and molecular levels. Glandular atrophy, hypertrophy, adenomyosis, and the separation of glands from the basal layer of the endometrium have all been observed surrounding myomas in otherwise normal endometrium [23]. Studies have shown altered expression of the HOXA-10 and HOXA-11 genes, which are hypothesized to be involved in the molecular events leading to implantation, in fibroids [24]. These changes, together with focal endometrial inflammation [19, 21], may impair implantation. Finally, vascular disturbances such as venous congestion and diminished endometrial perfusion may compromise nidation [25–27].

Medical Interventions

Until the recent introduction of selective progesterone receptor modulators, gonadotropin-releasing hormone (GnRH) agonists such as leuprolide acetate were considered the most effective medical option for management of symptomatic fibroids [28, 29]. In vitro studies show that GnRH agonists lead to increased expression of GnRHR1, COL1A1, fibronectin, and versican variant V0 in leiomyoma cells [30]. In addition, GnRH agonists inhibit the production of extracellular matrix proteins despite the presence of gonadal hormones [31]. A RCT comparing leuprolide plus iron with iron alone found a significant reduction in uterine and myoma volume with leuprolide treatment [29]. This finding is consistent across multiple similar studies [32–34] and confirmed by a Cochrane meta-analysis [35]. Unfortunately, menopausal side effects related to hypoestrogenism have been widely reported in the majority of leuprolide-treated patients in all studies and generally preclude long-term treatment [28, 29, 32–34]. Because this therapy is typically limited to short-term symptomatic treatment prior to surgery, it has not been explored as an alternative to surgery [36]. While the fertility outcomes of leuprolide therapy in management of myomas have never been tested, many have advocated for its use as an adjunct to surgical myomectomy in women who desire further fertility because of the decreased uterine trauma involved in excising smaller lesions [34, 37].

Selective progesterone receptor modulators, most notably ulipristal, have been evaluated as a nonsurgical option for fibroids [38]. A landmark double-blind non-inferiority study found that ulipristal was non-inferior to leuprolide in controlling bleeding from symptomatic fibroids, and significantly fewer (10 vs 40%) moderate to severe hot flashes were observed in the ulipristal group [28]. Although never studied as an intervention for infertility, multiple studies have demonstrated regression of fibroids after treatment with ulipristal with improvement of anemia and pelvic pain [28, 39, 40], suggesting that that medical management may reverse some of the endomyometrial changes that are hypothesized to diminish fertility. Ulipristal downregulates angiogenic factors and cell proliferation in leiomyoma cells but not normal myometrial cells by increasing the expression of caspase-3 and decreasing the expression of Bcl-2 [36, 41, 42]. Case series of pregnancies resulting from ulipristal treatment in infertile patients also have been reported, including two patients whose fibroid regression was significant enough to resolve previous cavitary distortion and permit a pregnancy without the need for surgery [43, 44].

Danazol is also frequently used to control bleeding from fibroids [36], but this therapy currently lacks reliable supporting evidence [45].

Surgical Intervention

The role of myomectomy for infertility varies based on the type, number, and size of fibroids, as well as other factors that affect a patient's fertility, including ovarian reserve and age [15]. Weak mechanistic evidence supporting the benefits of surgical intervention comes from a study of infertile patients with intramural leiomyomas (IM) not distorting the endometrial cavity that found that mRNA expression of HOXA-10 and HOXA-11 from mid-luteal endometrial biopsies had a trend toward decreased levels compared with fertile patients and that this expression significantly increased 3 months after myomectomy [46].

There is clear evidence that myomectomy for submucosal fibroids significantly improves fertility outcomes associated with both spontaneous conception and IVF. A meta-analysis reported that myomectomy doubled clinical IVF pregnancy rates compared with patients who did not undergo myomectomy (RR: 2.034, 95% CI: 1.081–3.826) [10]. Similarly, a prospective study evaluating 181 women with fibroids showed improved pregnancy rates in the year following myomectomy without additional fertility interventions [47]. Among patients with submucosal fibroids, 43.3% who underwent abdominal or hysteroscopic myomectomy achieved pregnancy, compared to 27.2% among patients who did not undergo surgery [47]. Overall, these data suggest an important role for myomectomy to improve fertility outcomes in patients planning to undergo IVF or pursue natural conception. The Society of Obstetricians and Gynecologists of Canada has issued clinical practice guidelines recommending the removal of submucosal fibroids to improve pregnancy rates in patients with otherwise unexplained infertility [48]. The benefits of myomectomy appear to be most pronounced in patients under the age of 35 with less than 3 years of infertility [49].

Although intramural fibroids appear to have a negative impact on fertility as well, there is no clear consensus on whether myomectomy for intramural myomas improves fertility outcomes. A prospective study evaluating spontaneous conception rates in 181 patients with fibroids showed improved pregnancy rates in patients with intramural fibroids in the year after myomectomy compared to patients who declined myomectomy (from 40.9 to 56.5%); however, this improvement did not reach statistical significance [47]. Another prospective cohort study evaluated IVF outcomes in patients with intramural or subserosal fibroids with at least one fibroid measuring >5 cm in diameter. These investigators showed significantly increased rates of clinical pregnancy and delivery across three IVF cycles among patients with fibroids who underwent myomectomy prior to IVF, as compared to those who did not [50]. Conversely, a 2012 Cochrane review including three randomized controlled trials found insufficient evidence to support an improvement in fertility outcomes after myomectomy for patients with intramural fibroids [51]. Given the lack of clear fertility benefit to myomectomy for intramural fibroids, decisions about when to pursue myomectomy can be challenging. The uncertain benefits of myomectomy must be balanced with the risks of surgery, including postoperative adnexal adhesions and uterine rupture during subsequent pregnancy [15]. The Society of Obstetricians and Gynecologists of Canada recommends against the removal of intramural fibroids in patients with unexplained infertility who have hysteroscopically confirmed normal endometrial cavity endometrium, regardless of the size of the fibroids [48]. However, large intramural myomas may increase the risk of pregnancy complications such as miscarriage, preterm delivery, malpresentation, outlet obstruction, postpartum hemorrhage, and pain from degeneration.

As there is no evidence for reduced fertility associated with subserosal fibroids, unless fibroids are large enough to obstruct the fallopian tubes or affect uterine growth, they should not be removed to optimize fertility outcomes [15, 48].

When myomectomy is indicated, there is little available data to suggest a benefit of one surgical approach over another. Resection of submucosal fibroids should be performed hysteroscopically when ≥50% of the myoma is intracavitary, as this is the least invasive mode of myomectomy. Expert opinion suggests that fibroids ≤5 cm in diameter can typically be resected hysteroscopically, though larger fibroids have successfully been removed using a hysteroscopic approach [48]. Two randomized trials compared reproductive outcomes after laparoscopic versus abdominal myomectomy. One study of 131 patients who underwent myomectomy showed no significant differences in the rates of pregnancy, miscarriage, cesarean delivery, or preterm delivery in the laparoscopic versus abdominal myomectomy groups [52]. Not surprisingly, the investigators reported a shorter hospital stay and a smaller postoperative hemoglobin drop in the laparoscopic compared with the abdominal group [52]. Another study of reproductive outcomes after minilaparotomy and laparoscopic myomectomy showed similar cumulative pregnancy, live birth, and miscarriage rates at 12 months [53]. Laparoscopic myomectomy is typically recommended for myomas <10–12 cm in size, less than 4 in number and for intramural myomas >3–5 cm in size with cavity distortion in cases of infertility [18, 38, 54]. Robotic-assisted laparoscopic myomectomy offers similar outcomes to laparoscopic myomectomy, but operative times and costs are increased [55].

Other Interventions

Uterine artery embolization (UAE) has been studied and effectively used to improve bulk symptoms and menorrhagia [56–59]. However, desire for future fertility is a contraindication to UAE given the poor reproductive and obstetric outcomes observed following the procedure. In an average follow-up of 33.4 months, only 1 in 31 women became pregnant after UAE [60]. A randomized controlled trial comparing UAE to myomectomy in 121 patients with intramural fibroids >4 cm revealed a significantly increased rate of miscarriage and a decreased rate of pregnancy in the UAE group compared to the myomectomy cohort [61]. Similarly, a cohort of 53 pregnancies after UAE and 139 pregnancies after laparoscopic myomectomy showed a higher rate of preterm delivery, fetal malpresentation, and cesarean section in the UAE group [62]. The most common complication reported in pregnancies after UAE is postpartum hemorrhage; however, cases of abnormal placentation have also been reported [63]. In addition, UAE may decrease ovarian reserve by compromising the ovarian blood supply through the utero-ovarian ligament, leading to a detectable increase in FSH and decrease in AMH compared with expected age-related changes [64]. Although pregnancy is possible following uterine artery embolization, the procedure should not be offered to patients seeking future fertility.

Magnetic resonance-guided focused ultrasound surgery (MRgFUS) has also been explored as an intervention for fibroids [65]. MRgFUS permits thermal ablation of fibroids while minimizing damage to nearby structures using mapping from T2-weighted MRI. Preliminary experience of fertility outcomes from this technique has been most extensively described by Rabinovici, who reported 54 pregnancies in 51 women after MRgFUS [66].

Preliminary studies of a recently approved laparoscopic radiofrequency volumetric thermal ablation device [67] have observed a significantly shorter hospital stay, and less intraoperative blood loss with this treatment than with laparoscopic myomectomy, although fertility outcomes are still unknown [68].

Polyps

Endometrial polyps are focal overgrowths of endometrial glands and stroma within the uterine cavity supplied by a single blood vessel [69]. The functional layer of the polyp endometrium may be asynchronous with the surrounding endometrium,

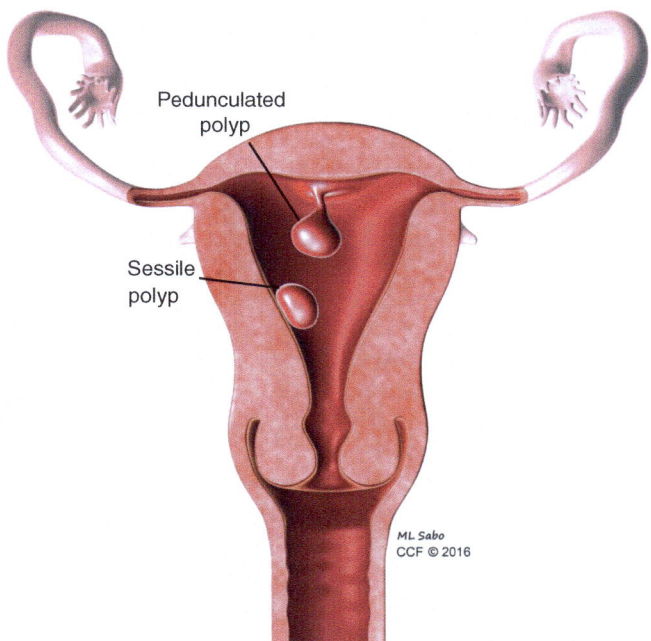

Fig. 10.2 Uterine polyps. Hysteroscopic resection of both pedunculated and sessile polyps is both technically straightforward and highly effective in improving IVF outcomes. ©ML Sabo CCF 2016

predisposing patients to symptoms of abnormal uterine bleeding [70]. Polyps are classified as sessile or pedunculated and can be found anywhere in the uterine cavity, but are particularly common near the fundus [71] (Fig. 10.2).

The overall prevalence of polyps in asymptomatic women undergoing treatment for infertility has ranged across studies from 6 to 32% [72, 73]. Polyps are more prevalent in women with unexplained infertility (15.6%) compared with those with a history of tubal ligation (3.2%) [70].

Pathophysiology

As with fibroids, mechanical distortion of the cavity impeding sperm or ovum transport is thought to play a role in reducing fertility [70]. Elevated nuclear factor kappa-B (NF-κB) expression and p65 immunoreactivity were observed in the endometrium of women with polyps compared with unexplained infertile and fertile controls [74]. In addition, elevated expression of progesterone receptor (PR) in the polyp stromal compartment and elevated Cox-2 and Bcl-2 in the glandular compartment were noted in obese females whose polyps were examined following resection [75]. Decreased LIF mRNA expression has been reported in women with abnormal uterine cavities (uterine submucosal myoma or an endometrial polyp) during the mid-secretory phase [76], and the presence of endometrial polyps is associated with decreased mid-secretory concentrations of IGFBP-1, TNF-α, and osteopontin [77]. These expression changes are reversed following surgical polypectomy [77]. These findings collectively suggest that inflammatory changes may contribute to polyp-associated infertility.

Surgical Intervention

In contrast to fibroids, there is consensus on the role of surgical intervention for endometrial polyps in the management of infertility. A systematic review reported that hysteroscopic polypectomy prior to IUI can increase clinical pregnancy rate compared with diagnostic hysteroscopy alone [78]. These findings are largely based on a single RCT of patients with polyps comparing hysteroscopic polypectomy with diagnostic hysteroscopy that found significantly higher pregnancy rates in the treatment group after up to four IUI cycles [79].

Expert opinion suggests that hysteroscopic polypectomy should be performed prior to IVF to optimize chances of successful implantation [80]. There remains some controversy about the true benefit of operative hysteroscopy in light of a meta-analysis of routine hysteroscopy prior to IVF that noted a benefit to hysteroscopy on pregnancy rates (RR, 1.44, 95% CI 1.08–1.92) that was not related to the degree of uterine pathology noted [81]. Nonetheless, evaluation of the uterine cavity and removal of any polyps remains the standard of care.

Intrauterine Adhesions

Intrauterine adhesions vary in extent from a single filmy adhesion to complete obliteration of the endometrial cavity [82, 83] (Fig. 10.3). They are most commonly the result of uterine instrumentation, particularly postpartum curettage [84]. Although the term Asherman syndrome is often used interchangeably with intrauterine adhesions, a distinction should be made between asymptomatic intrauterine adhesions and hysteroscopically confirmed adhesions associated with amenorrhea, hypomenorrhea, subfertility, recurrent pregnancy loss, or abnormal placentation including previa and accreta. The latter category is defined as Asherman syndrome [85].

Given a reported prevalence of adhesions of up to 38% in patients with early pregnancy loss [86] and 8% in infertile women [87], clinicians must be aware of the possibility of an adhesion among patients seeking infertility treatment even in the absence of secondary amenorrhea, a diagnosis associated with a 3% prevalence of adhesions [87].

Although hysteroscopy is the gold standard for diagnosis, hysterosalpingography and saline sonohysterography can also be used to evaluate for adhesions. However, hysteroscopy is required to determine the extent and location of adhesions [85].

Fig. 10.3 Uterine adhesions may completely obliterate the uterine cavity and replace functional endometrium. Clinical success in terms of restoring normal menstrual and reproductive function is based on the degree of cavity scarring and the ability of the remaining endometrium to cover the raw surfaces following adhesiolysis. ©ML Sabo CCF 2016

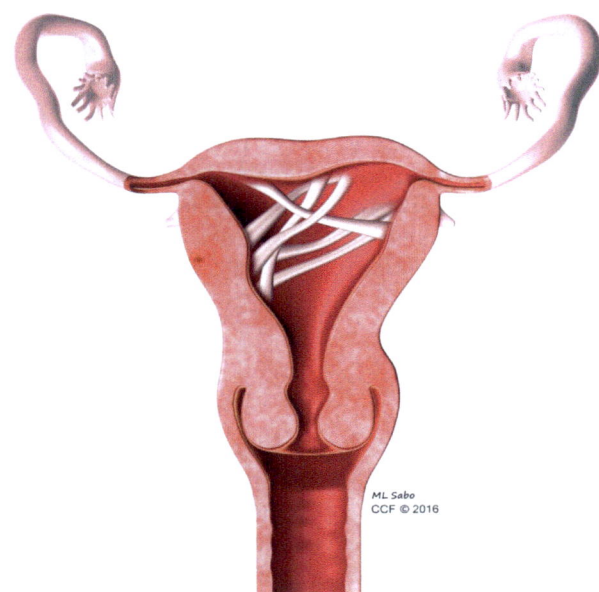

Pathophysiology

In a review of 1856 cases of intrauterine adhesions, over 90% were associated with a previous pregnancy [84]. Of the patients with a pregnancy-related adhesion, two thirds had undergone a post-abortion/miscarriage curettage [84]. A possible explanation for the susceptibility of the gravid uterus to Asherman is the low estrogen status at the time of instrumentation, given that the endometrium requires estrogen for regeneration [85]. Other rare causes in a non-gravid uterus were traced to a diagnostic curettage, myomectomy, polypectomy, placement of an IUD, exposure to radiation, and genital tuberculosis [84, 88]. In addition, intrauterine adhesions are widely reported to form following endometrial ablation procedures [89, 90], contraindicating use of this treatment modality in women desiring fertility [91].

Intrauterine adhesions are characterized by multiple histologic changes, including replacement of endometrial stroma with fibrous tissue, replacement of the functionalis and basalis layers with cubo-columnar epithelium, and adherence of opposing endometrial surfaces, obliterating the cavity [85, 92]. The epithelial monolayer that replaces the functional endometrial layer is not responsive to hormonal stimulation, and synechiae form across the cavity. The tissue is typically avascular. Calcification or ossification may occur in the stroma, and glands may be either inactive or cystically dilated [88]. Alterations to the vascularity of the endometrium have been shown using angiography, with a significant reduction in myometrial blood flow and vascular occlusion in patients with hypomenorrhea [93]. These changes are likely to adversely affect implantation, as hypotrophic endometrium is unreceptive to an embryo [88, 93]. While inflammation is thought to play a role, a study of women who underwent cesarean sections found that endometritis alone does not play a significant role in adhesion formation [94].

An evaluation of 2151 cases of Asherman syndrome showed an infertility rate of 43% [84]. This infertility may be a result of obstruction of the fallopian tubes, uterine cavity, or cervical canal due to adhesions [85]. The synechiae may negatively affect sperm transport and implantation [85]. Elevated rates of pregnancy loss among patients with Asherman syndrome may be secondary to insufficient endometrial tissue to support implantation and placental development and abnormal vascularization of remaining endometrial tissue due to fibrosis [85].

Treatment

No high-quality RCTs exist to support surgical correction of intrauterine adhesions to treat infertility [78, 82]. Nonetheless cohort studies strongly support hysteroscopic adhesiolysis for patients found to have intrauterine adhesions. Hysteroscopic lysis of adhesions has become the standard of care for treating Asherman syndrome and pregnancy rates after intervention range from 33 to 80% [85]. In a study of 187 patients treated surgically, 80% subsequently achieved a term pregnancy [95], while another study of 90 patients with recurrent pregnancy loss found that intervention improved the newborn delivery rate of treated patients from 18.3 to 64% [96]. Patients with Asherman syndrome who become pregnant after treatment remain at increased risk of miscarriage, preterm delivery, abnormal placentation, intrauterine growth restriction, and uterine rupture [85].

A number of methods have been evaluated to prevent the recurrence of adhesions after surgery. Among these are unmedicated IUDs, balloon catheters, exogenous estrogens, and hyaluronic acid [82, 85]. With the exception of hyaluronic acid gel, which is not available in the US, the other adjuvant treatments were ineffective.

Female Genital Tract Malformations

Congenital uterine malformations represent a broad range of developmental disorders and syndromes. Isolated uterine malformations are typically the result of failure of the mullerian ducts to fuse in the midline, resulting in arcuate, didelphic, bicornuate, or unicornuate uteri, or failure of resorption of the fused medial walls, leading to a uterine septum (Fig. 10.4). There are numerous classification systems for this spectrum of disorders. The American Fertility Society classification system from 1988 is perhaps the most popular [97].

Uterine malformations have been estimated to be present in 6.7% of the general population and 7.3% of the infertile population, suggesting an overall limited role for these factors in contributing to infertility [98]. The arcuate uterus is the most common anomaly in the general population, while a septate uterus is the most

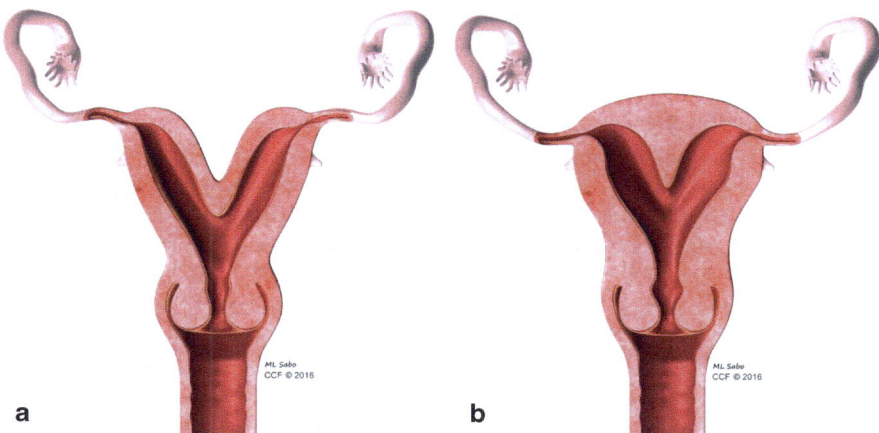

Fig. 10.4 Uterine anomalies including septate, arcuate, bicornuate, unicornuate, and didelphic uteri affect reproductive outcomes. (**a**) Bicornuate uterus. (**b**) Septate uterus. ©ML Sabo CCF 2016

Table 10.1 Effect of mullerian anomalies on reproduction

	Pregnancy	SAB	PTD	Malpresentation
Arcuate	1.0	1.4	1.5	2.5*
Septate	0.9*	2.9*	2.1*	6.2*
Bicornuate	0.9	3.4*	2.6*	5.4*
Unicornuate	0.7	2.2*	3.5*	2.7*
Didelphys	0.9	1.1	3.6*	3.7*

Meta-analysis of 9 controlled studies with 3805 patients
Relative risk compared to normal uterus, $*p < 0.05$
SAB spontaneous abortion, *PTD* preterm delivery
Modified from Chan et al. Ultrasound Obstet Gynecol 2011;38:31–82

common in the infertile population, suggesting that certain anomalies may introduce barriers to achieving fertility [98].

Congenital uterine anomalies have been most widely reported to occur in the recurrent miscarriage population, with an estimated prevalence of 13–17% [98–103]. Poor IVF and reproductive outcomes have been reported in patients with untreated uterine anomalies [104] (Table 10.1). An abnormal uterine cavity is thought to impair fertility by anatomical means, motivating surgery for restoration of normal anatomy [100]. Pregnancies resulting from anatomically distorted cavities are much more likely to result in breech presentation and necessitate Cesarean delivery than those in normal cavities [105]. A history of recurrent pregnancy losses is the primary indication for treatment of patients with uterine malformations [98, 106, 107]. Because no high-quality randomized controlled trials exist to support surgical correction of these anomalies in patients with recurrent pregnancy loss or infertility [78], there remains considerable debate in the field regarding appropriate management [108–110].

Uterine Septum

The septate uterus is the most common of the uterine anomalies and is the anomaly associated with the highest rates of pregnancy complications, including early abortion (44.3%), fetal malpresentation, intrauterine growth restriction, and preterm delivery (22.4%) [100]. A meta-analysis comparing women with septate uteri to normal controls noted reduced clinical pregnancy rates (RR 0.86), increased first-trimester miscarriage rates (RR 2.89), increased rates of preterm birth (RR 2.14), and an elevated risk of fetal malpresentation at delivery (RR 6.24) [111].

The association between the uterine septum and poor obstetric outcomes is not well understood. Several mechanisms are thought to underlie this association, including alterations in vascularity of the septum and changes in tissue composition and receptivity of the septum to steroids hormones [112–114]. A small study comparing the septal endometrium with endometrium from the lateral uterine wall showed altered differentiation and estrogenic maturation of septal endometrium, suggesting that the septum may be an unfit location for implantation [112]. A histopathologic study found increased muscular fibers in uterine septa compared to normal myometrium, leading the authors to theorize that irregular contractility from septum muscle fibers contributed to an increased spontaneous miscarriage rate [113]. mRNA expression of VEGF receptors was significantly lower in the endometrium lining the septum compared with the endometrium lining the walls of the normal uterus, suggesting that alterations in septum vascularity may contribute to poor obstetric outcomes [114].

Fortunately, the uterine septum is highly amenable to correction by hysteroscopic septoplasty. Abdominal metroplasty, i.e., Jones and Tomkins procedures, is of historic interest only [107]. Surgical intervention has been shown to improve reproductive outcomes in patients with uterine septa. A review of patients treated with hysteroscopic metroplasty found a significant decrease in abortion (16.4%) and preterm delivery rates (6.8%) compared with untreated controls [100]. Another study reported that the miscarriage rate decreased from 88% before metroplasty to 14% after, with an 80% live birth rate compared with a 4% preoperative rate [101]. Improved IVF implantation rates were reported following metroplasty [104], leading to the recommendation that it be performed prior to an embryo transfer [115]. A prospective trial comparing metroplasty in infertile patients with a septate uterus to expectant management in patients with unexplained infertility found a significantly higher pregnancy rate following surgical intervention (38.6 vs 20.4%), supporting the notion that a septum adversely impacts fertility [116]. These findings are supported by a meta-analysis noting that hysteroscopic resection of a uterine septum substantially reduced the probability of a spontaneous abortion (RR 0.37) compared with untreated patients [117]. A 2011 Cochrane review attempted to evaluate the impact of metroplasty in patients with recurrent pregnancy loss; however, no randomized controlled trials could be identified for inclusion [118]. A multicenter randomized trial known as the Randomized Uterine Septum Transection Trial (TRUST) is currently underway to evaluate reproductive outcomes after septoplasty in women with a history of recurrent miscarriage, infertility, or preterm birth.

Arcuate Uterus

Patients with an arcuate uterus have an 82.7% reported live birth rate [119], essentially comparable to unaffected patients. Early abortion (25.7%) and preterm delivery (7.5%) are relatively uncommon complications [100]. Existing literature has to date largely failed to demonstrate a significant association between an arcuate uterus and adverse fertility outcomes, and hysteroscopic intervention is not generally recommended [120]. However a recent meta-analysis finding increased rates of second-trimester miscarriage (RR 2.39) and fetal malpresentation at delivery (RR 2.53) in patients with arcuate uterus compared with normal controls may lead to a reevaluation of this question [111]. These latter findings may be due to inclusion of septate uteri as arcuate in the study classification.

Unicornuate Uterus

The live birth rate in patients with a unicornuate uterus has been reported to be approximately 54.2% [119]. Early abortion (36.5%) and preterm delivery (16.2%) are more common in this population compared with the arcuate uterus population [100]. Complications associated with a unicornuate uterus are more typically related to sustaining a pregnancy than to achieving one [121]. However, a 33% reduced implantation rate compared with normal anatomy controls has been observed in IVF transfers, suggesting that implantation may also be affected by unicornuate anatomy [104]. Because 13% of pregnancies in patients with a unicornuate uterus occur in a "noncommunicating" rudimentary horn due to sperm transmigration [103], surgical removal of a rudimentary horn has been recommended to prevent uterine rupture as well as address likely symptoms of dysmenorrhea [98, 115]. However, there is no evidence that such intervention improves reproductive outcomes [115].

Didelphic Uterus

A 40% live birth rate has been reported in patients with a didelphic uterus [119]. Early abortion (32.2%) and preterm delivery (28.3%) are also common [100]. In reproductive terms, the didelphic uterus is considered to have similar pregnancy outcomes to the unicornuate uterus because it can be viewed as a duplicated unicornuate uterus [100, 122]. However, a long-term follow-up of 49 cases of didelphic uterus did not find significant impairment in fertility (94% pregnancy rate, 75% fetal survival), although 84% ultimately delivered by cesarean section [123]. Highly unusual pregnancy outcomes have been reported in patients with didelphic uteri, including a multi-fetal gestation in separate uterine horns with a 72-day lapse between the delivery of one fetus and the other [124]. While surgical procedures to repair a didelphic uterus have been developed, none have been shown to improve reproductive outcome, and all carry risk of cervical incompetence [115].

Bicornuate Uterus

A 62.5% live birth rate has been reported in patients with a bicornuate uterus [119], and early abortion (36.0%) and preterm delivery (23%) rates are elevated compared with arcuate controls [100]. These adverse outcomes are related more to gestation than conception, leading many to reserve metroplasty (performed transabdominally) for patients who experience recurrent pregnancy loss or infertility [115]. However, in those treated with abdominal metroplasty for bicornuate uterus, fetal survival and term gestation rates approach 90% [125].

Hydrosalpinges

Hydrosalpinges are characterized by distal blockage of the fallopian tubes with fluid accumulation [126] (Fig. 10.5). The disease most commonly follows an ascending sexually transmitted infection [127]. Two large meta-analyses with approximately 6700 and 5600 patients undergoing fresh and frozen IVF cycles showed that the live birth rates were halved in women with uni- or bilateral hydrosalpinges [128, 129]. Implantation and pregnancy rates were also significantly reduced, and miscarriage rates significantly increased, in the presence of hydrosalpinges [128, 129].

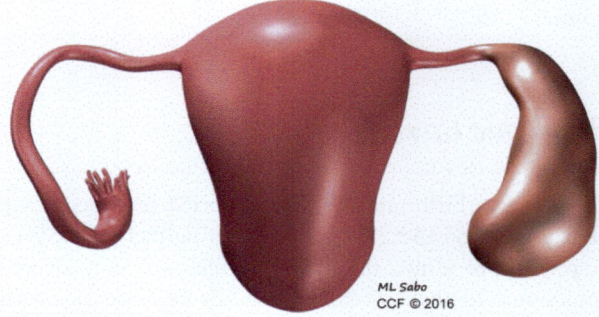

Fig. 10.5 Hydrosalpinx is characterized by distal blockage with fluid accumulation. It is treatable by salpingectomy, proximal tubal occlusion, or neosalpingostomy depending on the extent of the tubal damage. ©ML Sabo CCF 2016

Pathophysiology

Three potential mechanisms have been proposed to explain the detrimental effects of hydrosalpingeal fluid on embryo implantation. The mechanical factor suggests that reflux of the hydrosalpingeal fluid into the uterine cavity may flush out the embryo [130, 131] or create a fluid barrier to implantation [132]. Other mechanical effects are increased uterine peristalsis [133] and decreased endometrial perfusion [134].

The second mechanism is diminished endometrial receptivity through the alteration of various factors which may promote implantation. Leukemia inhibitory factor, integrin 3, and mucin 1 (MUC1) are significantly reduced in patients with hydrosalpinges [135]. Endometrial NF-κB is increased, and cystic fibrosis transmembrane conductance regulator and MUC1 are decreased with hydrosalpinges [136]. HOXA10 mRNA expression in endometrial cells is decreased when cultured with hydrosalpingeal fluid [137]. Some of these changes have been demonstrated to revert to normal following salpingectomy [138, 139].

The third mechanism is embryotoxicity which has been demonstrated in multiple studies in a mouse model but not in humans [133]. The adverse effects may be mediated by increased oxidative stress [140] or altered cytokine concentrations [141]. It is also possible that the embryotoxic effect is due to dilution of essential nutrients.

Treatment

A Cochrane review of prospective randomized studies concluded that salpingectomy for hydrosalpinges prior to IVF doubled the clinical pregnancy rate compared to untreated hydrosalpinges (OR 2.3, 95% CI 1.48–2.62), effectively negating the detrimental effects of hydrosalpinges on IVF success rates [142]. A randomized control trial comparing laparoscopic salpingectomy or tubal ligation with expectant management reported significant benefits with surgical intervention compared with the untreated control group [143]. There were no significant differences between the two treatment groups for ovarian response to stimulation, number of oocytes retrieved or embryos produced, clinical pregnancy rates, or live birth rates.

A retrospective study found that laparoscopic neosalpingostomy yielded comparable clinical pregnancy rates to salpingectomy for treating hydrosalpinges prior to IVF [144]. In patients who are poor candidates for laparoscopic treatment of hydrosalpinges, hysteroscopic placement of the Essure (Bayer, Whippany, NJ) device for proximal tubal occlusion may be considered. However, a randomized clinical trial comparing it to laparoscopic tubal ligation noted a significant reduction in implantation, clinical pregnancy, and live birth rates in the Essure group [145]. The spontaneous abortion rate was also doubled in the Essure group, though it did not reach statistical significance.

Ultrasound-guided aspiration of the hydrosalpinges fluid prior to IVF was also evaluated as a nonsurgical option. Unfortunately, the fluid rapidly reaccumulated, and no significant difference in clinical pregnancy rates compared with untreated controls was found in a randomized trial [146]. A subsequent study performed sclerotherapy by injecting 98% ethanol into the aspirated hydrosalpinges for 5–10 min, eliminating the problem of recurrence [134]. In this prospective nonrandomized trial comparing sclerotherapy to untreated hydrosalpinges, sclerotherapy significantly increased both the implantation and clinical pregnancy rates. In addition, the non-treated hydrosalpinges group had decreased endometrial perfusion based on Doppler ultrasound parameters. While it can be concluded from all of the above that hydrosalpinges impair implantation and that treating them by various means restores IVF success rates, it remains uncertain whether all hydrosalpinges behave the same. Specifically, it remains unknown if small hydrosalpinges that are not visible by transvaginal ultrasonography are a clinical concern and warrant treatment prior to initiating an IVF cycle.

Conclusions

Recurrent implantation failure with IVF may be due to anatomic disorders such as myomas, endometrial polyps, intrauterine adhesions, mullerian anomalies, and hydrosalpinges. In most cases, a detailed mechanistic understanding of how these conditions impair implantation remains elusive. Furthermore, evidence to support the effectiveness of surgical treatment on improving IVF outcomes is often limited by few studies with small sample sizes, inconsistent classification of the condition, lack of an appropriate control group, and variable follow-up intervals. Clearly, there is a need for research to address these knowledge deficiencies. In the meantime, the best available evidence favors myomectomy for myomas distorting the endometrial cavity. Hysteroscopic polypectomy, adhesiolysis, and septoplasty are also recommended prior to initiating an IVF cycle. In addition, salpingectomy, proximal tubal occlusion, or neosalpingostomy, in selected cases, should be performed for hydrosalpinges in order to restore optimal IVF success rates.

References

1. Marshall LM, et al. Variation in the incidence of uterine leiomyoma among premenopausal women by age and race. Obstet Gynecol. 1997;90:967–73.
2. Munro MG, Critchley HOD, Fraser IS. The FIGO classification of causes of abnormal uterine bleeding in the reproductive years. Fertil Steril. 2011;95:2204–8, 2208.e1–3
3. Munro MG. Abnormal uterine bleeding. Cambridge: Cambridge University Press; 2010.
4. Munro MG, Critchley HOD, Broder MS, Fraser IS. FIGO classification system (PALM-COEIN) for causes of abnormal uterine bleeding in nongravid women of reproductive age. Int J Gynaecol Obstet. 2011;113:3–13.

5. Mehine M, et al. Characterization of uterine leiomyomas by whole-genome sequencing. N Engl J Med. 2013;369:43–53.
6. Mäkinen N, et al. MED12, the mediator complex subunit 12 gene, is mutated at high frequency in uterine leiomyomas. Science. 2011;334:252–5.
7. Dou Q, et al. Suppression of transforming growth factor-beta (TGF beta) and TGF beta receptor messenger ribonucleic acid and protein expression in leiomyomata in women receiving gonadotropin-releasing hormone agonist therapy. J Clin Endocrinol Metab. 1996;81:3222–30.
8. Mas A, et al. Stro-1/CD44 as putative human myometrial and fibroid stem cell markers. Fertil Steril. 2015;104:225–34.e3.
9. Klatsky PC, Tran ND, Caughey AB, Fujimoto VY. Fibroids and reproductive outcomes: a systematic literature review from conception to delivery. Am J Obstet Gynecol. 2008;198:357–66.
10. Pritts EA, Parker WH, Olive DL. Fibroids and infertility: an updated systematic review of the evidence. Fertil Steril. 2009;91:1215–23.
11. Somigliana E, et al. Fibroids and female reproduction: a critical analysis of the evidence. Hum Reprod Update. 2007;13:465–76.
12. Check JH, Choe JK, Lee G, Dietterich C. The effect on IVF outcome of small intramural fibroids not compressing the uterine cavity as determined by a prospective matched control study. Hum Reprod. 2002;17:1244–8.
13. Surrey ES, Lietz AK, Schoolcraft WB. Impact of intramural leiomyomata in patients with a normal endometrial cavity on in vitro fertilization-embryo transfer cycle outcome. Fertil Steril. 2001;75:405–10.
14. Benecke C, Kruger TF, Siebert TI, Van der Merwe JP, Steyn DW. Effect of fibroids on fertility in patients undergoing assisted reproduction. A structured literature review. Gynecol Obstet Investig. 2005;59:225–30.
15. Brady PC, Stanic AK, Styer AK. Uterine fibroids and subfertility: an update on the role of myomectomy. Curr Opin Obstet Gynecol. 2013;25:255–9.
16. Practice Committee of American Society for Reproductive Medicine in Collaboration with Society of Reproductive Surgeons. Myomas and reproductive function. Fertil Steril. 2008;90:S125–30.
17. Yoshino O, et al. Decreased pregnancy rate is linked to abnormal uterine peristalsis caused by intramural fibroids. Hum Reprod. 2010;25:2475–9.
18. Donnez J, Jadoul P. What are the implications of myomas on fertility? A need for a debate? Hum Reprod. 2002;17:1424–30.
19. Hunt JE, Wallach EE. Uterine factors in infertility–an overview. Clin Obstet Gynecol. 1974;17:44–64.
20. Vollenhoven BJ, Lawrence AS, Healy DL. Uterine fibroids: a clinical review. Br J Obstet Gynaecol. 1990;97:285–98.
21. Ingersoll FM. Fertility following myomectomy. Fertil Steril. 1963;14:596–602.
22. Yoshino O, et al. Myomectomy decreases abnormal uterine peristalsis and increases pregnancy rate. J Minim Invasive Gynecol. 2012;19:63–7.
23. Deligdish L, Loewenthal M. Endometrial changes associated with myomata of the uterus. J Clin Pathol. 1970;23:676–80.
24. Rackow BW, Taylor HS. Submucosal uterine leiomyomas have a global effect on molecular determinants of endometrial receptivity. Fertil Steril. 2010;93:2027–34.
25. Buttram VC, Reiter RC. Uterine leiomyomata: etiology, symptomatology, and management. Fertil Steril. 1981;36:433–45.
26. Farrer-Brown G, Beilby JO, Tarbit MH. Venous changes in the endometrium of myomatous uteri. Obstet Gynecol. 1971;38:743–51.
27. Farrer-Brown G, Beilby JO, Tarbit MH. The vascular patterns in myomatous uteri. J Obstet Gynaecol Br Commonw. 1970;77:967–75.
28. Donnez J, et al. Ulipristal acetate versus leuprolide acetate for uterine fibroids. N Engl J Med. 2012;366:421–32.

29. Stovall TG, Muneyyirci-Delale O, Summitt RL, Scialli AR. GnRH agonist and iron versus placebo and iron in the anemic patient before surgery for leiomyomas: a randomized controlled trial. Leuprolide Acetate Study Group. Obstet Gynecol. 1995;86:65–71.
30. Britten JL, et al. Gonadotropin-releasing hormone (GnRH) agonist leuprolide acetate and GnRH antagonist cetrorelix acetate directly inhibit leiomyoma extracellular matrix production. Fertil Steril. 2012;98:1299–307.
31. Malik M, et al. Gonadotropin-releasing hormone analogues inhibit leiomyoma extracellular matrix despite presence of gonadal hormones. Fertil Steril. 2016;105:214–24.
32. Watanabe Y, et al. Efficacy of a low-dose leuprolide acetate depot in the treatment of uterine leiomyomata in Japanese women. Fertil Steril. 1992;58:66–71.
33. Friedman AJ, Hoffman DI, Comite F, Browneller RW, Miller JD. Treatment of leiomyomata uteri with leuprolide acetate depot: a double-blind, placebo-controlled, multicenter study. The Leuprolide Study Group. Obstet Gynecol. 1991;77:720–5.
34. Cirkel U, et al. Experience with leuprorelin acetate depot in the treatment of fibroids: a German multicentre study. Clin Ther. 1992;14(Suppl A):37–50.
35. Lethaby A, Vollenhoven B, Sowter M. Pre-operative GnRH analogue therapy before hysterectomy or myomectomy for uterine fibroids. Cochrane Database Syst Rev. 2001;2:CD000547. https://doi.org/10.1002/14651858.CD000547.
36. Trefoux Bourdet A, Luton D, Koskas M. Clinical utility of ulipristal acetate for the treatment of uterine fibroids: current evidence. Int J Womens Health. 2015;7:321–30.
37. Coddington CC, et al. Short term treatment with leuprolide acetate is a successful adjunct to surgical therapy of leiomyomas of the uterus. Surg Gynecol Obstet. 1992;175:57–63.
38. Donnez J, Donnez O, Dolmans M-M. With the advent of selective progesterone receptor modulators, what is the place of myoma surgery in current practice? Fertil Steril. 2014;102:640–8.
39. Kalampokas T, Kamath M, Boutas I, Kalampokas E. Ulipristal acetate for uterine fibroids: a systematic review and meta-analysis. Gynecol Endocrinol. 2016;32:91–6.
40. Donnez J, et al. Ulipristal acetate versus placebo for fibroid treatment before surgery. N Engl J Med. 2012;366:409–20.
41. Chwalisz K, et al. Selective progesterone receptor modulator development and use in the treatment of leiomyomata and endometriosis. Endocr Rev. 2005;26:423–38.
42. Maruo T, et al. Effects of progesterone on growth factor expression in human uterine leiomyoma. Steroids. 2003;68:817–24.
43. Luyckx M, et al. First series of 18 pregnancies after ulipristal acetate treatment for uterine fibroids. Fertil Steril. 2014;102:1404–9.
44. Luyckx M, et al. Long-term nonsurgical control with ulipristal acetate of multiple uterine fibroids, enabling pregnancy. Am J Obstet Gynecol. 2016;214(6):756.e1–2. https://doi.org/10.1016/j.ajog.2016.02.049.
45. Ke L-Q, Yang K, Li J, Li C-M. Danazol for uterine fibroids. Cochrane Database Syst Rev. 2009;3:CD007692. https://doi.org/10.1002/14651858.CD007692.pub2.
46. Unlu C, Celik O, Celik N, Otlu B. Expression of endometrial receptivity genes increase after myomectomy of intramural leiomyomas not distorting the endometrial cavity. Reprod Sci. 2016;23:31–41.
47. Casini ML, Rossi F, Agostini R, Unfer V. Effects of the position of fibroids on fertility. Gynecol Endocrinol. 2006;22:106–9.
48. Carranza-Mamane B, et al. The management of uterine fibroids in women with otherwise unexplained infertility. J Obstet Gynaecol Can. 2015;37:277–88.
49. Dessolle L, et al. Determinants of pregnancy rate and obstetric outcome after laparoscopic myomectomy for infertility. Fertil Steril. 2001;76:370–4.
50. Bulletti C, De Ziegler D, Polli V, Flamigni C. The role of leiomyomas in infertility. J Am Assoc Gynecol Laparosc. 1999;6:441–5.
51. Metwally M, Cheong YC, Horne AW. Surgical treatment of fibroids for subfertility. Cochrane Database Syst Rev. 2012;11:CD003857.

52. Seracchioli R, et al. Fertility and obstetric outcome after laparoscopic myomectomy of large myomata: a randomized comparison with abdominal myomectomy. Hum Reprod. 2000;15:2663–8.
53. Palomba S, et al. A multicenter randomized, controlled study comparing laparoscopic versus minilaparotomic myomectomy: reproductive outcomes. Fertil Steril. 2007;88:933–41.
54. Thomas RL, Winkler N, Carr BR, Doody KM, Doody KJ. Abdominal myomectomy–a safe procedure in an ambulatory setting. Fertil Steril. 2010;94:2277–80.
55. Iavazzo C, Mamais I, Gkegkes ID. Robotic assisted vs laparoscopic and/or open myomectomy: systematic review and meta-analysis of the clinical evidence. Arch Gynecol Obstet. 2016;294:5–17.
56. van der Kooij SM, Bipat S, Hehenkamp WJK, Ankum WM, Reekers JA. Uterine artery embolization versus surgery in the treatment of symptomatic fibroids: a systematic review and meta-analysis. Am J Obstet Gynecol. 2011;205:317.e1–18.
57. Moss JG, et al. Randomised comparison of uterine artery embolisation (UAE) with surgical treatment in patients with symptomatic uterine fibroids (REST trial): 5-year results. BJOG. 2011;118:936–44.
58. Jun F, et al. Uterine artery embolization versus surgery for symptomatic uterine fibroids: a randomized controlled trial and a meta-analysis of the literature. Arch Gynecol Obstet. 2012;285:1407–13.
59. Ananthakrishnan G, et al. Randomized comparison of uterine artery embolization (UAE) with surgical treatment in patients with symptomatic uterine fibroids (REST trial): subanalysis of 5-year MRI findings. Cardiovasc Intervent Radiol. 2013;36:676–81.
60. Torre A, et al. Uterine artery embolization for severe symptomatic fibroids: effects on fertility and symptoms. Hum Reprod. 2014;29:490–501.
61. Mara M, et al. Midterm clinical and first reproductive results of a randomized controlled trial comparing uterine fibroid embolization and myomectomy. Cardiovasc Intervent Radiol. 2008;31:73–85.
62. Goldberg J, et al. Pregnancy outcomes after treatment for fibromyomata: uterine artery embolization versus laparoscopic myomectomy. Am J Obstet Gynecol. 2004;191:18–21.
63. Berkane N, Moutafoff-Borie C. Impact of previous uterine artery embolization on fertility. Curr Opin Obstet Gynecol. 2010;22:242–7.
64. Hehenkamp WJK, et al. Loss of ovarian reserve after uterine artery embolization: a randomized comparison with hysterectomy. Hum Reprod. 2007;22:1996–2005.
65. Clark NA, Mumford SL, Segars JH. Reproductive impact of MRI-guided focused ultrasound surgery for fibroids: a systematic review of the evidence. Curr Opin Obstet Gynecol. 2014;26:151–61.
66. Rabinovici J, et al. Pregnancy outcome after magnetic resonance-guided focused ultrasound surgery (MRgFUS) for conservative treatment of uterine fibroids. Fertil Steril. 2010;93:199–209.
67. Berman JM, et al. Three-year outcome of the Halt trial: a prospective analysis of radiofrequency volumetric thermal ablation of myomas. J Minim Invasive Gynecol. 2014;21:767–74.
68. Brucker SY, et al. Laparoscopic radiofrequency volumetric thermal ablation of fibroids versus laparoscopic myomectomy. Int J Gynaecol Obstet. 2014;125:261–5.
69. Peterson WF, Novak ER. Endometrial polyps. Obstet Gynecol. 1956;8:40–9.
70. Shokeir TA, Shalan HM, El-Shafei MM. Significance of endometrial polyps detected hysteroscopically in eumenorrheic infertile women. J Obstet Gynaecol Res. 2004;30:84–9.
71. Salim S, Won H, Nesbitt-Hawes E, Campbell N, Abbott J. Diagnosis and management of endometrial polyps: a critical review of the literature. J Minim Invasive Gynecol. 2011;18:569–81.
72. Hinckley MD, Milki AA. 1000 office-based hysteroscopies prior to in vitro fertilization: feasibility and findings. JSLS. 2004;8:103–7.
73. Fatemi HM, et al. Prevalence of unsuspected uterine cavity abnormalities diagnosed by office hysteroscopy prior to in vitro fertilization. Hum Reprod. 2010;25:1959–65.

74. Bozkurt M, Şahin L, Ulaş M. Hysteroscopic polypectomy decreases NF-κB1 expression in the mid-secretory endometrium of women with endometrial polyp. Eur J Obstet Gynecol Reprod Biol. 2015;189:96–100.
75. Pinheiro A, et al. Expression of hormone receptors, Bcl-2, Cox-2 and Ki67 in benign endometrial polyps and their association with obesity. Mol Med Rep. 2014;9:2335–41.
76. Hasegawa E, et al. Expression of leukemia inhibitory factor in the endometrium in abnormal uterine cavities during the implantation window. Fertil Steril. 2012;97:953–8.
77. Ben-Nagi J, Miell J, Yazbek J, Holland T, Jurkovic D. The effect of hysteroscopic polypectomy on the concentrations of endometrial implantation factors in uterine flushings. Reprod Biomed Online. 2009;19:737–44.
78. Bosteels J, et al. Hysteroscopy for treating subfertility associated with suspected major uterine cavity abnormalities. Cochrane Database Syst Rev. 2015;2:CD009461.
79. Pérez-Medina T, et al. Endometrial polyps and their implication in the pregnancy rates of patients undergoing intrauterine insemination: a prospective, randomized study. Hum Reprod. 2005;20:1632–5.
80. Kodaman PH. Hysteroscopic polypectomy for women undergoing IVF treatment: when is it necessary? Curr Opin Obstet Gynecol. 2016;28(3):184–90. https://doi.org/10.1097/GCO.0000000000000277.
81. Pundir J, Pundir V, Omanwa K, Khalaf Y, El-Toukhy T. Hysteroscopy prior to the first IVF cycle: a systematic review and meta-analysis. Reprod Biomed Online. 2014;28:151–61.
82. Bosteels J, et al. Anti-adhesion therapy following operative hysteroscopy for treatment of female subfertility. Cochrane Database Syst Rev. 2015;11:CD011110.
83. Evans-Hoeker EA, Young SL. Endometrial receptivity and intrauterine adhesive disease. Semin Reprod Med. 2014;32:392–401.
84. Schenker JG, Margalioth EJ. Intrauterine adhesions: an updated appraisal. Fertil Steril. 1982;37:593–610.
85. Yu D, Wong Y-M, Cheong Y, Xia E, Li T-C. Asherman syndrome–one century later. Fertil Steril. 2008;89:759–79.
86. Wang X, Li Z, A YN, Zou S. Hysteroscopy for early abortion after IVF-ET: clinical analysis of 84 cases. Zhonghua Nan Ke Xue. 2011;17:52–4.
87. Thomson AJM, Abbott JA, Deans R, Kingston A, Vancaillie TG. The management of intrauterine synechiae. Curr Opin Obstet Gynecol. 2009;21:335–41.
88. Deans R, Abbott J. Review of intrauterine adhesions. J Minim Invasive Gynecol. 2010;17:555–69.
89. Leung PL, Tam WH, Yuen PM. Hysteroscopic appearance of the endometrial cavity following thermal balloon endometrial ablation. Fertil Steril. 2003;79:1226–8.
90. Taskin O, et al. Long-term histopathologic and morphologic changes after thermal endometrial ablation. J Am Assoc Gynecol Laparosc. 2002;9:186–90.
91. Mukul LV, Linn JG. Pregnancy complicated by uterine synechiae after endometrial ablation. Obstet Gynecol. 2005;105:1179–82.
92. Schenker JG. Etiology of and therapeutic approach to synechia uteri. Eur J Obstet Gynecol Reprod Biol. 1996;65:109–13.
93. Foix A, et al. The pathology of postcurettage intrauterine adhesions. Am J Obstet Gynecol. 1966;96:1027–33.
94. Polishuk WZ, Anteby SO, Weinstein D. Puerperal endometritis and intrauterine adhesions. Int Surg. 1975;60:418–20.
95. Valle RF, Sciarra JJ. Intrauterine adhesions: hysteroscopic diagnosis, classification, treatment, and reproductive outcome. Am J Obstet Gynecol. 1988;158:1459–70.
96. Katz Z, Ben-Arie A, Lurie S, Manor M, Insler V. Reproductive outcome following hysteroscopic adhesiolysis in Asherman's syndrome. Int J Fertil Menopausal Stud. 1996;41:462–5.
97. The American Fertility Society classifications of adnexal adhesions, distal tubal occlusion, tubal occlusion secondary to tubal ligation, tubal pregnancies, müllerian anomalies and intrauterine adhesions. Fertil Steril. 1988;49:944–55.

98. Saravelos SH, Cocksedge KA, Li T-C. Prevalence and diagnosis of congenital uterine anomalies in women with reproductive failure: a critical appraisal. Hum Reprod Update. 2008;14:415–29.
99. Patton PE. Anatomic uterine defects. Clin Obstet Gynecol. 1994;37:705–21.
100. Grimbizis GF, Camus M, Tarlatzis BC, Bontis JN, Devroey P. Clinical implications of uterine malformations and hysteroscopic treatment results. Hum Reprod Update. 2001;7:161–74.
101. Homer HA, Li TC, Cooke ID. The septate uterus: a review of management and reproductive outcome. Fertil Steril. 2000;73:1–14.
102. Kupesic S. Clinical implications of sonographic detection of uterine anomalies for reproductive outcome. Ultrasound Obstet Gynecol. 2001;18:387–400.
103. Letterie G. Structural abnormalities and reproductive failure: effective techniques for diagnosis and management. New York: Blackwell Science; 1998.
104. Lavergne N, Aristizabal J, Zarka V, Erny R, Hedon B. Uterine anomalies and in vitro fertilization: what are the results? Eur J Obstet Gynecol Reprod Biol. 1996;68:29–34.
105. Heinonen PK, Saarikoski S, Pystynen P. Reproductive performance of women with uterine anomalies. An evaluation of 182 cases. Acta Obstet Gynecol Scand. 1982;61:157–62.
106. DeCherney AH, Russell JB, Graebe RA, Polan ML. Resectoscopic management of müllerian fusion defects. Fertil Steril. 1986;45:726–8.
107. Fayez JA. Comparison between abdominal and hysteroscopic metroplasty. Obstet Gynecol. 1986;68:399–403.
108. Devi Wold AS, Pham N, Arici A. Anatomic factors in recurrent pregnancy loss. Semin Reprod Med. 2006;24:25–32.
109. Propst AM, Hill JA. Anatomic factors associated with recurrent pregnancy loss. Semin Reprod Med. 2000;18:341–50.
110. Bailey AP, Jaslow CR, Kutteh WH. Minimally invasive surgical options for congenital and acquired uterine factors associated with recurrent pregnancy loss. Womens Health. 2015;11:161–7.
111. Chan YY, et al. Reproductive outcomes in women with congenital uterine anomalies: a systematic review. Ultrasound Obstet Gynecol. 2011;38:371–82.
112. Fedele L, et al. Ultrastructural aspects of endometrium in infertile women with septate uterus. Fertil Steril. 1996;65:750–2.
113. Sparac V, Kupesic S, Ilijas M, Zodan T, Kurjak A. Histologic architecture and vascularization of hysteroscopically excised intrauterine septa. J Am Assoc Gynecol Laparosc. 2001;8:111–6.
114. Raga F, Casañ EM, Bonilla-Musoles F. Expression of vascular endothelial growth factor receptors in the endometrium of septate uterus. Fertil Steril. 2009;92:1085–90.
115. Taylor E, Gomel V. The uterus and fertility. Fertil Steril. 2008;89:1–16.
116. Mollo A, et al. Hysteroscopic resection of the septum improves the pregnancy rate of women with unexplained infertility: a prospective controlled trial. Fertil Steril. 2009;91:2628–31.
117. Venetis CA, et al. Clinical implications of congenital uterine anomalies: a meta-analysis of comparative studies. Reprod Biomed Online. 2014;29:665–83.
118. Kowalik CR, et al. Metroplasty versus expectant management for women with recurrent miscarriage and a septate uterus. Cochrane Database Syst Rev. 2011;6:CD008576. https://doi.org/10.1002/14651858.CD008576.pub3.
119. Raga F, et al. Reproductive impact of congenital Müllerian anomalies. Hum Reprod. 1997;12:2277–81.
120. Mucowski SJ, Herndon CN, Rosen MP. The arcuate uterine anomaly: a critical appraisal of its diagnostic and clinical relevance. Obstet Gynecol Surv. 2010;65:449–54.
121. Reichman D, Laufer MR, Robinson BK. Pregnancy outcomes in unicornuate uteri: a review. Fertil Steril. 2009;91:1886–94.
122. Buttram VC. Müllerian anomalies and their management. Fertil Steril. 1983;40:159–63.
123. Heinonen PK. Clinical implications of the didelphic uterus: long-term follow-up of 49 cases. Eur J Obstet Gynecol Reprod Biol. 2000;91:183–90.

124. Mashiach S, Ben-Rafael Z, Dor J, Serr DM. Triplet pregnancy in uterus didelphys with delivery interval of 72 days. Obstet Gynecol. 1981;58:519–21.
125. Papp Z, Mezei G, Gávai M, Hupuczi P, Urbancsek J. Reproductive performance after transabdominal metroplasty: a review of 157 consecutive cases. J Reprod Med. 2006;51:544–52.
126. Chu J, et al. Salpingostomy in the treatment of hydrosalpinx: a systematic review and meta-analysis. Hum Reprod. 2015;30:1882–95.
127. Bahamondes L, et al. Identification of main risk factors for tubal infertility. Fertil Steril. 1994;61:478–82.
128. Zeyneloglu HB, Arici A, Olive DL. Adverse effects of hydrosalpinx on pregnancy rates after in vitro fertilization-embryo transfer. Fertil Steril. 1998;70:492–9.
129. Camus E, et al. Pregnancy rates after in-vitro fertilization in cases of tubal infertility with and without hydrosalpinx: a meta-analysis of published comparative studies. Hum Reprod. 1999;14:1243–9.
130. Mansour RT, Aboulghar MA, Serour GI, Riad R. Fluid accumulation of the uterine cavity before embryo transfer: a possible hindrance for implantation. J In Vitro Fert Embryo Transf. 1991;8:157–9.
131. Andersen AN, Lindhard A, Loft A, Ziebe S, Andersen CY. The infertile patient with hydrosalpinges–IVF with or without salpingectomy? Hum Reprod. 1996;11:2081–4.
132. Vandromme J, et al. Hydrosalpinges in in-vitro fertilization: an unfavourable prognostic feature. Hum Reprod. 1995;10:576–9.
133. Strandell A, Lindhard A. Why does hydrosalpinx reduce fertility? The importance of hydrosalpinx fluid. Hum Reprod. 2002;17(5):1141.
134. Jiang H, Pei H, Zhang W, Wang X. A prospective clinical study of interventional ultrasound sclerotherapy on women with hydrosalpinx before in vitro fertilization and embryo transfer. Fertil Steril. 2010;94:2854–6.
135. Li L, et al. Effects of hydrosalpinx on pinopodes, leukaemia inhibitory factor, integrin beta3 and MUC1 expression in the peri-implantation endometrium. Eur J Obstet Gynecol Reprod Biol. 2010;151:171–5.
136. Song Y, et al. NF κB expression increases and CFTR and MUC1 expression decreases in the endometrium of infertile patients with hydrosalpinx: a comparative study. Reprod Biol Endocrinol. 2012;10:86.
137. Daftary GS, et al. Salpingectomy increases peri-implantation endometrial HOXA10 expression in women with hydrosalpinx. Fertil Steril. 2007;87:367–72.
138. Seli E, et al. Removal of hydrosalpinges increases endometrial leukaemia inhibitory factor (LIF) expression at the time of the implantation window. Hum Reprod. 2005;20:3012–7.
139. Bildirici I, Bukulmez O, Ensari A, Yarali H, Gurgan T. A prospective evaluation of the effect of salpingectomy on endometrial receptivity in cases of women with communicating hydrosalpinges. Hum Reprod. 2001;16:2422–6.
140. Bedaiwy MA, et al. Relationship between oxidative stress and embryotoxicity of hydrosalpingeal fluid. Hum Reprod. 2002;17:601–4.
141. Bedaiwy MA, et al. Relationship between cytokines and the embryotoxicity of hydrosalpingeal fluid. J Assist Reprod Genet. 2005;22:161–5.
142. Johnson N, van Voorst S, Sowter MC, Strandell A, Mol BWJ. Surgical treatment for tubal disease in women due to undergo in vitro fertilisation. Cochrane Database Syst Rev. 2010;1:CD002125. https://doi.org/10.1002/14651858.CD002125.pub3.
143. Kontoravdis A, et al. Proximal tubal occlusion and salpingectomy result in similar improvement in in vitro fertilization outcome in patients with hydrosalpinx. Fertil Steril. 2006;86:1642–9.
144. Chanelles O, et al. Hydrosalpinx and infertility: what about conservative surgical management? Eur J Obstet Gynecol Reprod Biol. 2011;159:122–6.
145. Dreyer K, et al. Hysteroscopic proximal tubal occlusion versus laparoscopic salpingectomy as a treatment for hydrosalpinges prior to IVF or ICSI: an RCT. Hum Reprod. 2016. https://doi.org/10.1093/humrep/dew050.
146. Hammadieh N, et al. Ultrasound-guided hydrosalpinx aspiration during oocyte collection improves pregnancy outcome in IVF: a randomized controlled trial. Hum Reprod. 2008;23:1113–7.

Chapter 11
Microbiome in Embryonic Implantation and Implantation Failure

Jason M. Franasiak, Inmaculada Moreno, and Carlos Simon

Introduction

The Human Microbiome

The human microbiome is the sum of microorganisms, together with their genomes, which inhabit the human body, and represents a large entity. In fact, the human body is colonized with an order of magnitude more bacteria than human cells in the body [1]. Its impact and influence on the reproductive process existed even prior to a full understanding of its existence in the nineteenth century. The Hungarian physician Ignaz Semmelweis who lived from 1818 to 1865 intently studied "puerperal childbed fever"—a disease we know of today as postpartum endometritis. At the time, maternal mortality from the disease ranged from 7 to 15%. These studies led to his proposal in 1847 that hand washing in a hypochlorite solution could nearly

*Co-First Authors

J.M. Franasiak*, MD, HCLD (✉)
Sidney Kimmel Medical College, Thomas Jefferson University Philadelphia, Philadelphia, PA, USA

IVI-RMA of New Jersey, Basking Ridge, NJ, USA
e-mail: jfranasiak@rmanjs.com

I. Moreno*, PhD
Research Department, Igenomix, Valencia, Spain

Department of Obstetrics and Gynecology, School of Medicine, Stanford University, Stanford, CA, USA
e-mail: Inmaculada.moreno@igenomix.com

C. Simon, MD, PhD
Department of Pediatrics, Obstetrics and Gynecology, University of Valencia/INCLIVA, Spain, Igenomix, Valencia, Spain

Department of Obstetrics and Gynecology, Stanford University, Stanford, CA, USA

Department of Obstetrics and Gynecology, Baylor College of Medicine, Houston, TX, USA
e-mail: carlos.simon@igenomix.com

© Springer International Publishing AG 2018
J.M. Franasiak, R.T. Scott Jr. (eds.), *Recurrent Implantation Failure*,
https://doi.org/10.1007/978-3-319-71967-2_11

175

eliminate the risk of puerperal fever. This along with germ theory findings proposed by Pasteur forever entwined reproductive health with the human microbiome.

However, the progression of our understanding of the role of the microbiome in both physiologic and pathophysiologic reproductive processes has been somewhat protracted. The advent of culture and microscopy were of great importance to a more complete characterization; however, the limits of these technologies have become apparent. Indeed, many microorganisms are not readily detected by traditional cultivation techniques, and thus their role in physiologic and pathophysiologic processes remains incompletely understood. A recent study in the surgical literature shows that more than 50% of the dominant pathogens and 85% of major pathogens in wound infections will not be identified by standard culture techniques [2]. However, new technologies and techniques have begun to revolutionize the way that we think of our microbiome.

The majority of published medical literature focuses on the subset of the microbiome which is involved in pathogenesis, while only a subset focuses on the physiologic role the microbiome plays. The importance of this physiologic role was prominently recognized as the human genome project was published in 2001 [3]. The scientists involved called for a "second human genome project" that would investigate the normal microbiome colonies at various sites in order to understand the synergistic interactions between the microbiome and its host [4, 5]. Several initiatives commenced worldwide, and in the United States the Human Microbiome Project (HMP) led by the National Institutes of Health (NIH) was launched in 2007 which utilized high-throughput sequencing technologies to characterize the human microbiome in normal, healthy volunteers at several different body sites which included the vagina [1].

This scientific revolution has been initiated by implementing new technologies such as DNA fingerprinting, microarrays, and targeted or whole genome sequencing that have in turn empowered the field of metagenomics—the study of genetic material recovered directly from environmental samples, in this case, the human reproductive tract. Indeed, work through the HMP and other investigators utilizing this technology have revealed that sites in the body traditionally thoughts to be sterile, such as the uterine cavity and the placenta, are in fact colonized with their own unique microbiome [6, 7]. These molecular techniques take advantage of the 16S rRNA gene which is unique to bacterial and contains a number of hypervariable regions which act like "fingerprints." These fingerprint sequences can then be used to identify genus and species based on a reference sequence. In addition to the sequencing technology, the field has seen great improvement in the bioinformatics that process this data. Indeed, bioinformatics research in the microbiome is at this point evolving faster than the molecular techniques which generate the data.

The Human Microbiome in Reproduction

Much of the data surrounding the normal or healthy microbiome of the reproductive tract comes from the gynecology literature which characterized the vaginal microbiome as it changed through puberty, during the menstrual cycle, and in menopause [8]. There was further characterization of dysbiosis as seen in a number of reproductive tract pathologies, as is seen in pelvic inflammatory disease caused by organisms such as *C. trachomatis*. The reproductive tract is dominated by *Lactobacilli* species, and this dominance is often altered in disease. These alterations in the microbiome may also be impactful on the reproductive potential of patients with implantation failure. Further, the physiologic alterations of the microbiome due to fluctuating estrogen levels have implications on controlled ovarian hyperstimulation in which supraphysiologic estrogen levels are achieved followed by a fresh embryo transfer. A greater understanding of this fluctuation in assisted reproduction may lead to more personalized treatment strategies.

It is important to note that the physiologic role of the microbiome in reproduction extends beyond the important implantation phase and into the health of the gestational phase as well. Thus, since our goal is healthy, full-term live birth, the role of the microbiome and its alteration in the pre- and peri-implantation phase may have much more wide-reaching implications. Indeed, dysbiosis in obstetrics has been linked to inflammatory states which result in spontaneous preterm birth, among other adverse obstetric outcomes [9].

As excitement for exploration of the "second human genome" has increased, our understanding of how the microbiome affects reproductive competence and implantation has evolved [6]. Data has been gathered on the microbiome at every stage of human reproduction from the ovary, follicle, and oocyte, to the testes and semen/spermatozoa, to the fallopian tube, uterus, cervix, and vagina. Both the male and female reproductive tracts exhibit complexity and diversity only realized within the last decade, and the microbiome is integrally involved in the process of human reproduction (Fig. 11.1).

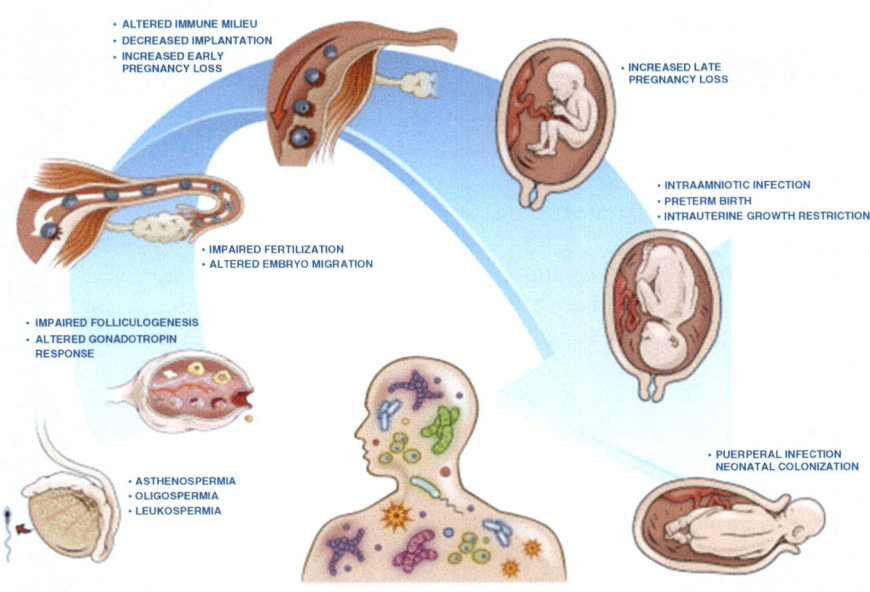

The Microbiome in Human Reproduction

Fig. 11.1 The microbiome's involvement in human reproduction. Used with permission [10]

Characterization of the Reproductive Tract Microbiome

The human microbiome's definition—the totality of microorganisms and their collective genetic material present in or on the human body—was attributed to the American molecular biologist Joshua Lederberg in 2001 [11]. Of great importance to this definition is how the metagenomics data is procured. It is important to recognize that microbiome data are procured in one of two ways: culture-based or sequencing-based technology. Much of the early work describing the human microbiome comes from culture-based approaches utilizing the 16S rRNA analysis of highly conserved genes as a way to identify organisms in mixtures [12, 13].

However, data from cultivation-independent techniques suggests that many organisms cannot be identified utilizing culture-based techniques which results in an underestimate of the diversity of the ecosystem as well as failing to identify potentially important organisms when describing their relation to health and disease [14, 15]. Indeed, work which has followed in the wake of the HMP has utilized the advances of culture-independent approaches in order to confirm that places traditionally thoughts to be sterile, such as the uterine cavity and the placenta, are in fact colonized with their own unique microbiome. Thus, culture-based data, while still foundational and informative, must be interpreted within the limits of the technology.

The major goal of the HMP launched in 2007 by the NIH was to investigate the relationship between disease and changes in the human microbiome. It utilized high-throughput sequencing of the 16S rRNA gene. Specifically, the sequencing focuses on hypervariable regions within the gene which serves as a molecular fingerprint down to the genus and species level [16, 17]. Although data in regards to the microbiome of the reproductive tract has not utilized it extensively to date, metagenomics has also become an increasingly widespread approach to describing the microbiome [18]. Using this method, also termed community genomics, analysis of microorganisms occurs by direct extraction and cloning of DNA from a grouping of organisms. It allows for analysis which extends beyond phylogenetic descriptions and makes attempts as studying the physiology and ecology of the microbiome.

For the purpose of metagenomic analysis with high-throughput sequencing, biologic specimens can be simply collected. There is no need for complex care leading to specific culture conditions. DNA extraction and microbial DNA purification steps are performed. Subsequently, one of several molecular genetics techniques is then applied. The most common are fingerprinting, DNA microarrays, targeted sequencing, and whole genome sequencing (Fig. 11.2).

The various techniques available in metagenomics supply both strengths and weaknesses depending upon the primary purpose of the analysis. For example, fingerprinting, which utilizes the 16S rRNA gene to cluster bacterial communities, is relatively inexpensive, but lacks specificity. Targeted sequencing and microarray data focus on the hypervariable regions of the 16S rRNA and allow for greater specificity down to the genus and species level. However, this technique relies on bioinformatics processing which maps reads to a known or reference genome. Thus,

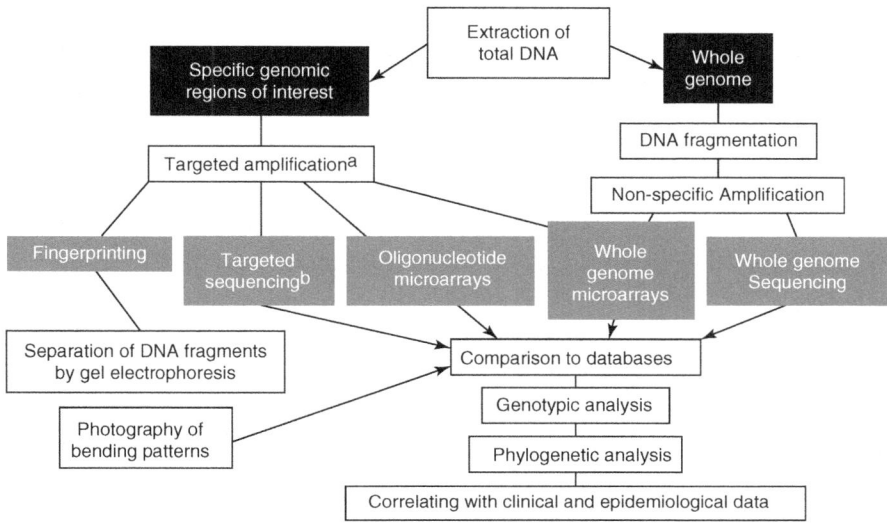

Fig. 11.2 Molecular techniques utilized when characterizing the human microbiome. Used with permission [11]

they are reliant upon mapping to previously identified sequences or species. Although costly, whole genome sequencing allows for full discovery of an organisms genome and may yield information about functional differences of bacteria in a community.

Metagenomic sample sequencing produces read lengths of 200–300 bp paired-end reads up to 1000 bp reads depending on what sequencing platform is utilized. Read lengths and read depths—the number of reads per colony—are important in accurate characterization. The data generated by the sequencing must be processed and organized into clusters termed operational taxonomic units (OTUs). This is accomplished by mapping the 16S sequence to publically available taxonomic databases. OTUs are then utilized to determine sample composition and diversity. Several open-source software packages, for example, QIIME (Quantitative Insight Into Microbial Ecology), assist with the bioinformatics processing and analysis.

Microbiome Characterization: Limitations

We have discussed the limitations of cultivation-dependent techniques as compared to cultivation-independent techniques in terms of accurate characterization of biodiversity. However, it is important to note some of the limitations of the technologies described above which are unique to the high-throughput sequencing approach.

Sequencing metagenomics samples allows the investigator to determine presence or absence of microbial genetic material. There is not data provided regarding the vitality of the microorganisms. Further, although read counts can be helpful in this regard, quantification of a particular organism in a sample can be challenging. This read count clustering, also known as "binning," can be performed when known sequences exit; however it becomes much more challenging and less accurate when analyzing novel species [19].

Further limitations relate to clinical functionality. For example, while sequencing can give insight into the makeup of the microbiome, it does not give information about its biologic function, like resistance or susceptibility to antibiotics. Further there is a growing body of data which suggest that these microorganisms are not simply free-floating on the surface of tissue but form their own three-dimensional biofilms with inner and outer layers. This adds an additional complexity which could be of great importance but has been explored very little. The fact that these biofilms exist from the vagina to the fallopian tubes allows complex and dynamic interactions between the gametes and embryo as well as the maternal tissue interface [20, 21].

The Female Reproductive Tract Microbiome in Health and Disease

The Microbiome in the Vagina and Uterus in Health

The vast majority of data reporting the characterization of the normal state of the reproductive tract microbiome come from studies analyzing vaginal samples, due to the outdated belief that the uterine cavity was a sterile site. In this line, it has been widely reported that the normal vaginal microbiome in healthy women is generally dominated by *Lactobacilli* species [22], although it is subject to important variations along women's lifetime depending on age, changes in hormonal levels, as well as sexual activity and hygiene habits [23]. The vaginal microbiota during the infancy is characterized by a mixture of aerobic and anaerobic bacterial populations including *Prevotella*, *Peptostreptococcus*, *Enterobacteria*, *Streptococcus*, and *Staphylococcus* species [24]. In the pubertal period, the pH of the vagina decreases, and glycogen production increases in response to the estrogen rise, promoting the colonization of *Lactobacilli* species which are able to grow in acidic environments and displace other kinds of bacteria. A vaginal microbiota dominated by *Lactobacillus* genus has tradi-tionally been associated with vaginal health during the woman's reproductive life, as the production of lactic acid by these bacteria would prevent the growth of potential pathogens that could produce vaginal or urinary infections, as well as sexually trans-mitted infections [25–27]. During menopause, estrogens levels decrease again together with the dominance of *Lactobacillus*, while high percentage of *Lactobacillus* is recovered in women receiving hormone replacement therapy [28, 29].

The analysis of the vaginal microbiome using molecular techniques has revealed that five vaginal community state types (CSTs) can be found in healthy reproductive-age women based on their bacterial composition. More than 70% of the women demonstrated vaginal microbiota dominated by *L. crispatus*, *L. gasseri*, *L. iners*, or

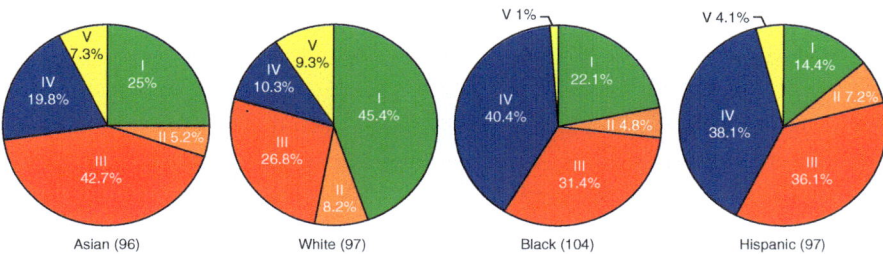

Fig. 11.3 The vaginal bacterial community state types differ in women from different ethnicities. Number of women analyzed in each ethnic group is shown in parentheses. Used with permission [22]

L. jensenii, corresponding to CST-I, CST-II, CST-III, and CST-V, respectively. A small but yet important proportion of women presented CST-IV vaginal microbiota, characterized by lower percentage of *Lactobacilli* and dominance of anaerobic bacteria including *Aerococcus, Atopobium, Dialister, Gardnerella, Megasphaera, Prevotella*, and *Sneathia* species [22].

Interestingly, the vaginal microbiome is influenced by myriad factors and is dependent on its relationship with the host. One example is the influence of the ethnic background on the vaginal microbiota (Fig. 11.3); while Caucasian and Asian populations present a higher prevalence for *Lactobacilli*-dominated CST-I and CST-III, respectively, the non-*Lactobacilli*-dominated CST-IV microbiota is much more prevalent in Hispanic and African-American women [22].

Knowledge about the normal upper genital tract microbiome is much more scarce, as the uterine cavity has been historically considered to be sterile [30], and the isolation of bacteria from endometrial samples had been long considered to come from patients suffering overt uterine infections or through contamination of the sample [31, 32]. The existence of bacterial communities in the upper genital tract has been corroborated by qPCR detection of bacteria in 95% of endometrial samples obtained from asymptomatic women undergoing hysterectomy for benign indications [33]. Due to the limited number of targeted bacteria analyzed, no comprehensive endometrial microbiota data was available from these women, but it shows that the uterine cavity presents bacterial colonization that is quantitatively and qualitatively different from that of the vaginal microbiome from the same women [33].

Recently, a study conducted using next-generation sequencing of the 16S rRNA gene has compared the vaginal and endometrial microbiota of asymptomatic and fertile nonpregnant women [34]. Consistent with the work by Mitchell and coworkers, bacterial communities were detected in 100% of the subjects analyzed, showing that *Lactobacillus* was the most represented genus in endometrial fluid samples followed by *Gardnerella, Prevotella, Atopobium*, and *Sneathia*, which have been also identified in vagina. However, in approximately 20% of the women analyzed, the bacteria community identified in the vagina was dramatically different from the one in the endometrium, showing that, although closely related, endometrial and vaginal microbiota are not identical in each woman [34].

Pathological Shifts of the Female Reproductive Tract Microbiome

The comprehensive understanding of the human microbiota in the reproductive tract, as well as other body sites, has revolutionized the traditional concept of bacterial pathogens. As mentioned above, *Lactobacillus*-deficient communities dominated by anaerobic bacteria, usually associated with a disease state, have been identified in the genital tract of otherwise healthy and asymptomatic women. In this scenario, the definition of a pathogenic microbiota should be revisited to evaluate not only the intrinsic virulence of a specific microorganism by itself but also its impact in the surrounding bacterial community and finally the impact on the host [35]. In this case, in the absence of symptoms, a non-*Lactobacillus*-dominated microbiota would be considered as "normal" even if it is made up of bacteria classically associated with human genital infections. Despite this, dysbiotic deviation from the "normal/healthy" *Lactobacillus*-dominated microbiota may produce imbalances in the homeostasis of the reproductive tract that may increase the susceptibility for acquiring bacterial or viral infections and other gynecological diseases [36].

Bacterial Vaginosis

Bacterial vaginosis (BV) is a clinical microbiological syndrome caused by the shift from a *Lactobacillus*-dominated vaginal microbiota to a polymicrobial population including *Atopobium vaginalis*, *Gardnerella vaginalis*, *Dialister* spp., *Megasphaera* spp., *Prevotella* spp., *Sneathia* spp., and/or the so-called BV-associated bacteria (BVAB), among others. The prevalence of BV in the USA has been estimated to be 29.2% in the last decade [37]. Oral metronidazole in combination with vaginal clindamycin is the current treatment for BV, but relapse infection within a year is observed in 50% of the treated patients due to resistant bacterial strains [38].

BV has been associated with a higher risk of pelvic inflammatory disease [39], HIV-1 [40], and obstetrical complications such as late miscarriage and preterm delivery [41–43]. The implications of BV on infertility and IVF success remain unclear [44]. Of note, there is a high prevalence of BV in infertile patients occurring in as many as 40% of women receiving assisted reproductive treatment [42].

Chronic Endometritis

Chronic endometritis (CE) is a persistent inflammatory condition of the endometrial mucosa produced by infection of the uterine cavity with common bacteria such as *Corynebacterium*, *Enterococcus faecalis*, *Escherichia coli*, *Gardnerella vaginalis*, *Klebsiella pneumoniae*, *Proteus* spp., *Pseudomonas aeruginosa*, *Staphylococcus* spp., and *Streptococcus* spp.; genital pathogens as *Neisseria gonorrhoeae*, *Chlamydia trachomatis*, and *Ureaplasma urealyticum*; and yeasts like *Saccharomyces cerevisiae* and *Candida* spp. [45–47]. The general prevalence of CE is 19%, but this percentage can be underestimated as it is often asymptomatic and thus, rarely suspected or diagnosed [48]. The current treatment for CE consists of a combination of ceftriaxone, metronidazole, and doxycycline (according to the Center for Disease Control), but relapse is a common feature in patients. Because of the frequent lack of symptoms and the fact that CE is not detectable through transvaginal ultrasound, the diagnosis is the most challenging feature its assessment. Traditional diagnosis methods include the histological observation of infiltrated plasma cells in endometrial stromal compartment, followed by classical microbiological culture, while observation of micropolyps, edema, and hyperemia through hysteroscopy has been lately accepted as a reliable method for the diagnosis of CE [49].

The prevalence of CE ranges from 2.8 to 29% in IVF patients depending on the diagnostic method used [49–56]. Although the impact of CE on IVF outcomes has been described to be minimal [50], retrospective studies have pointed out to an implication in repeated implantation failure (RIF) [55, 57, 58] and recurrent miscarriage (RM) [59]. These correlations have been corroborated in asymptomatic patients diagnosed by hysteroscopy that significantly improved their reproductive outcomes after receiving antibiotic treatment for CE [57, 59].

Microbiome in Assisted Reproductive Technology

In order to give a full picture of the microbiome in reproduction, we have discussed the importance of the role of the microbiome in the physiology and pathophysiology of the gynecologic tract and will discuss its importance during gestation. Indeed, these areas have been foremost in the research to date. However, given the connections between the microbiome, host immunity, and infertility, it is quite clear that the vaginal and uterine microbiomes play a role in the physiology and pathophysiology of human reproduction.

Vaginal Microbiome in ART

The vaginal microbiome has been characterized to a great degree through the HMP. Perhaps some of the most interesting data which came from this analysis was the analysis of diversity. The vaginal tract exhibited some of the lowest alpha (within samples from the same subject) and beta (comparison between subjects) diversity when classified using phylotypes compared to other sites such as the mouth or the skin [60] (Fig. 11.4). Indeed, when samples were taken at the vaginal introitus, midpoint, and posterior fornix, the variation of species was not great, and *Lactobacillus* spp. dominated all sites. The fact that vaginal communities is normal,

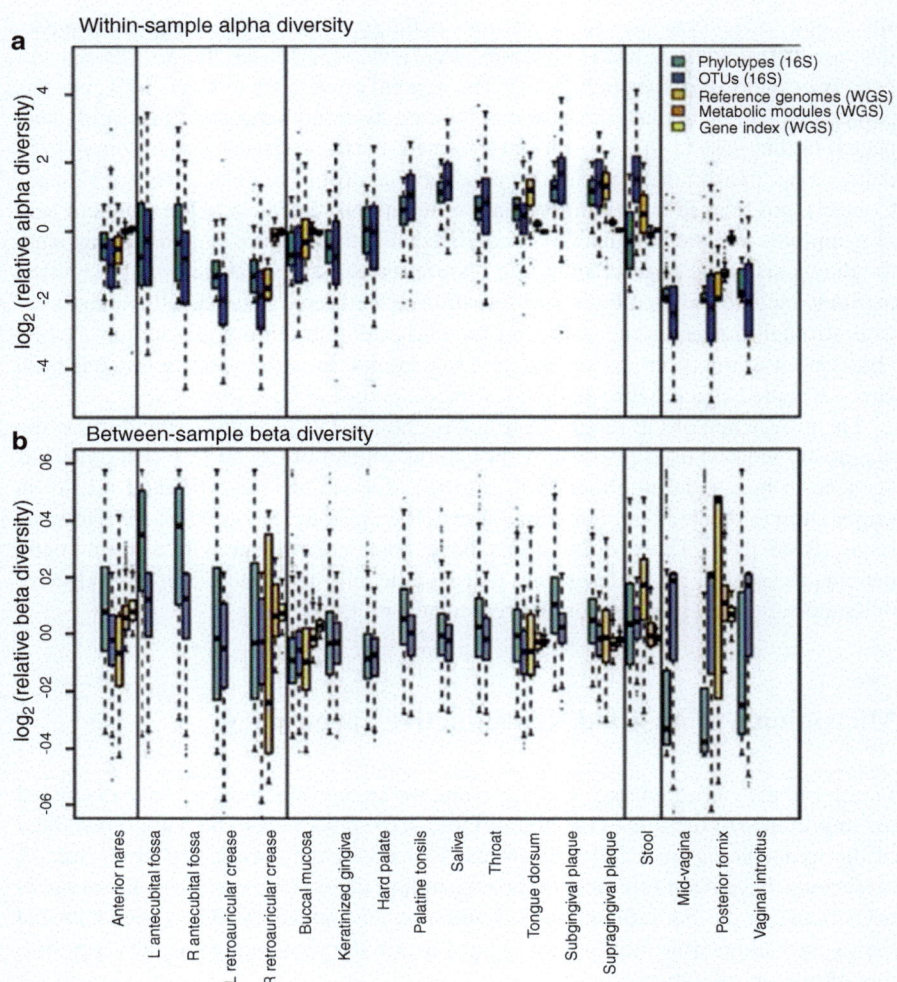

Fig. 11.4 The Human Microbiome Project utilized 16S rRNA sequencing to identify diversity at various body sites. The alpha and beta diversity of the female reproductive tract is low when compared to other body sites. Used with permission [60]

healthy volunteers is relatively simple as compared to other sites of the body means that characterization of health and disease states could be informative in clearly defining shifts in the microbiome—in other words, simplicity of normality allows for easier identification of abnormality.

The vaginal microbiome as it pertains to ART has been investigated several ways. Utilizing culture-based technology, certain bacteria, such as *Enterobacteriaceae* and *Staphylococcus*, found at the time of embryo transfer on the transfer catheter were associated with poorer outcomes [61]. More robust studies utilizing sequencing techniques and analyzing diversity indices found that lower diversity indices had better outcomes—as one would hypothesize given the fact the "normal state" has low diversity with *Lactobacilli* dominance [62].

Of note regarding stimulation, the vaginal microbiome has been shown to change during the normal menstrual cycle with varied estrogen levels in the physiologic range [17]. It is thus reasonable to assume the controlled ovarian stimulation required to achieve success in IVF would also impact the vaginal microbiome. This may represent yet another reason, in addition to embryo and endometrial synchrony and implantation failure discussed elsewhere in this book, that certain circumstances may dictate improved outcomes in terms of implantation when a physiologic state which more approximates nature is procured.

Endometrial Microbiome and Embryonic Implantation

Although in present day the revelation is not so profound, it was only recently that the upper genital tract colonization could be deemed anything but pathologic [63–67]. There are a number of barriers in terms of cervical mucus and alterations of inflammatory milieu which may dictate that the microbiome in the upper tract would differ from the lower tract, but to think it was sterile would be difficult given that spermatozoa must traverse the same path. Indeed, studies which employed radiolabeled albumin spheres placed in the vagina found they ascended into the uterus in as little as 2 min [68].

The microbiological state of the endometrium at the time of embryo transfer has been long considered of particular interest as it could impact embryo implantation. Accumulated evidence from studies reporting bacterial isolates recovered upon microbiological culture of the embryo transfer catheter tip have linked the presence of endometrial pathogens to poor reproductive outcomes in IVF patients. Concretely, the isolation of *Enterobacteriaceae*, *Streptococcus* spp., *Staphylococcus* spp., *E. coli*, and Gram-negative bacteria from the transfer catheter tip is associated with significantly reduced implantation and pregnancy rates [61, 69–73].

In the "microbiome era," the attribution of negative IVF outcome to a specific isolated bacterium is not suitable anymore. The entire microbial community needs to be addressed in order to draw conclusions. To do so, all the efforts are now focused on the identification of an endometrial microbiome signature responsible for reproductive failure or success. In this regard, only few studies have been undertaken to characterize the endometrial microbiome in infertile patients.

Verstraelen and collaborators have reported the endometrial microbiome of 19 Caucasian patients with RIF, recurrent miscarriage (RM), or both [74]. The endometrial microbiota in those patients was formed by 183 bacterial phylotypes, being the *Bacteroides* and *Proteobacteria* phyla the most represented, although they found one patient with endometrial microbiota dominated by *Lactobacillus crispatus* and one patient presenting a polymicrobial community including *Prevotella* spp., *A. vaginae, Mobiluncus curtisii, Porphyromonas, Dialister* spp., and *Peptostreptococcus* spp. phylotypes [74]. The results of this work are consistent with previous evidences showing dysbiotic shifts from a *Lactobacillus*-dominated microbiome in the reproductive tract are more frequent in subfertile population [44].

The endometrial microbiome of infertile patients and its functional impact on reproductive outcome have been recently assessed in two different studies. In the first study, 33 patients of different ethnicities (26 Caucasian, 5 Asian, 1 African-American, and 1 Hispanic) were interrogated for their endometrial microbiota at the time of embryo transfer of a single euploid embryo, and these results were correlated with their IVF outcomes [7]. The core endometrial microbiota in this patients was made of 278 genera, being *Flavobacterium* and *Lactobacillus* the most abundant genera in both patients with ongoing and non-ongoing pregnancies, and no other taxa was significantly identified as differential between women with or without ongoing pregnancies, mainly due to the large number of variables in the study that was not able to survive correction for multiple comparison in the statistical analysis [7]. The latest work has analyzed the impact of endometrial microbiome on reproductive outcome in endometrial fluid from 35 infertile Caucasian patients presenting RIF despite of having receptive endometrium assessed by molecular analysis [34]. The endometrial microbiota was made of 108 components being *Lactobacillus* spp. the most abundant bacteria detected. The results of this study show that endometrial microbiota profile can be classified according to the structure and relative abundance of the bacteria identified in endometrial fluid, as *Lactobacillus* dominated or non-*Lactobacillus* dominated with a cutoff value of *Lactobacillus* relative abundance ≥90% as the only significant variable able to predict reproductive success. Thus, a non-*Lactobacillus*-dominated (<90%) endometrial microbiota significantly correlates with adverse reproductive outcomes—measured as implantation, pregnancy, ongoing pregnancy, and miscarriage rates—when compared to subjects presenting a *Lactobacillus*-dominated (≥90%) endometrial microbiota (Fig. 11.5) pointing to the importance of endometrial bacteria in reproductive health [34].

The Immune System, the Microbiome, and Implantation

A full detail of the immune systems interaction with implantation physiology and pathophysiology is discussed elsewhere in this book. It is important to note here however that the microbiome is integrally involved with the immune systems and thus the permissive environment required for successful implantation. Indeed, a complex microenvironment is created by the cytokines involved in both endometrial receptivity as well as embryo development and is influenced by nutrition, stress, injury, and infection and inflammation [75].

In addition to direct inhibition, production of H_2O_2 and bacteriocins, and modulation of epithelial receptivity, the microbiome has been implicated in directly modulating the immune system, in particular T lymphocytes [76]. T helper (Th) cells have also been shown to influence ART outcomes. In particular, there is a focus on

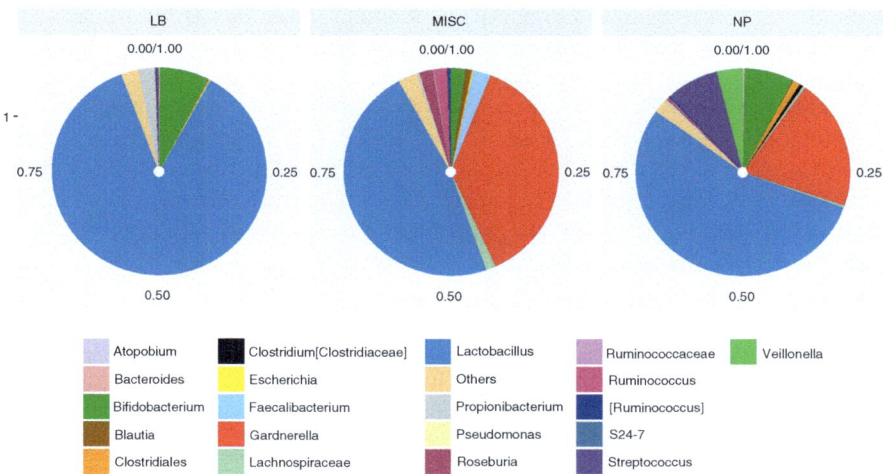

Fig. 11.5 Low abundance of *Lactobacillus* in endometrial microbiota is associated with poor reproductive outcomes in IVF patients. *LB* live birth, *MISC* miscarriage, *NP* no pregnancy. Adapted from [34]

the ratio of Th1 cells, which produce interferon-gamma (IFN) and lymphotoxin, and Th2 cells, which produce IL-4, IL-5, IL-13, IL-25, and GM-CSF. Both cells produce GM-CSF, TNF, IL-2, and IL-3 [77]. The Th2 cells predominate during normal pregnancy, whereas Th1 is more predominate in women with pregnancy losses [78–81]. The Th1/Th2 ratio construct has been expanded to the Th1/Th2 as well as the Th17 and regulatory T cell construct. The Th17 cells secrete IL-17 which is pro-inflammatory and the T regulatory cells work to induce immune tolerance [82, 83]. Similar to Th1/Th2 ratios, studies have shown increased rates of unexplained spontaneous abortion with an increase in Th17 and decrease in regulatory T cells [84, 85].

The complex interaction between the microbiome, immune modulators, and implantation and reproductive competence is evolving rapidly. Once the physiologic state of the reproductive tract microbiome is better characterized, we will be able to determine more concretely how this microbiome changes the immune milieu and affects the process of immune tolerance.

Antimicrobials and ART

Although the vaginal and uterine microbiome is incompletely understood in terms of its relationship to reproductive outcomes, there is a long history of attempting to influence it using prophylactic antibiotics at the time of procedures during ART. Given that antiseptics are often toxic, antibiotics have been utilized as a method of manipulating the microbiome since the studies in the late 1970s which showed that contamination during ART procedures could negatively impact outcomes [86, 87]. Indeed, given concern for embryo transfer catheter tip contamination and inoculating of the upper tract, antibiotics are often prescribed leading up to the embryo transfer. This is of concern as wide-spectrum prophylactic antibiotics have the potential to interfere with the "healthy" microbiome which exists at the time of embryo transfer as well as impact those bacteria which are pathologic.

A recent Cochrane Database Systematic Review analyzed randomized controlled trials in the literature which investigated antibiotics at embryo transfer [88]. Only four potential studies were identified, of which three were excluded. The remaining study reported on clinical pregnancy rates as the primary outcome. Although administration reduced microbial contamination as defined by culture of embryo transfer catheter tips, the clinical pregnancy rate in those receiving antibiotics was 36%, and those not receiving was 35.5% (OR 1.02, 95% CI 0.66 to 1.58) [89]. The reviewers concluded more evidence is needed with live birth as the primary outcome [88].

One possible explanation for the lack of clear benefit of antimicrobial use at the time of embryo transfer is that, while the antibiotics successfully decrease the load of bacteria which are alive and can be cultured, it does not decrease the burden of bacterial remnants which still serve to modulate the immune system [89, 90]. This modulation of the immune system by the microbiome may indeed play the most critical role in the connection with ART outcomes.

Although at the present time, data on antimicrobial use has not shown clear benefit, there are other ways in which the microbiome might be altered. Rather than eliminating pathogenic bacteria, perhaps bacteria with beneficial profiles could be replaced. Probiotics have been investigated as a way to treat vaginal infections such as bacterial vaginosis with success [91]. This same approach may be a way to positively affect ART outcomes in the future, although more metagenomic data is needed to more fully characterize the physiologic state prior to intervention attempts.

The Impact of the Microbiome on Pregnancy Outcomes

Non-gravid vs. Gravid Vaginal Microbiome

The vaginal microbiome has been shown to be distinct in pregnant versus nonpregnant women in terms of structure and stability. Contrary to that observed in nonpregnant women, vaginal microbiota of pregnant women is very stable, and shifts in endometrial microbiota only occur between *Lactobacillus*-dominated CSTs. As a result gravid vaginal microbiota is most often dominated by *L. crispatus*, *L. jensenii*, and *L. gasseri* in women delivering at term, while taxa associated to CST-IV are very rarely observed in pregnant women regardless of their ethnicity [92]. When the spatiotemporal dynamics of the vaginal microbiota has been interrogated, results have shown that the diversity and richness of this microbiota decrease with gestational age and proximity to the uterus [93]. However, a destabilization of the vaginal microbiota is commonly observed within few weeks preceding delivery and remains altered for approximately 1 year after delivery, showing certain similarities to the communities typically colonizing the gut [93, 94]. The relevance of *Lactobacillus* spp. in the vaginal microbiota during pregnancy and the mechanisms leading to this dominance remain unknown. However, some hypothesis points to the protective role that *Lactobacilli* could play in the reproductive tract against potential ascending infection which represents a risk factor for many obstetrical conditions [95].

Placental Microbiome

The isolation of bacteria from placentas of healthy women delivering at term was reported for the first time in 1988 [96], challenging the general believe of a sterile onset of life. Nowadays, it is well accepted that the placenta harbors a low abundance but unique microbiome that is not the result of uterine infections or chorioamnionitis. The placental microbiome is composed of commensal bacteria belonging to *Proteobacteria, Actinobacteria, Firmicutes, Bacteroidetes, Tenericutes,* and *Fusobacteria* phyla [97]. Only a small set of taxa as *Burkholderia, Streptosporangium,* and *Roseovarius* are increased in placentas of women delivering preterm. Many different models have been proposed to explain the bacterial seeding of the placenta, from ascension from the lower genital tract to the contamination during delivery. However, the vast similarity observed between the community population of the placenta and the oral microbiome of nonpregnant women suggests that these bacteria may reach the placenta through hematogenous spread early in pregnancy, at the time of vascularization and placentation [97].

Preterm Birth

Preterm birth (PTB) is defined as an early birth before 37 weeks of gestation. This very prevalent obstetrical complication has been linked to intrauterine infection with pathogenic microorganisms colonizing the fetal membranes, amniotic fluid, cord blood, placental, and fetus [98]. It is generally believed that this intrauterine infection could be originated in the lower genital tract by ascension of the pathogenic microorganisms producing the preterm premature rupture of membranes leading to PTB. This hypothesis is supported by evidences showing an association of BV with PTB [99]. Another hypothesis, given the placental microbiome's similarity to the oral cavity microbiome, is the hematogenous spread from periodontal infections. This would explain the high correlation observed between PTB and periodontal disease [100]. However, despite the mechanism of infection, the microorganisms causing PTB are well defined and include *Ureaplasma urealyticum, Ureaplasma parvum, Mycoplasma hominis, E. coli, Bacteroides* spp., *G. vaginalis, Sneathia sanguinegens*, *Streptococcus* spp., and *Fusobacterium nucleatum* [101, 102] as well as with a decrease or lack of *L. crispatus* in the urogenital tract [94, 103].

Summary

The microbiome in health and human disease, in particular in relation to the success or failure of human reproduction, is beginning to be unraveled. Given the abilities of new technologies and techniques for sampling and analyzing the microbiome in the reproductive tract, this knowledge is now growing at an unprecedented rate. As the reproductive tract dysbiosis is better characterized and understood, we may be better equipped to manipulate it more expertly and depart from the practice of broad-spectrum, indiscriminant antibiotic use which has been the mainstay of therapy.

References

1. Peterson J, Garges S, Giovanni M, McInnes P, Wang L, Schloss JA, et al. The NIH human microbiome project. Genome Res. 2009;19(12):2317–23.
2. Rhoads DD, Cox SB, Rees EJ, Sun Y, Wolcott RD. Clinical identification of bacteria in human chronic wound infections: culturing vs. 16S ribosomal DNA sequencing. BMC Infect Dis. 2012;12:321.
3. Venter JC, Adams MD, Myers EW, Li PW, Mural RJ, Sutton GG, et al. The sequence of the human genome. Science. 2001;291(5507):1304–51.
4. Davies J. In a map for human life, count the microbes, too. Science. 2001;291(5512):2316.
5. Relman DA, Falkow S. The meaning and impact of the human genome sequence for microbiology. Trends Microbiol. 2001;9(5):206–8.
6. Franasiak JM, Scott RT. Reproductive tract microbiome in assisted reproductive technologies. Fertil Steril. 2015;104(6):1364–71.
7. Franasiak JM, Werner MD, Juneau CR, Tao X, Landis J, Zhan Y, et al. Endometrial microbiome at the time of embryo transfer: next-generation sequencing of the 16S ribosomal subunit. J Assist Reprod Genet. 2016;33(1):129–36.
8. Green KA, Zarek SM, Catherino WH. Gynecologic health and disease in relation to the microbiome of the female reproductive tract. Fertil Steril. 2015;104(6):1351–7.
9. Fox C, Eichelberger K. Maternal microbiome and pregnancy outcomes. Fertil Steril. 2015;104(6):1358–63.
10. Franasiak JM, Scott RT. Introduction: microbiome in human reproduction. Fertil Steril. 2015;104(6):1341–3.
11. Mor A, Driggers PH, Segars JH. Molecular characterization of the human microbiome from a reproductive perspective. Fertil Steril. 2015;104(6):1344–50.
12. Giovannoni SJ, Britschgi TB, Moyer CL, Field KG. Genetic diversity in Sargasso Sea bacterioplankton. Nature. 1990;345(6270):60–3.
13. Dymock D, Weightman AJ, Scully C, Wade WG. Molecular analysis of microflora associated with dentoalveolar abscesses. J Clin Microbiol. 1996;34(3):537–42.
14. Verhelst R, Verstraelen H, Claeys G, Verschraegen G, Delanghe J, Van Simaey L, et al. Cloning of 16S rRNA genes amplified from normal and disturbed vaginal microflora sug-

gests a strong association between Atopobium vaginae, Gardnerella vaginalis and bacterial vaginosis. BMC Microbiol. 2004;4:16.

15. Zhou X, Bent SJ, Schneider MG, Davis CC, Islam MR, Forney LJ. Characterization of vaginal microbial communities in adult healthy women using cultivation-independent methods. Microbiology. 2004;150(Pt 8):2565–73.

16. Eckburg PB, Bik EM, Bernstein CN, Purdom E, Dethlefsen L, Sargent M, et al. Diversity of the human intestinal microbial flora. Science. 2005;308(5728):1635–8.

17. Hyman RW, Fukushima M, Diamond L, Kumm J, Giudice LC, Davis RW. Microbes on the human vaginal epithelium. Proc Natl Acad Sci U S A. 2005;102(22):7952–7.

18. Handelsman J. Metagenomics: application of genomics to uncultured microorganisms. Microbiol Mol Biol Rev. 2004;68(4):669–85.

19. Alneberg J, Bjarnason BS, de Bruijn I, Schirmer M, Quick J, Ijaz UZ, et al. Binning metagenomic contigs by coverage and composition. Nat Methods. 2014;11(11):1144–6.

20. Swidsinski A, Verstraelen H, Loening-Baucke V, Swidsinski S, Mendling W, Halwani Z. Presence of a polymicrobial endometrial biofilm in patients with bacterial vaginosis. PLoS One. 2013;8(1):e53997.

21. Trinidad A, Ibanez A, Gomez D, Garcia-Berrocal J, Ramierz-Camacho R. Application of environmental scanning electron microscopy for study of biofilms in medical devices. In: Méndez-Vilas A, Díaz J, editors. Microscopy: science, technology, applications and education. Badajoz: Formatex Research Centre; 2010. p. 204–10.

22. Ravel J, Gajer P, Abdo Z, Schneider GM, Koenig SSK, McCulle SL, et al. Vaginal microbiome of reproductive-age women. Proc Natl Acad Sci U S A. 2011;108(Suppl 1):4680–7.

23. Gajer P, Brotman RM, Bai G, Sakamoto J, Schütte UME, Zhong X, et al. Temporal dynamics of the human vaginal microbiota. Sci Transl Med. 2012;4(132):132ra52.

24. Huang B, Fettweis JM, Brooks JP, Jefferson KK, Buck GA. The changing landscape of the vaginal microbiome. Clin Lab Med. 2014;34(4):747–61.

25. O'Hanlon DE, Moench TR, Cone RA. Vaginal pH and microbicidal lactic acid when lactobacilli dominate the microbiota. PLoS One. 2013;8(11):e80074.

26. Donders GG, Bosmans E, Dekeersmaecker A, Vereecken A, Van Bulck B, Spitz B. Pathogenesis of abnormal vaginal bacterial flora. Am J Obstet Gynecol. 2000;182(4):872–8.

27. Cohen J. Infectious disease. Vaginal microbiome affects HIV risk. Science. 2016;353(6297):331.

28. Pabich WL, Fihn SD, Stamm WE, Scholes D, Boyko EJ, Gupta K. Prevalence and determinants of vaginal flora alterations in postmenopausal women. J Infect Dis. 2003;188(7):1054–8.

29. Brotman RM, Shardell MD, Gajer P, Fadrosh D, Chang K, Silver MI, et al. Association between the vaginal microbiota, menopause status, and signs of vulvovaginal atrophy. Menopause. 2014;21(5):450–8.

30. Romero R, Espinoza J, Mazor M. Can endometrial infection/inflammation explain implantation failure, spontaneous abortion, and preterm birth after in vitro fertilization? Fertil Steril. 2004;82(4):799–804.

31. Hemsell DL, Obregon VL, Heard MC, Nobles BJ. Endometrial bacteria in asymptomatic, nonpregnant women. J Reprod Med. 1989;34(11):872–4.

32. Møller BR, Kristiansen FV, Thorsen P, Frost L, Mogensen SC. Sterility of the uterine cavity. Acta Obstet Gynecol Scand. 1995;74(3):216–9.

33. Mitchell CM, Haick A, Nkwopara E, Garcia R, Rendi M, Agnew K, et al. Colonization of the upper genital tract by vaginal bacterial species in nonpregnant women. Am J Obstet Gynecol. 2015;212(5):611.e1–9.

34. Moreno I, Codoñer FM, Vilella F, Martínez-Blanch JF, Valbuena D, Jimenez-Almazán J, Alonso R, Alamá P, Remohí J, Pellicer A, Ramón D, Simón C. Evidence that the endometrial microbiota has an effect on implantation success or failure. Am J Obstet Gynecol. 2016;215(6):684–703.

35. Larsen B, Monif GR. Understanding the bacterial flora of the female genital tract. Clin Infect Dis. 2001;32(4):e69–77.

36. Schwebke JR. Abnormal vaginal flora as a biological risk factor for acquisition of HIV infection and sexually transmitted diseases. J Infect Dis. 2005;192(8):1315–7.
37. Koumans EH, Sternberg M, Bruce C, McQuillan G, Kendrick J, Sutton M, et al. The prevalence of bacterial vaginosis in the United States, 2001–2004; associations with symptoms, sexual behaviors, and reproductive health. Sex Transm Dis. 2007;34(11):864–9.
38. Bradshaw CS, Morton AN, Hocking J, Garland SM, Morris MB, Moss LM, et al. High recurrence rates of bacterial vaginosis over the course of 12 months after oral metronidazole therapy and factors associated with recurrence. J Infect Dis. 2006;193(11):1478–86.
39. Ness RB, Kip KE, Hillier SL, Soper DE, Stamm CA, Sweet RL, et al. A cluster analysis of bacterial vaginosis-associated microflora and pelvic inflammatory disease. Am J Epidemiol. 2005;162(6):585–90.
40. Atashili J, Poole C, Ndumbe PM, Adimora AA, Smith JS. Bacterial vaginosis and HIV acquisition: a meta-analysis of published studies. AIDS. 2008;22(12):1493–501.
41. Hillier SL, Nugent RP, Eschenbach DA, Krohn MA, Gibbs RS, Martin DH, et al. Association between bacterial vaginosis and preterm delivery of a low-birth-weight infant. The vaginal infections and prematurity study group. N Engl J Med. 1995;333(26):1737–42.
42. Leitich H, Bodner-Adler B, Brunbauer M, Kaider A, Egarter C, Husslein P. Bacterial vaginosis as a risk factor for preterm delivery: a meta-analysis. Am J Obstet Gynecol. 2003;189(1):139–47.
43. Romero R, Chaiworapongsa T, Kuivaniemi H, Tromp G. Bacterial vaginosis, the inflammatory response and the risk of preterm birth: a role for genetic epidemiology in the prevention of preterm birth. Am J Obstet Gynecol. 2004;190(6):1509–19.
44. van Oostrum N, De Sutter P, Meys J, Verstraelen H. Risks associated with bacterial vaginosis in infertility patients: a systematic review and meta-analysis. Hum Reprod. 2013;28(7):1809–15.
45. Greenwood SM, Moran JJ. Chronic endometritis: morphologic and clinical observations. Obstet Gynecol. 1981;58(2):176–84.
46. Cicinelli E, De Ziegler D, Nicoletti R, Colafiglio G, Saliani N, Resta L, et al. Chronic endometritis: correlation among hysteroscopic, histologic, and bacteriologic findings in a prospective trial with 2190 consecutive office hysteroscopies. Fertil Steril. 2008;89(3):677–84.
47. Cicinelli E, De Ziegler D, Nicoletti R, Tinelli R, Saliani N, Resta L, et al. Poor reliability of vaginal and endocervical cultures for evaluating microbiology of endometrial cavity in women with chronic endometritis. Gynecol Obstet Investig. 2009;68(2):108–15.
48. Yoshii N, Hamatani T, Inagaki N, Hosaka T, Inoue O, Yamada M, et al. Successful implantation after reducing matrix metalloproteinase activity in the uterine cavity. Reprod Biol Endocrinol. 2013;11:37.
49. Cicinelli E, Resta L, Nicoletti R, Tartagni M, Marinaccio M, Bulletti C, et al. Detection of chronic endometritis at fluid hysteroscopy. J Minim Invasive Gynecol. 2005;12(6):514–8.
50. Kasius JC, Fatemi HM, Bourgain C, Sie-Go DMDS, Eijkemans RJC, Fauser BC, et al. The impact of chronic endometritis on reproductive outcome. Fertil Steril. 2011;96(6):1451–6.
51. Kasius JC, Broekmans FJM, Sie-Go DMDS, Bourgain C, Eijkemans MJC, Fauser BC, et al. The reliability of the histological diagnosis of endometritis in asymptomatic IVF cases: a multicenter observer study. Hum Reprod. 2012;27(1):153–8.
52. Polisseni F, Bambirra EA, Camargos AF. Detection of chronic endometritis by diagnostic hysteroscopy in asymptomatic infertile patients. Gynecol Obstet Investig. 2003;55(4):205–10.
53. Féghali J, Bakar J, Mayenga JM, Ségard L, Hamou J, Driguez P, et al. Systematic hysteroscopy prior to in vitro fertilization. Gynecol Obstet Fertil. 2003;31(2):127–31.
54. Oliveira FG, Abdelmassih VG, Diamond MP, Dozortsev D, Nagy ZP, Abdelmassih R. Uterine cavity findings and hysteroscopic interventions in patients undergoing in vitro fertilization-embryo transfer who repeatedly cannot conceive. Fertil Steril. 2003;80(6):1371–5.
55. Johnston-MacAnanny EB, Hartnett J, Engmann LL, Nulsen JC, Sanders MM, Benadiva CA. Chronic endometritis is a frequent finding in women with recurrent implantation failure after in vitro fertilization. Fertil Steril. 2010;93:437–41.

56. Matteo M, Cicinelli E, Greco P, Massenzio F, Baldini D, Falagario T, et al. Abnormal pattern of lymphocyte subpopulations in the endometrium of infertile women with chronic endometritis. Am J Reprod Immunol. 2009;61(5):322–9.
57. Cicinelli E, Matteo M, Tinelli R, Lepera A, Alfonso R, Indraccolo U, et al. Prevalence of chronic endometritis in repeated unexplained implantation failure and the IVF success rate after antibiotic therapy. Hum Reprod. 2015;30(2):323–30.
58. Yang R, Du X, Wang Y, Song X, Yang Y, Qiao J. The hysteroscopy and histological diagnosis and treatment value of chronic endometritis in recurrent implantation failure patients. Arch Gynecol Obstet. 2014;289(6):1363–9.
59. Cicinelli E, Matteo M, Tinelli R, Pinto V, Marinaccio M, Indraccolo U, et al. Chronic endometritis due to common bacteria is prevalent in women with recurrent miscarriage as confirmed by improved pregnancy outcome after antibiotic treatment. Reprod Sci. 2014;21(5):640–7.
60. Human Microbiome Project Consortium. Structure, function and diversity of the healthy human microbiome. Nature. 2012;486(7402):207–14.
61. Selman H, Mariani M, Barnocchi N, Mencacci A, Bistoni F, Arena S, et al. Examination of bacterial contamination at the time of embryo transfer, and its impact on the IVF/pregnancy outcome. J Assist Reprod Genet. 2007;24(9):395–9.
62. Hyman RW, Herndon CN, Jiang H, Palm C, Fukushima M, Bernstein D, et al. The dynamics of the vaginal microbiome during infertility therapy with in vitro fertilization-embryo transfer. J Assist Reprod Genet. 2012;29(2):105–15.
63. Hein M, Petersen AC, Helmig RB, Uldbjerg N, Reinholdt J. Immunoglobulin levels and phagocytes in the cervical mucus plug at term of pregnancy. Acta Obstet Gynecol Scand. 2005;84(8):734–42.
64. Ulcova-Gallova Z. Immunological and physicochemical properties of cervical ovulatory mucus. J Reprod Immunol. 2010;86(2):115–21.
65. Lieberman JA, Moscicki A-B, Sumerel JL, Ma Y, Scott ME. Determination of cytokine protein levels in cervical mucus samples from young women by a multiplex immunoassay method and assessment of correlates. Clin Vaccine Immunol. 2008;15(1):49–54.
66. Ming L, Xiaoling P, Yan L, Lili W, Qi W, Xiyong Y, et al. Purification of antimicrobial factors from human cervical mucus. Hum Reprod. 2007;22(7):1810–5.
67. Ansbacher R, Boyson WA, Morris JA. Sterility of the uterine cavity. Am J Obstet Gynecol. 1967;99(3):394–6.
68. Zervomanolakis I, Ott HW, Hadziomerovic D, Mattle V, Seeber BE, Virgolini I, et al. Physiology of upward transport in the human female genital tract. Ann N Y Acad Sci. 2007;1101:1–20.
69. Egbase PE, Al-Sharhan M, Al-Othman S, Al-Mutawa M, Udo EE, Grudzinskas JG. Incidence of microbial growth from the tip of the embryo transfer catheter after embryo transfer in relation to clinical pregnancy rate following in-vitro fertilization and embryo transfer. Hum Reprod. 1996;11:1687–9.
70. Fanchin R, Harmas A, Benaoudia F, Lundkvist U, Olivennes F, Frydman R. Microbial flora of the cervix assessed at the time of embryo transfer adversely affects in vitro fertilization outcome. Fertil Steril. 1998;70:866–70.
71. Egbase PE, Udo EE, Al-Sharhan M, Grudzinskas JG. Prophylactic antibiotics and endocervical microbial inoculation of the endometrium at embryo transfer. Lancet. 1999;354(9179):651–2.
72. Moore DE, Soules MR, Klein NA, Fujimoto VY, Agnew KJ, Eschenbach DA. Bacteria in the transfer catheter tip influence the live-birth rate after in vitro fertilization. Fertil Steril. 2000;74(6):1118–24.
73. Salim R, Ben-Shlomo I, Colodner R, Keness Y, Shalev E. Bacterial colonization of the uterine cervix and success rate in assisted reproduction: results of a prospective survey. Hum Reprod. 2002;17(2):337–40.
74. Verstraelen H, Vilchez-Vargas R, Desimpel F, Jauregui R, Vankeirsbilck N, Weyers S, et al. Characterisation of the human uterine microbiome in non-pregnant women through deep sequencing of the V1-2 region of the 16S rRNA gene. PeerJ. 2016;4:e1602.

75. Robertson SA, Chin PY, Glynn DJ, Thompson JG. Peri-conceptual cytokines – setting the trajectory for embryo implantation, pregnancy and beyond. Am J Reprod Immunol. 2011;66:2–10.
76. Petrova MI, van den Broek M, Balzarini J, Vanderleyden J, Lebeer S. Vaginal microbiota and its role in HIV transmission and infection. FEMS Microbiol Rev. 2013;37(5):762–92.
77. Commins SP, Borish L, Steinke JW. Immunologic messenger molecules: cytokines, interferons, and chemokines. J Allergy Clin Immunol. 2010;125(2 Suppl 2):S53–72.
78. Hudić I, Fatusić Z. Progesterone-induced blocking factor (PIBF) and Th(1)/Th(2) cytokine in women with threatened spontaneous abortion. J Perinat Med. 2009;37(4):338–42.
79. Kalu E, Bhaskaran S, Thum MY, Vishwanatha R, Croucher C, Sherriff E, et al. Serial estimation of Th1:th2 cytokines profile in women undergoing in-vitro fertilization-embryo transfer. Am J Reprod Immunol. 2008;59(3):206–11.
80. Kwak-Kim JY, Gilman-Sachs A, Kim CE. T helper 1 and 2 immune responses in relationship to pregnancy, nonpregnancy, recurrent spontaneous abortions and infertility of repeated implantation failures. Chem Immunol Allergy. 2005;88(1660–2242 (Print)):64–79.
81. Kwak-Kim JYH, Chung-Bang HS, Ng SC, Ntrivalas EI, Mangubat CP, Beaman KD, et al. Increased T helper 1 cytokine responses by circulating T cells are present in women with recurrent pregnancy losses and in infertile women with multiple implantation failures after IVF. Hum Reprod. 2003;18(4):767–73.
82. Milner JD. IL-17 producing cells in host defense and atopy. Curr Opin Immunol. 2011;23(6):784–8.
83. Peterson RA. Regulatory T-cells: diverse phenotypes integral to immune homeostasis and suppression. Toxicol Pathol. 2012;40(2):186–204.
84. Ernerudh J, Berg G, Mjösberg J. Regulatory T helper cells in pregnancy and their roles in systemic versus local immune tolerance. Am J Reprod Immunol. 2011;66(Suppl 1):31–43.
85. Wang W-J, Hao C-F, null Y-L, Yin G-J, Bao S-H, Qiu L-H, et al. Increased prevalence of T helper 17 (Th17) cells in peripheral blood and decidua in unexplained recurrent spontaneous abortion patients. J Reprod Immunol. 2010;84(2):164–70.
86. Czernobilsky B. Endometritis and infertility. Fertil Steril. 1978;30(2):119–30.
87. van Os HC, Roozenburg BJ, HAB J-C, Leerentveld RA, MCW S, Zeilmaker GH, et al. Vaginal disinfection with povidone iodine and the outcome of in-vitro fertilization. Hum Reprod. 1992;7(3):349–50.
88. Kroon B, Hart RJ, Wong BMS, Ford E, Yazdani A. Antibiotics prior to embryo transfer in ART. Cochrane Database Syst Rev. 2012;3:CD008995.
89. Brook N, Khalaf Y, Coomarasamy A, Edgeworth J, Braude P. A randomized controlled trial of prophylactic antibiotics (co-amoxiclav) prior to embryo transfer. Hum Reprod. 2006;21(11):2911–5.
90. Klebanoff MA, Carey JC, Hauth JC, Hillier SL, Nugent RP, Thom EA, et al. Failure of metronidazole to prevent preterm delivery among pregnant women with asymptomatic Trichomonas vaginalis infection. N Engl J Med. 2001;345(7):487–93.
91. Recine N, Palma E, Domenici L, Giorgini M, Imperiale L, Sassu C, et al. Restoring vaginal microbiota: biological control of bacterial vaginosis. A prospective case–control study using Lactobacillus rhamnosus BMX 54 as adjuvant treatment against bacterial vaginosis. Arch Gynecol Obstet. 2015:1–7.
92. Lamont RF, Sobel JD, Akins RA, Hassan SS, Chaiworapongsa T, Kusanovic JP, et al. The vaginal microbiome: new information about genital tract flora using molecular based techniques. BJOG. 2011;118:533–49.
93. Aagaard K, Riehle K, Ma J, Segata N, Mistretta TA, Coarfa C, et al. A metagenomic approach to characterization of the vaginal microbiome signature in pregnancy. PLoS One. 2012;7:e36466.
94. DiGiulio DB, Callahan BJ, McMurdie PJ, Costello EK, Lyell DJ, Robaczewska A, et al. Temporal and spatial variation of the human microbiota during pregnancy. Proc Natl Acad Sci U S A. 2015;112(35):11060–5.

95. Romero R, Hassan SS, Gajer P, Tarca AL, Fadrosh DW, Nikita L, et al. The composition and stability of the vaginal microbiota of normal pregnant women is different from that of non-pregnant women. Microbiome. 2014;2(1):4.
96. Hillier SL, Martius J, Krohn M, Kiviat N, Holmes KK, Eschenbach DA. A case-control study of chorioamnionic infection and histologic chorioamnionitis in prematurity. N Engl J Med. 1988;319(15):972–8.
97. Aagaard K, Ma J, Antony KM, Ganu R, Petrosino J, Versalovic J. The placenta harbors a unique microbiome. Sci Transl Med. 2014;6(237):237ra65.
98. Goldenberg RL, Culhane JF, Iams JD, Romero R. Epidemiology and causes of preterm birth. Lancet. 2008;371:75–84.
99. McGregor JA, French JI. Bacterial vaginosis and preterm birth. N Engl J Med. 1996;334(20):1337–9.
100. Madianos PN, Bobetsis YA, Offenbacher S. Adverse pregnancy outcomes (APOs) and periodontal disease: pathogenic mechanisms. J Periodontol. 2013;84:S170–80.
101. Jefferson KK. The bacterial etiology of preterm birth. Adv Appl Microbiol. 2012;80:1–22.
102. Combs CA, Gravett M, Garite TJ, Hickok DE, Lapidus J, Porreco R, et al. Amniotic fluid infection, inflammation, and colonization in preterm labor with intact membranes. Am J Obstet Gynecol. 2014;210(2):125.e1–125.e15.
103. Prince AL, Ma J, Kannan PS, Alvarez M, Gisslen T, Harris RA, et al. The placental membrane microbiome is altered among subjects with spontaneous preterm birth with and without chorioamnionitis. Am J Obstet Gynecol. 2016;214(5):627.e1–627.e16.

Chapter 12
Psychosocial Implications of Recurrent Implantation Failure

Andrea Mechanick Braverman and Keren Sofer

Introduction

Infertility has often been described as an emotional roller coaster as intended parents have sought medical treatment to resolve their fertility problems. Concerns that infertility problems are rooted in psychological issues are reflected in the oft-heard advice of "just relax and you'll get pregnant." Historically, psychological theories were developed as models to explain infertility [1]. Sigmund Freud posited a theory of infertility as a consequence of a fear of impregnation. Later on, Berg and Wilson addressed this psychogenic model more broadly, looking at psychopathology as contributing to or causing infertility [2]. Thus the investigation of psychopathology as contributing to or causing infertility has reflected the lay belief that stress or other psychogenic difficulties are implicated in infertility.

In the past several decades, these psychogenic models have been challenged by the increased ability to diagnose the physiological causes for male and female infertility. Scientific methods and diagnostic means have led to a dramatic change in the understanding of infertility as doctors can now identify many of the physical factors that cause infertility. As a result of this shift, psychosocial research began to focus on the relationship between various aspects of psychosocial functioning on overall success rates in infertility treatment. The hope was that if psychosocial functioning was associated with implantation or endometrial development, it would create opportunities to improve pregnancy outcomes. This research has faced the formidable challenge of controlling for the myriad of intervening variables that could

A.M. Braverman, PhD (✉)
Sidney Kimmel Medical College of Thomas Jefferson University, Philadelphia, PA, USA
e-mail: Andrea.Braverman@jefferson.edu

K. Sofer, PsyD
Independent Practice, Philadelphia, PA, USA
e-mail: keren.L.sofer@gmail.com

© Springer International Publishing AG 2018
J.M. Franasiak, R.T. Scott Jr. (eds.), *Recurrent Implantation Failure*,
https://doi.org/10.1007/978-3-319-71967-2_12

contribute to findings of significance or non-significance, resulting in a body of contradictory results.

Psychosocial research has since expanded in breadth, with studies seeking to uncover not only potential links between various psychological factors and pregnancy outcomes but also ways in which psychosocial challenges impact the course of infertility treatment, compliance with treatment protocols, and treatment dropout. These links become all the more relevant with repeated implantation failure, as patients undergo multiple cycles of in vitro fertilization (IVF) and must contend with the stress of IVF on a prolonged basis along with the distress of failure.

This chapter will review the research focused on the scope of psychosocial challenges that infertility patients may experience before, during, and following interventions such as IVF, factors that increase an infertile couple's risk for psychosocial difficulties and the potential impact of psychosocial functioning on pregnancy outcomes. Additionally, an overview of researched psychosocial and psychotropic interventions will provide an examination of treatments which can decrease the psychological burden and prevent poor psychosocial outcomes for infertile couples.

Psychosocial Functioning of Infertility Patients

Researchers and clinicians continue to show interest in the psychosocial functioning of infertility patients for a multitude of reasons. Psychosocial functioning encompasses management of stress, attributions of sources of difficulties, and utilization of relationships in dealing with stress. Understanding an individual's level of psychosocial functioning can assist medical teams in determining which psychosocial interventions would be most pertinent and effective at a given time. Additionally, awareness of infertility patients' coping strategies can help clinicians predict which individuals are more likely to discontinue treatment, adjust poorly, display inconsistent compliance to medication or monitoring, and develop contentious relationships with medical staff.

The stress-diathesis model is useful in understanding the course of psychosocial functioning with infertility. Infertility patient undergo enormous emotional, physical, relational, and sometimes spiritual stressors, putting strain on their coping abilities. The core assertion of this model is that individuals are influenced by both stress and diathesis, the former referring to difficult life events and traumatic experiences and the latter referring to genetics, personality traits, or other qualities that are largely fixed during one's lifetime. As the quantity and significance of stressors increase, in combination with genetic predisposition to mental illness, certain personality traits, and prior losses or adverse experiences, one becomes more vulnerable to mental health setbacks [3]. Infertility can present a perfect storm of many stressors which, coupled with certain predispositions, can leave the individual more vulnerable to an emotional or mental health challenge during treatment.

Functioning of Infertility Patients Before and During Treatment

As the stress-diathesis model would assert, pretreatment functioning can influence an infertility patient's coping and psychosocial adjustment as she begins treatment. Her functioning at the commencement of treatment, however, may not reflect how she functioned before her infertility diagnosis or attempts to conceive. Prior to a diagnosis of infertility, a patient may have contended with fertility issues for years [4], and as such her infertility can be seen as a chronic stressor that has already been present for some time [5].

Even in the absence of information on functioning prior to the infertility diagnosis, assessment of infertility patients' functioning as they are about to begin treatment is valuable for a few reasons. First, this information can shed light on what increased vulnerability one may have to developing a psychiatric disorder or other adverse responses during and after interventions. Additionally, an examination of how an infertility patient continues to adjust during and after treatment can assist in well-timed referrals for mental health treatment or referrals for other coping resources.

Prevalence of Psychiatric Disorders Prior to Commencing Medical Interventions

A number of studies have examined pretreatment functioning of infertility patients and its impact on their adjustment throughout and beyond infertility treatment. In their review of 25 years of research, Verhaak et al. [6] found nine studies among those accepted into the review that considered the impact of pretreatment functioning. One area of investigation in these studies was of state anxiety which develops due to stress and threats, in contrast to trait anxiety which reflects ongoing high anxiety that is embedded in one's personality. The levels of state anxiety among the infertility patients differed between studies, which the researchers hypothesized may have been due to cultural differences based on the countries where the various studies were conducted.

The Verhaak review [6] found, perhaps surprisingly, that overall women did not appear to have levels of depression higher than control groups prior to treatment in most studies. They suggested that the lack of elevated rates of depression pretreatment might be indicative of the hopefulness of starting treatment and taking action to solve the problem. However, this finding is contradicted in other research. For example, one study, not included in this review, found that prior to beginning treatment, 33% of infertile Chinese women endorsed depressive symptoms according to the General Health Questionnaire, a self-report measure [7].

Studies included in the review differed in their methodologies, which could help explain the varying prevalence rates of psychiatric disorders or symptoms prior to beginning interventions [6]. Approaches to determining pretreatment functioning differed between studies included in the review; some studies only looked at anxiety [8, 9], while others looked at both anxiety and depression [10–12]. Researchers were selective regarding the types of psychiatric difficulties they looked for, typically focusing on anxiety and depression and excluding diagnostic categories such as substance abuse and other conditions such as bipolar disorder.

An additional obstacle to determining rates of psychiatric difficulties in infertility patients was addressed by Williams et al. [13]. They determined in their review examining mood disorders among infertility patients that "only a few studies that investigate depressive symptoms in newly diagnosed infertility patients actually use diagnostically valid and reliable criteria for confirming a mood disorder." Many studies employ methodologies which lack a rigorous diagnostic element, limiting the ability to confirm the presence of diagnosable conditions and more details regarding participants' psychosocial functioning.

In fact, only three studies using more diagnostically valid criteria to determine rates of depression in infertility patients before commencing treatment were identified in the review by Williams et al. [13]. However, those studies' results lack consistency [14, 15]. One study did not find a difference between infertility patients and controls on measures of mood disorders, while another study did find a significant difference, with infertility patients scoring higher on a depression scale as compared with healthy controls.

A study conducted in Taiwan also used more in-depth methodology for diagnosis. Their approach encompassed administration of the Mini International Neuropsychiatric Interview and the Hospital Anxiety and Depression Scale by a board-certified psychiatrist, rather than a more general self-report questionnaire [16]. The overall rate of psychiatric disorders among 112 infertile women who were attending a reproductive health clinic prior to beginning treatment was 40.2%. The conditions that comprised the highest proportion were anxiety disorders, followed closely by depressive disorders. The high rate of generalized anxiety disorder (26.2%) found in the Chen study is consistent with the Verhaak [6] review's finding that state anxiety was higher than control groups in most of the studies they examined.

While the studies and reviews detailed above reveal a mixed picture regarding prevalence of pretreatment psychosocial difficulties among infertility patients, taken together they illustrate that the presence of such difficulties in some infertility patients is undeniable. These difficulties have the potential to intensify throughout treatment and impact the course of treatment.

Prevalence of Psychiatric Disorders During Treatment

A number of studies have been conducted to determine how infertility patients manage psychologically during treatment. Swedish couples undergoing IVF were found to exhibit high rates of psychiatric disorders at the onset of one round of IVF treatment [17]. The researchers administered an initial screening measure followed up by a comprehensive telephone assessment for those who showed psychological distress on the initial screening. Their findings showed that full criteria were met for DSM IV diagnoses in almost 20% of women and over 7% of men, with major depressive disorder being the most common diagnosis, while another 11% of women and 2.9% of men met a subthreshold diagnosis. Similarly, [18], using two standardized depression scales, found 37% of infertile women undergoing treatment had symptoms of depression, as compared to healthy controls, who had about half that rate.

Another study found that both men and women undergoing IVF who met criteria for a psychiatric diagnosis were more likely to report physical symptoms, with women reporting higher rates of "fatigue, headache, nausea and abdominal pain whereas fatigue and insomnia were the physical symptoms most commonly reported by men with a psychiatric diagnosis [17]." This demonstrates the intersecting nature of mind and body, with both reciprocally influencing the other, sometimes in ways that are difficult to disentangle. As such, psychiatric and physical symptoms can manifest in a variety of ways during treatment, impacting treatment compliance and even willingness to continue treatment.

Factors Influencing Psychosocial Adjustment During and Following Treatment

Investigation into the risk factors that may increase the likelihood of an infertility patient developing psychosocial difficulties has important implications for timely mental health interventions. Not surprisingly, there is evidence that infertility patients who have had major depressive disorder (MDD) in their lifetime are at risk for developing MDD during infertility treatment. A 2016 study, and the only one to date to examine this issue, demonstrated that a diagnosis of MDD prior to commencing treatment was found to be the single largest predictor of MDD during infertility treatment, while controlling for other factors such as partner support, and baseline levels of anxiety and depression [19]. It is clear that some symptoms of MDD, such as sad or irritable mood, poor concentration, decreased motivation, disrupted sleep, and decreased energy levels, have the potential to seriously impact the course of infertility treatment for some patients.

Other variables such as age of woman, amount of time dealing with infertility, the diagnosis itself, and number of IVF or intracytoplasm sperm injection (ICSI) treatments may not present as risk factors for the development of psychosocial difficulties [20]. In this same study, which was conducted among patients in the United States, it was demonstrated that demographic factors such as age and years married were not related to infertility patients' experience of stress. Factors that do appear to impact stress included attitudes, number of tests received, and treatment cost [20].

Van den Broeck et al. [21] investigated factors that contribute to the distress experienced by male and female infertility patients. The factors they found that played a role in exacerbation of distress were those that would also contribute to the development of psychiatric disorders in the general population. More specifically, they identified the personality dimensions of dependency and self-criticism, poor quality of attachment in their spousal relationship, and poor social support, as having greater significance than specific infertility concerns and characteristics related to the infertility experience. They write that "in this way, the infertility-specific concerns and characteristics might only be secondary expressions of basic psychological dimensions."

Volgsten et al. [22] studied a range of demographic variables and risk factors for the development of psychiatric disorders in infertile couples. They concluded that, for the development of a mood disorder, a previous pregnancy and obesity were independent risk factors for women, while unexplained infertility was a risk factor for men. Interestingly, for women, there were no independent risk factors associated with anxiety disorders, and the sample size for men was too small to draw any conclusions. Despite looking at a very broad range of potential risk factors—age, smoking status, native language, socioeconomic status, economic status, and fertility history—none were significantly related to psychiatric diagnosis, with the exception of previous pregnancy. The researchers noted some surprise at the dearth of identified risk factors, as many of the ones they investigated have been identified as risk factors for the development of psychiatric conditions in the general population. With regard to the socioeconomic and economic factors, these infertility patients were receiving free treatment, as Sweden has universal healthcare that covers up to three IVF cycles. In this context, the particular factors related to finances did not impact the development of depressive or anxiety disorders.

Lack of success in giving birth following infertility treatment may present as a risk factor for poor adjustment in the long term. While there is a dearth of longitudinal studies looking at long-term adjustment to failure to conceive after IVF, researchers have found some evidence of increased depressive symptoms in those patients that fail to conceive, while patients who were successful experienced a resolution in psychiatric symptoms [6].

One large Swedish cohort study by Baldur-Felskov et al. [23] looked at rates of psychiatric hospitalization for women following successful versus failed infertility treatment. They found that those who did not give birth were more likely to have been hospitalized for certain mental disorders including alcohol or drug abuse, psychotic disorders, and other diagnoses, in years to come. An obvious limitation of this study is that it only examined hospitalizations, which represent the most severe manifestation of mental illnesses, but even so, it demonstrates a possibility of elevated risk following treatment failure.

Impact of Psychosocial Functioning on Pregnancy Outcomes

Reproductive doctors and patients want to understand how psychosocial functioning may influence pregnancy outcomes. A 2004 study examined hypotheses for ways in which a patient's experience of stress might influence her reproductive functioning (Cwikel et al.). For example, they reviewed research showing how various neurochemical pathways related to stress intertwine with the function of the gonadal axis, possibly impacting fertility outcomes. Cortisol, a hormone released in response to stress, was demonstrated to not impact pregnancy outcome in IVF in one study they reviewed, but anticipatory cortisol, the cortisol released right before IVF, appeared to have an impact.

Overall, they indicated that while there appear to be some possible links between the ways in which the physiology of stress may interfere with reproductive processes, researchers have not yet identified clear pathways. However, it is not unreasonable to conclude that the experience of stress has an impact on one's physiology in ways that may impact the outcome of fertility treatment. The study posited a theory based on the research that psychological distress (i.e., depression and anxiety) impacts various physiological systems which in turn may decrease the chances of a successful outcome from IVF or other treatments.

Treatment Burden and Dropout

Repeated implantation failure is a significant part of the treatment burden. Research has shown that undergoing multiple cycles of IVF is associated with negative effects such as depression, hopelessness, and stress and has demonstrated that the waiting period post-embryo transfer is perceived as the time of greatest distress for many, if not most, patients [24]. With repeated implantation failure, it is easy to see that the waiting period, referred to on patient Internet discussion groups as the "two weeks waiting," has the potential to become a time of greatest distress.

Does treatment burden or psychopathology lead to treatment dropout? A 2012 meta-analysis reviewed 22 studies that included 21,453 patients from eight countries [24]. The three most frequently cited reasons for treatment dropout among the studies were postponement of treatment, physical and psychological burden, and relationship and personal problems. Reasons varied across stages of treatment although some were stage-specific. Psychological burden was found to be common across treatment stages and found to be the main reason for discontinuation of treatment across all treatment stages.

Interventions for Managing the Burden of Treatment

Screening Tools

Several tools have been developed to screen for patient distress. SCREEN IVF was developed to specifically screen for infertility distress and successfully identified 75% of patients at risk for depression and anxiety [25]. At their pretreatment and again at 3–4 weeks post-pregnancy test, 279 women were administered the SCREEN IVF instrument comprised of 34 items on general and infertility-specific psychological factors. The purpose of the tool was to give clinicians a way to identify patients in distress or with a vulnerability to emotional distress so that interventions or referrals could be offered.

The Fertility Quality of Life (FertiQoL) questionnaire is the only internationally developed questionnaire which evaluates the quality of life for men and women experiencing infertility [26]. The self-administered questionnaire has 36 items that assess core (24 items) and treatment-related quality of life (QoL) (10 items) and overall life and physical health (2 items); the reliability measures were satisfactory. Overall, it covers four domains: emotional, mind-body, social, and relational. It is currently available for free in 39 languages. FertiQoL is becoming the gold standard for infertility screening, and the relational factor scores are shown to be useful in assessing relationship adjustment to identify patients undergoing ART who are more likely to report poor or good relationship quality [27]. FertiQoL may be a useful tool in measuring and understanding the impact of repeated implantation failure both in individuals and for couples.

To date other measures that have been developed have had local or convenience samples. One of the more widely used instruments, the Fertility Problem Inventory, was developed on primarily Caucasian Canadians who were involved in infertility treatment [28]. Other instruments available have also had other limitations that limit their general utility. None has been developed to look at neither the specific stress of repeated implantation failure nor specifics of treatment such as the waiting period between embryo transfer and pregnancy test.

Pursuit of Mental Health Treatment by Infertility Patients

Although treatment, such as repeated implantation, create many demands and burdens on patients, most women and men experiencing infertility do not seek psychosocial professional support, even those who are showing psychosocial distress. Verhaak et al. [5] found that though over 30% of women undergoing IVF and 10% of men in their study met criteria for at least one psychiatric disorder or subthreshold diagnoses, only about 11% of them participated in counseling at that time. This low rate surprised the researchers, as counseling was offered and available to all participants at the initial appointment. A low rate of mental health treatment was also noted by Chen et al. [16], in which only 6.7% of those with a psychiatric diagnosis had sought psychiatric treatment in the past. This puts patients at risk for an exacerbation of symptoms, poor treatment compliance, potential disruptions in their relationships, as well as overall decline in their quality of life.

Several hypotheses exist as to why, despite endorsement of symptoms, infertility patients do not pursue psychological support in high numbers even when it is offered to them. One reason is that they are so focused on their fertility needs and thus perceive their emotional needs as beyond the scope of treatment. Patients do not necessarily connect their psychological well-being with their ability to comply with medical treatment protocols and ability to function in other domains in their lives.

Some might fear judgment by medical professionals who may deem them incapable of tolerating treatment or, ultimately, handling parenthood. Chen et al. [16] wrote that "the effort to be a good patient, although a proper way to cope with the stress of an assisted reproduction treatment, may prevent participants from revealing psychological distress to their clinicians" (p 5). A theme that emerges from these hypotheses is that of secrecy, one that still shrouds those struggling with infertility. In a sense, then, the secrecy of a couple's emotional struggles due to infertility becomes yet another dimension of their perceived inadequacy and the accompanying shame.

Chen et al. [16] suggest that some patients may lack an awareness of their own emotional functioning and that "it is possible that estimation based on the subjects' self-assessment of whether or not they are depressed may underestimate these psychiatric disorders" (p 5). Patients may view their suffering as "normal" and thus believe there is nothing that can be done to improve their quality of life or coping. This can pose a risk because in the face of deteriorating psychological health, one may begin to make poor decisions and suffer consequences in relationships. Some researchers have suggested that patients do not seek out psychological counseling because they feel they can handle their stress and view that distress asinherent in the infertility process rather than a pathology that needs intervention [29]. A patient may perceive a referral to psychological counseling as a belief on the part of the medical provider that he or she has "failed" to cope adequately, rather than as an opportunity to increase coping strategies while undergoing treatment.

It should not be understated that acknowledging psychological difficulties continues to carry enormous stigma [30]. For some fertility patients, who are already likely carrying the burden of frustration, shame, and grief, acknowledging psychological problems in a direct way to their doctors may prove to be too much for them to bear, particularly when doctors do not directly ask about this domain of their lives. Patients may be concerned that any stigma attached to the need for psychological support has the potential to limit or deny access to infertility treatment.

Uptake of psychological services was found to be most heavily influenced by three factors: comfort level with consulting with a mental health professional, coping resources, and practical concerns about arranging a meeting with a psychologist/counselor [31]. Patients indicated that their distress level needed to exceed their coping resources, such as social support from family and friends, in order to seek out counseling services. In other words, just because many infertility patients experience distress, it may be a small but distinct porportion whose distress levels tax their coping to the point of pursuing counseling.

Boivin et al. [31] cited two models they believed explained the findings of their study looking at low rates of counseling among infertility patients: the hierarchical-compensatory model [32] and the health belief model [33]. The hierarchical-compensatory model proposes that individuals seek out support in a hierarchical fashion, first seeking it from those close to them, then from professionals; this is consistent with the findings in this study, in that participants tended to seek social support first and the majority found it sufficient for their needs and so did not seek out professional support. The health belief model puts forth the hypothesis that individuals determine the extent of their distress that would warrant them seeking out professional services. In other words, patients may only seek help if they feel their distress is intense enough. The most highly distressed patients in this study tended to cite logistical concerns as a barrier to obtaining treatment, even though services had been offered to them and had been advertised through the clinic where they were being treated.

This introduces questions around why these high-distress patients struggled to obtain the professional support they needed despite it being made available to them. The researchers suggest some possible reasons, such as high levels of distress making it difficult for patients to take in practical information about initiating services [34] and the need in those cases for counseling staff to do more to facilitate the provision of services to those high-distress patients.

Psychosocial Interventions

Myriad behavioral and cognitive interventions for coping with treatment burden have been explored in various studies. Early studies looked at the impact of group psychological interventions [35] and found that group interventions made a significant difference in pregnancy rates, but later studies have not replicated those findings [36]. Further studies looked at mind-body approaches for managing the burden of treatment and found them effective at reducing symptoms of depression and stress and increasing a sense of social support [37] in contrast to the earlier studies which focused on whether interventions increased pregnancy rates.

A recent meta-analysis reviewed 14 different types of interventions that were included in 20 randomized controlled studies [38]. The interventions were classified into five categories: cognitive behavioral therapy (CBT) ($n = 3$), mind-body intervention (MBI) ($n = 3$), counseling ($n = 4$), positive reappraisal coping therapy ($n = 2$), and other psychosocial interventions ($n = 8$) which included hypnosis, Internet-based interventions, crisis interventions, expressive writing, harp therapy, written emotional disclosure, telephone emotional support, and group psychotherapy. The genre of skills taught involved psychoeducation, skill training, emotional support, and cognitive restructuring. This review found that cognitive behavioral therapy, mind-body interventions, counseling, and coping therapy are the most frequently adopted psychological interventions for infertile women and men. However, the review did not find that counseling interventions showed positive effects. The authors recommend that new therapeutic approaches with proven efficacy be the focus to support individuals and couples going through infertility with particular attention to the "two weeks waiting" time prior to the pregnancy test, an area which has been inadequately researched.

Cognitive approaches with positive cognitive reappraisal have been found to lead to modest gains in easing the psychological burden but have not been found to increase pregnancy rates [39]. Patients were randomized into either a control or treatment group prior to the start of their IVF cycle. The treatment group was given a set of ten statements which facilitate positive thinking and diminish dwelling on negative aspects. Researchers found that the exercise did not diminish treatment dropout or increase pregnancy rates, though it was perceived as helpful.

As patients are getting more information and support online, online interventions have been developed for psychoeducational support [40]. A total of 190 women were randomized into two experimental and two no-treatment control groups. After the e-health module, trends were observed for utility in several psychological domains: decreased global stress ($P = 0.10$), sexual concerns ($P = 0.059$), distress related to child-free living ($P = 0.063$), increased infertility self-efficacy ($P = 0.067$), and decision-making clarity ($P = 0.079$). Easy access to online e-health modules could be adapted for patients experiencing repeated implantation failure. Sub-modules could address managing the specific burden of repeated implantation failure.

Psychotropic Medication Management

A more recent area of investigation is the use of antidepressants or anxiolytics and pregnancy outcome [41]. Although there is an existing and emerging body of literature on pharmacological interventions with pregnant and postpartum women, very few studies have examined the relationship of pharmacological interventions with the infertile population. Estimates are that more than half of women pursuing infertility treatment take antidepressants [42]. In a recent analysis of a Swedish birth registry from 2007 to 2012 of women who went through IVF, researchers found that women who were using antidepressants before IVF were found to have slightly reduced odds of pregnancy and live birth [42]. Women with depression and/or anxiety who were not taking antidepressants had a more pronounced reduction in odds for pregnancy. The analysis was unable to identify or speculate what the mechanism might be for the reduction, e.g., is it the underlying disease impacting on egg or embryo quality, mechanisms for implantation, or some other factor?

Research has explored whether psychotropic medication such as antidepressants is effective in the treatment of depression, and many studies conclude that the efficacy and risk do not warrant their use [43]. However, other reviews have concluded that the use of antidepressants is relatively safe and their use is warranted for both maternal and fetal health [44].

As a result of the controversy around psychotropic medication's efficacy and whether it may decrease chances of success for pregnancy, along with the potential for risks during pregnancy to the developing fetus, there has been a call for a reduction or a cessation of use for infertility patients [45]. Clinicians were urged to refer to known effective treatments for depression and anxiety such as cognitive behavioral therapy which has none of the medication risks. Those researchers who have not concluded that there is a significant risk do endorse using medication during treatment and pregnancy citing that that there are significant risks from the depression that must be taken into consideration.

Reducing treatment burden is argued to enhance infertility treatment care for both patients and providers [46]. Patient distress can impact and contribute to the stress load for staff which can impact treatment. It is easy to see how additive cycles of implantation failure can be mitigated if staff are aware of and responsive to patient distress.

Conclusion

The literature around the psychosocial impact of infertility and repeated implantation failure is full of inconsistencies and methodological challenges. There is not a clear consensus regarding the role of interventions for coping with the emotional challenges and its impact on treatment outcome. However, research is showing promising strategies for coping with the emotional impact which may help foster resilience, thus allowing patients to remain in treatment to maximize their biological potential. Certainly, repeated implantation can impact expectations and hope which can influence treatment compliance. These promising strategies yield increased quality of life for individuals and couples pursuing treatment. Collaborative care for the infertile patient remains the gold standard for best practices for patient care.

References

1. Boivin J, Gameiro S. Evolution of psychology and counseling in infertility. Fertil Steril. 2015;104(2):251–9.
2. Berg BJ, Wilson JF. Psychological functioning across stages of treatment for infertility. J Behav Med. 1991;14(1):11–26.
3. Ingram RE, Luxton DD. Vulnerability-stress models. In: Development of psychopathology: a vulnerability-stress perspective. Thousand Oaks: Sage; 2005. p. 32–46.
4. Mazure CM, Greenfeld DA. J Assist Reprod Genet. 1989;6:242–56. https://doi.org/10.1007/BF01132873.
5. Verhaak CM, Smeenk JM, Evers AW, van Minnen A, Kremer JA, Kraaimaat FW. Predicting emotional response to unsuccessful fertility treatment: a prospective study. J Behav Med. 2005;28(2):181–90.
6. Verhaak CM, Smeenk JM, Evers AW, Kremer JA, Kraaimaat FW, Braat DD. Women's emotional adjustment to IVF: a systematic review of 25 years of research. Hum Reprod Update. 2007;13(1):27–36.
7. Lok IH, Lee DTS, Cheung LP, Chung WS, Lo WK, Haines CJ. Psychiatric morbidity amongst infertile Chinese women undergoing treatment with assisted reproductive technology and the impact of treatment failure. Gynecol Obstet Investig. 2002;53(4):195–9.
8. Mori E, Nadaoka T, Morioka Y, Saito H. Anxiety of infertile women undergoing IVF-ET: relation to the grief process. Gynecol Obstet Investig. 1997;44(3):157–62.
9. Visser AP, Haan G, Haan G, Wouters I. Psychosocial aspects of in vitro fertilization. J Psychosom Obstet Gynecol. 1994;15(1):35–43.
10. Edelmann RJ, Connolly KJ, Bartlett H. Coping strategies and psychological adjustment of couples presenting for IVF. J Psychosom Res. 1994;38(4):355–64.

11. Hearn MT, Yuzpe AA, Brown SE, Casper RF. Psychological characteristics of in vitro fertilization participants. Am J Obstet Gynecol. 1987;156(2):269–74.
12. Verhaak CM, Smeenk JM, Eugster A, van Minnen A, Kremer JA, Kraaimaat FW. Stress and marital satisfaction among women before and after their first cycle of in vitro fertilization and intracytoplasmic sperm injection. Fertil Steril. 2001;76(3):525–31.
13. Williams KE, Marsh WK, Rasgon NL. Mood disorders and fertility in women: a critical review of the literature and implications for future research. Hum Reprod Update. 2007;13(6):607–16.
14. Downey J, Yingling S, McKinney M, Husami N, Jewelewicz R, Maidman J. Mood disorders, psychiatric symptoms, and distress in women presenting for infertility evaluation. Fertil Steril. 1989;52(3):425–32.
15. Fassino S, Piero A, Boggio S, Piccioni V, Garzaro L. Anxiety, depression and anger suppression in infertile couples: a controlled study. Hum Reprod. 2002;17(11):2986–94.
16. Chen TH, Chang SP, Tsai CF, Juang KD. Prevalence of depressive and anxiety disorders in an assisted reproductive technique clinic. Hum Reprod. 2004;19(10):2313–8.
17. Volgsten H, Svanberg AS, Ekselius L, Lundkvist Ö, Poromaa IS. Prevalence of psychiatric disorders in infertile women and men undergoing in vitro fertilization treatment. Hum Reprod. 2008;23(9):2056–63.
18. Domar AD, et al. Psychological improvement in infertile women after behavioral treatment: a replication. Fertil Steril. 1992;58(1):144–7.
19. Holley SR, Pasch LA, Bleil ME, Gregorich S, Katz PK, Adler NE. Prevalence and predictors of major depressive disorder for fertility treatment patients and their partners. Fertil Steril. 2015;103(5):1332–9.
20. Abbey A, Halman LJ, Andrews FM. Psychosocial, treatment, and demographic predictors of the stress associated with infertility. Fertil Steril. 1992;57(1):122–8.
21. Van den Broeck U, D'Hooghe T, Enzlin P, Demyttenaere K. Predictors of psychological distress in patients starting IVF treatment: infertility-specific versus general psychological characteristics. Hum Reprod. 2010;25(6):1471–80.
22. Volgsten H, Svanberg AS, Ekselius L, Lundkvist Ö, Poromaa IS. Risk factors for psychiatric disorders in infertile women and men undergoing in vitro fertilization treatment. Fertil Steril. 2010;93(4):1088–96.
23. Baldur-Felskov B, Kjaer SK, Albieri V, Steding-Jessen M, Kjaer T, Johansen C, Dalton SO, Jensen A. Psychiatric disorders in women with fertility problems: results from a large Danish register-based cohort study. Hum Reprod. 2013;28(3):683–90.
24. Gameiro S, Boivin J, Peronace L, Verhaak CM. Why do patients discontinue fertility treatment? A systematic review of reasons and predictors of discontinuation in fertility treatment. Hum Reprod Update. 2012;18(6):652–69.
25. Verhaak CM, Lintsen AM, Evers AW, Braat DD. Who is at risk of emotional problems and how do you know? Screening of women going for IVF treatment. Hum Reprod. 2010;25(5):1234–40.
26. Boivin J, Takefman J, Braverman A. The fertility quality of life (FertiQoL) tool: development and general psychometric properties. Fertil Steril. 2011a;96(2):409–15.
27. Donarelli Z, Coco GL, Gullo S, Salerno L, Marino A, Sammartano F, Allegra A. The fertility quality of life questionnaire (FertiQoL) relational subscale: psychometric properties and discriminant validity across gender. Hum Reprod. 2016;31:2061.
28. Newton CR, Sherrard W, Glavac I. The Fertility Problem Inventory: measuring perceived infertility-related stress. Fertil Steril. 1999;72(1):54–62.
29. Boivin J. Is there too much emphasis on psychosocial counseling for infertile patients? J Assist Reprod Genet. 1997;14(4):184–6.
30. Parcesepe AM, Cabassa LJ. Public stigma of mental illness in the United States: a systematic literature review. Adm Policy Ment Health Ment Health Serv Res. 2013;40(5):384–99.
31. Boivin J, Scanlan LC, Walker SM. Why are infertile patients not using psychosocial counselling? Hum Reprod. 1999;14(5):1384–91.

32. Cantor MH. Neighbors and friends: an overlooked resource in the informal support system. Res Aging. 1979;1(4):434–63.
33. Rosenstock IM. Why people use health services. Milbank Q. 2005;83(4):Online-only.
34. Suls J, Wan CK. Effects of sensory and procedural information on coping with stressful medical procedures and pain: a meta-analysis. J Consult Clin Psychol. 1989;57(3):372.
35. Domar AD, Clapp D, Slawsby E, Kessel B, Orav J, Freizinger M. The impact of group psychological interventions on distress in infertile women. Health Psychol. 2000;19(6):568.
36. Boivin J, Griffiths E, Venetis CA. Emotional distress in infertile women and failure of assisted reproductive technologies: meta-analysis of prospective psychosocial studies. BMJ. 2011b;342:d223.
37. Psaros C, Kagan L, Shifren JL, Willett J, Jacquart J, Alert MD, Macklin EA, Styer AK, Denninger JW, LaRoche KL, Park ER. Mind–body group treatment for women coping with infertility: a pilot study. J Psychosom Obstet Gynecol. 2015;36(2):75–83.
38. Ying L, Wu LH, Loke AY. The effects of psychosocial interventions on the mental health, pregnancy rates, and marital function of infertile couples undergoing in vitro fertilization: a systematic review. J Assist Reprod Genet. 2016;33:689–701.
39. Domar AD, Gross J, Rooney K, Boivin J. Exploratory randomized trial on the effect of a brief psychological intervention on emotions, quality of life, discontinuation, and pregnancy rates in in vitro fertilization patients. Fertil Steril. 2015;104(2):440–51.
40. Cousineau TM, Green TC, Corsini E, Seibring A, Showstack MT, Applegarth L, Davidson M, Perloe M. Online psychoeducational support for infertile women: a randomized controlled trial. Hum Reprod. 2008;23(3):554–66.
41. Akioyamen LE, Minhas H, Holloway AC, Taylor VH, Akioyamen NO, Sherifali D. Effects of depression pharmacotherapy in fertility treatment on conception, birth, and neonatal health: a systematic review. J Psychosom Res. 2016;84:69–80.
42. Cesta CE, Viktorin A, Olsson H, Johansson V, Sjölander A, Bergh C, Skalkidou A, Nygren KG, Cnattingius S, Iliadou AN. Depression, anxiety, and antidepressant treatment in women: association with in vitro fertilization outcome. Fertil Steril. 2016;105(6):1594–602.
43. Urato AC. Are the SSRI antidepressants safe in pregnancy? Understanding the debate. Int J Risk Saf Med. 2015;27(2):93–9.
44. Kalra S, Born L, Sarkar M, Einarson A. The safety of antidepressant use in pregnancy. Expert Opin Drug Saf. 2005;4(2):273–84.
45. Domar AD, Moragianni VA, Ryley DA, Urato AC. The risks of selective serotonin reuptake inhibitor use in infertile women: a review of the impact on fertility, pregnancy, neonatal health and beyond. Hum Reprod. 2013;28:160.
46. Gameiro S, Boivin J, Domar A. Optimal in vitro fertilization in 2020 should reduce treatment burden and enhance care delivery for patients and staff. Fertil Steril. 2013;100(2):302–9.

Index

The manufacturer's authorised representative in the EU is Springer
Nature Customer Service Centre GmbH, Europaplatz 3, 69115 Heidelberg,
Germany. If you have any concerns regarding our products, please
contact ProductSafety@springernature.com

Printed and bound by CPI Group (UK) Ltd, Croydon, CR0 4YY
29/04/2026
02099451-0004